# MEASUREMENT WITH PERSONS

**SCIENTIFIC PSYCHOLOGY SERIES**

*Edited by Stephen W. Link, University of California, San Diego and James T. Townsend, Indiana University*

*Measurement With Persons: Theory, Methods, and Implementation Areas* edited by Birgitta Berglund, Giovanni B. Rossi, James T. Townsend and Leslie R. Pendrill

*Information-Processing Channels in the Tactile Sensory System* by George A. Gescheider, John H. Wright and Ronald T. Verrillo

*Unified Social Cognition* by Norman H. Anderson

*Introduction to the Theories of Measurement and Meaningfulness and the Use of Symmetry in Science* by Louis Narens

*Measurement and Representation of Sensations* edited by Hans Colonius and Ehtibar N. Dzhafarov

*Psychophysics Beyond Sensation* edited by Christian Kaernbach, Erich Schroger, and Hermann Muller

*Theories of Meaningfulness* by Louis Narens

*Empirical Direction in Design and Analysis* by Norman H. Anderson

*Computational, Geometric, and Process Perspectives on Facial Cognition* edited by Michael J. Wenger and James T. Townsend

*Utility of Gains and Losses* by R. Duncan Luce

*Toward a New Behaviorism. The Case against Perceptual Reductionism* by William R. Uttal

*The War Between Mentalism and Behaviorism* by William R. Uttal

*Recent Progress in Mathematical Psychology* edited by Cornelia E. Dowling, Fred S. Roberts, and Peter Theuns

*Localist Connectionist Approaches To Human Cognition* edited by Jonathan Grainger and Arthur M. Jacobs

*Adaptive Spatial Alignment* by Gordon M. Redding and Benjamin Wallace

*Sensation and Judgment* by John Baird

*Signal Detection Theory and Roc Analysis in Psychology and Diagnostics* by John Swets

*The Swimmer* by William R. Uttal, Gary Bradshaw, Sriram Dayanand, Robb Lovell, Thomas Shepherd, Ramakrishna Kakarala, Kurt Skifsted, and Greg Tupper

*Multidimensional Models of Perception and Cognition* by Gregory F. Ashby

*Cognition, Information Processing, and Psychophysics* edited by Hans-Georg Geissler, Stephen W. Link, and James T. Townsend

*The Wave Theory of Difference and Similarity* by Stephen W. Link

# MEASUREMENT WITH PERSONS

## Theory, Methods, and Implementation Areas

Edited by
BIRGITTA BERGLUND
GIOVANNI B. ROSSI
JAMES T. TOWNSEND
LESLIE R. PENDRILL

Psychology Press
Taylor & Francis Group
New York London

Psychology Press
Taylor & Francis Group
711 Third Avenue
New York, NY 10017

Psychology Press
Taylor & Francis Group
27 Church Road
Hove, East Sussex BN3 2FA


Psychology Press is an imprint of Taylor & Francis Group, an Informa business

Printed in the United States of America on acid-free paper
10 9 8 7 6 5 4 3 2 1

International Standard Book Number: 978-1-84872-939-1 (Hardback)



**Library of Congress Cataloging-in-Publication Data**

Measurements with persons : theory, methods, and implementation areas / editors, Birgitta Berglund ... [et al.].
p. cm. -- (Scientific psychology series)
Includes bibliographical references and index.
ISBN 978-1-84872-939-1 (hardback)
1. Perception--Mathematical models. 2. Senses and sensation--Mathematical models. 3. Human information processing--Mathematical models. I. Berglund, Birgitta. II. Title. III. Series.

BF311.M4325 2011
153.7028'7--dc22 2011008495

**Visit the Taylor & Francis Web site at**
**http://www.taylorandfrancis.com**

**and the Psychology Press Web site at**
**http://www.psypress.com**

*on ne voit bien qu'avec le coeur*

*l'essentiel est invisible pour les yeux*

**Antoine de Saint-Exupéry,** ***Le Petit Prince***

# Contents

# Preface

Measurement with persons involves human perception and interpretation for measuring complex holistic quantities and qualities. These are perceived or created by the human brain and mind. Providing the means for reproducible measurement of parameters such as pleasure and pain has important implications in evaluating all kinds of products, services, and conditions. Progress in this area requires the interlinking of related developments across a variety of disciplines, embracing the physical, biological, psychological, and social sciences. Moreover, it faces an ever-increasing demand for valid measurements as the basis for decision making.

A significant hurdle to surmount is the historical division that arose in the middle of the twentieth century between physicists and psychologists. The two sides disagreed strongly on the meaning of measurement and the possibility of "measuring" sensory events. This led to parallel developments in measurement science within the two separate camps. Both went on to generate remarkable results, but the lack of communication between them prevented coherent and interactive progress.

This book inaugurates a new era for this subject. Here a large board of scholars and scientists from physical, psychological, biological, and social sciences has accepted the challenge of working together to reach a common understanding of the theory of measurement and the methods. The aim is to provide what seems to be the first book ever issued covering the topic of measurement with persons by multi-, inter-, and transdisciplinary approaches. That means that the complementary aspects of general theory, measurement methods, instrumentation, and modeling are treated together in an integral way by world-renowned scientists in the fields of psychophysics and general psychology, measurement theory, metrology and instrumentation, neurophysiology, engineering, biology, and chemistry. Such a comprehensive approach is developed in general terms in the first part of the book and then demonstrated in frontier implementations in the second part.

This (so far) unparalleled coordination effort has been possible thanks to the European Framework Programme Seven, Coordination Action MINET: Measuring the Impossible Network, chaired by Birgitta Berglund, which has provided the opportunity, and funding from the European Commission (Contract no. 043297). The book results from an International Training Course for senior scientists held in June 2008 in Genova, Italy, and organized in the MINET environment. B. Berglund and G. B. Rossi chaired the course, and it was attended by researchers and advanced students from 14 different countries.

The book is organized in two parts. In the first part, generic theoretical and methodological issues are treated, including the conceptual basis of measurement in the various fields involved; the development of formal, representational, and probabilistic theories; the approach to experimentation; and the theories, models, and methods for multifaceted problems. In the second part, several implementation areas are presented, including sound, visual, and skin perception; functional brain imaging; body language and emotions; and, finally, the use of measurement in decision making.

**B. Berglund, G. B. Rossi, J. T. Townsend, and L. R. Pendrill**

# Contributors

**Birgitta Berglund**
Department of Psychology
Stockholm University
and
Institute of Environmental Medicine
Karolinska Institutet
Stockholm, Sweden

**Devin Burns**
Department of Psychology
Indiana University Bloomington
Bloomington, Indiana, USA

**Frans Cornelissen**
University Medical Centre Groningen
Groningen, The Netherlands

**Beatrice de Gelder**
Cognitive and Affective Neuroscience Laboratory
Faculty of Social and Behavioural Sciences
Tilburg University
Tilburg, The Netherlands

**Pasquale Anthony Della Rosa**
Department of Neuroscience
Università Vita Salute San Raffaele
Milan, Italy

**Ehtibar N. Dzhafarov**
Department of Psychological Studies
Purdue University
West Lafayette, Indiana, USA
and
Swedish Collegium for Advanced Study in the Social Sciences
Uppsala, Sweden

**Christian Eitzinger**
Profactor GmbH
Steyr-Gleink, Austria

**Ragne Emardson**
SP Technical Research Institute of Sweden
Borås, Sweden

**Jan-Mark Geusebroek**
Institute of Informatics
University of Amsterdam
Amsterdam, The Netherlands

**Teresa Goodman**
National Physical Laboratory
Teddington, United Kingdom

**Sven-Thomas Graupner**
Applied Cognitive Research Unit
Department of Psychology
Dresden University of Technology
Dresden, Germany

**Riitta Hari**
Brain Research Unit LTL
Helsinki University of Technology
Espoo, Finland

**Wolfgang Heidl**
Profactor GmbH
Steyr-Gleink, Austria

**Rupert Hölzl**
Otto-Selz Institute for Applied Psychology
University of Mannheim
Mannheim, Germany

**Dieter Kleinböhl**
Otto-Selz Institute for Applied Psychology
University of Mannheim
Mannheim, Germany

**Mariska E. Kret**
Cognitive and Affective Neuroscience Laboratory
Faculty of Social and Behavioural Sciences
Tilburg University
Tilburg, The Netherlands
and
Psychology Department
University of Amsterdam
Amsterdam, The Netherlands

**Guillaume Lemaitre**
Institut de Recherche et de Coordination Acoustique/Musique
Paris, France

**Stephen Link**
Department of Psychology
University of California, San Diego
La Jolla, California, USA

**Jan Bernard Marsman**
University Medical Centre Groningen
Groningen, The Netherlands

**Stephen McAdams**
CIRMMT
Schulich School of Music
McGill University
Montréal, Québec, Canada

**Sebastian Pannasch**
Applied Cognitive Research Unit
Department of Psychology
Dresden University of Technology
Dresden, Germany

**Lei Pei**
Department of Psychology
Indiana University Bloomington
Bloomington, Indiana, USA

**Leslie R. Pendrill**
SP Technical Research Institute of Sweden
Borås, Sweden

**Daniela Perani**
Department of Neuroscience
Università Vita Salute San Raffaele
Milan, Italy

**Fred S. Roberts**
Center for Discrete Mathematics and Theoretical Computer Science
Rutgers University
Piscataway, New Jersey, USA

**Giovanni Battista Rossi**
DIMEC
Università degli Studi di Genova
Genova, Italy

**Sergey A. Shevchik**
Institute of Cognitive Studies
National Research Center "Kurchatov Institute"
Moscow, Russia

**Charlotte B.A. Sinke**
Cognitive and Affective Neuroscience Laboratory
Faculty of Social and Behavioural Sciences
Tilburg University
Tilburg, The Netherlands

**Patrick Susini**
Institut de Recherche et de Coordination Acoustique/Musique
Paris, France

**James T. Townsend**
Department of Psychology
Indiana University Bloomington
Bloomington, Indiana, USA

**Jörg Trojan**
Central Institute of Mental Health
Department of Cognitive and Clinical Neuroscience
Mannheim, Germany

**Gerie W.A.M. van der Heijden**
Biometris
Wageningen University and Research Centre
Wageningen, The Netherlands

**Boris M. Velichkovsky**
Applied Cognitive Research Unit
Department of Psychology
Dresden University of Technology
Dresden, Germany

**Andrew Wallard**
Bureau International des Poids et Mesures
Sèvres, France

# 1 Measurement across physical and behavioral sciences

*Birgitta Berglund,[1] Giovanni Battista Rossi,[2] and Andrew Wallard[3]*

[1]Department of Psychology
Stockholm University
and
Institute of Environmental Medicine, Karolinska Institutet
Stockholm, Sweden

[2]DIMEC
Università degli Studi di Genova
Genova, Italy

[3]Bureau International des Poids et Mesures
Sèvres, France

## 1.1 The origins

Although measurement has been a key factor in the development of modern science, studies on its foundations appeared relatively late, in the second half of the nineteenth century. They concerned, at the same time, both physical and behavioral sciences and they paralleled the constitution of the international system of metrology, with the signing of the Metre Convention. It is important to be aware of such common roots for understanding and putting in the right perspective what happened later, up to the present day. So, a historical overview of these crucial nineteenth century developments is presented in the first part of this chapter, up to the division that arose among the two communities—physicists and engineers on the one side, psychological and behavioral scientists on the other—in the first part of the twentieth century. With lack of communication such division led to an essentially parallel development on the two sides. Nevertheless, noteworthy developments in measurement science and technology, as well as recent measurement needs emerging in science and society, call for a common effort toward reaching a common view, enabling interdisciplinary collaboration and ensuring a common development. This is the subject of the second part of the chapter. Lastly, in the third and final part, new trends are presented and discussed and research needs addressed.

## 1.2. In search of a theory for physical measurement

### *1.2.1 Helmholtz: The analogy between measuring and counting*

Helmholtz, in a *Memoire* published in 1887 (Helmholtz, 1971), investigated "the objective meaning of the fact that we express as quantities, through concrete numbers, situations of real objects" and he wanted to discuss "under what circumstances we are allowed to do so." "Concrete numbers," in his language, are those arising from the counting of real objects. He found a brilliant solution to the problem by establishing an analogy between measurement and counting.

The key idea is that, in many cases, the characteristic we want to measure is a *quantity*, in that it is the amount of something, and thus it may be thought of as the sum of a number of elementary parts, or units, of that something. In those cases *measurement is equivalent to the counting of such units*. From this analogy it is possible to derive the conditions that must be met in order for measurement to make sense, that is, the conditions for measurability. Counting is possible thanks to the properties of natural numbers, which undergo an order, based on the relation "greater than or equal to," and may be added to each other. Similarly, measurement is possible and well founded whenever it is possible to identify the empirical counterparts of the order relation and of the addition operation for the objects carrying the characteristic of interest. For example, in the case of mass measurement, order may be established by comparing objects by an equal-arms balance and addition of two objects consists in putting them on the same pan of the balance. Thanks to these properties it is possible to construct a measurement scale, which supports the practice of measurement, as we soon show. An important question is now whether it is possible to establish the above properties for all kinds of measurement. Helmholtz admits it is not and mentions an indirect approach as an approach. This idea was developed afterwards by Campbell, yielding the distinction between fundamental and derived quantities.

### *1.2.2 Campbell: The foundation of physical measurement*

The first organic presentation of a theory for physical measurement was by Campbell, in the second part of his book, *Physics—The Elements*, published in 1920 (Campbell, 1957). Like Helmholtz, he considers the problem of

> … why can and do we measure some properties of bodies while we do not measure others?… I have before my table [he writes] a tray containing several similar crystals. These crystals possess many properties among which may be included the following: Number, weight, density, hardness, colour, beauty. The first three of these qualities are undoubtedly capable of measurement—unless it be judged the number is to be excluded as being more fundamental than any measurement; concerning hardness it is difficult to say whether or not it can be measured, for though various systems of measuring hardness are in common use, it is generally felt that none of them are wholly satisfactory. Colour cannot be measured as the others can, that is to say it is impossible to denote the colour

> of an object by a single number *which can be determined with the same freedom from arbitrariness which characterises the assigning of a number to represent weight or density.* The last property, beauty, can certainly not be measured, unless we accept the view which is so widely current that beauty is determined by the market value. *What is the difference between the properties which determine the possibility or impossibility of measuring them?* (Campbell, 1957)

To answer this question, he considers two kinds of quantities,

- Fundamental (e.g., mass)
- Derived (e.g., density)

Both of these require an empirical property of *order*, which is (according to Helmholtz) the basic requirement for measurement. But fundamental quantities allow for a physical-addition operation also. Why is this operation so important? Because it is key in permitting the general procedure for fundamental measurement to be applied. Such a procedure consists in constructing a *measurement scale*, that is, a series *of* standards with properly assigned numerical values, and then in comparing any unknown object $r$ to it, in order to select the element in the series that is equivalent to it. Then it will be possible to assign to $r$ the same number (measure) as the selected element.

Let us see this in more detail, considering again the mass-measurement case. For the construction of the measurement scale, we first arbitrarily select one object, $u$, which will serve as the unit of the scale, and we assign the number 1 to it, that is, $m(u) = 1$, where $m$ is the *measure* function. Then we look for another element $u'$, equivalent to $u$, such that, put in the opposite pan of the balance, it will balance it. We now sum the two elements by putting them on the same pan of the balance and we look for a third element that balances with them. Clearly, we may assign the number 2. So we have constructed a multiple of the unit, and we may proceed similarly for the other multiples. Submultiples may also be constructed in a similar way. Once the scale is available, mass measurement may be performed by comparing an unknown object $r$, with the elements of the scale, with the balance, up to finding the element of the series, say $s$, equivalent to it: then we assign $m(r) = m(s)$. The scheme of the direct-measurement procedure just considered may be depicted as in Figure 1.1.

Noteworthy, in the process of construction of the scale, the only arbitrary choice concerns the selection of the unitary element; afterwards, the values to be assigned to the other elements are fully constrained by the need for conformity with the results

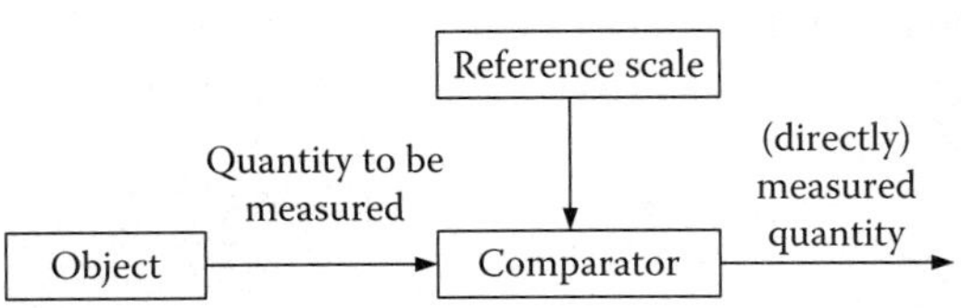


*Figure 1.1* Basic scheme for the direct measurement of a quantity.

of the summing operation. As a consequence of this, the measure may be interpreted as the ratio between the value of the characteristic in object $r$ and in the unitary element $u$. In other words, $m(r) = p/q$ implies that the sum of $q$ "copies" of $r$ balances with the sum of $p$ unitary elements. Note that $q$ copies of $r$ may be realized by proper amplification devices, for example, by using an unequal-arm balance, with arms in a ratio $q$:1 to each other.

Now we may understand Campbell's statement that only qualities "which can be determined with the same freedom from arbitrariness which characterises the assigning of a number to represent weight" fully qualify as measurable, and we may also comprehend the rationale behind it. What has been considered so far applies to fundamental quantities, yet there is another way of measuring something, the way that applies to derived quantities. Consider the case of density, $\rho$. For this quantity we may find a meaningful criterion for order, because we may say that $a$ is denser than $b$, if we may find a liquid in which $b$ floats, whereas $a$ sinks, but we do not have any criterion of empirical summation. Yet density "can be determined with the same freedom from arbitrariness which characterises the assigning of a number to represent weight," because we may identify density as the ratio of mass to volume: $\rho = M/V$, and we can measure mass and volume. So, given an object $a$, assuming we are able to measure its mass, obtaining $m_M(a)$, and its volume, obtaining $m_v(a)$, we may assign a measure to its density as $m_\rho(a) = m_M(a)/m_v(a)$. The other way to found measurement—the way that applies to derived quantities—thus consists in finding some physical law that allows expressing the measure of the characteristic of our interest as a function of the measure of other quantities whose measurability has already been assessed.

To sum up, Campbell holds that measurability may be established first by proving that the characteristic under investigation involves an empirical order relation and then either by finding a physical addition operation that allows the construction of a reference measurement scale and the performing of measurement by comparison with it, or by finding some physical law that allows the measure to be expressed as a function of other quantities. The first procedure applies to fundamental quantities, the second to derived ones and is illustrated in Figure 1.2.

In the case of derived measurement the foundation of measurement is subject to the physical (more generally we could say "natural") law that is invoked. In this regard, we may consider two possibilities: either it is also possible to measure the quantity directly, and so we only have to check whether the direct and the indirect approaches produce consistent results, or the law has an intrinsic validity and, if the same magnitude appears in two or more laws accepted in the same scientific domain, the consistency of the system may be invoked to support the measurability of the quantity under consideration and so plays a foundational role.

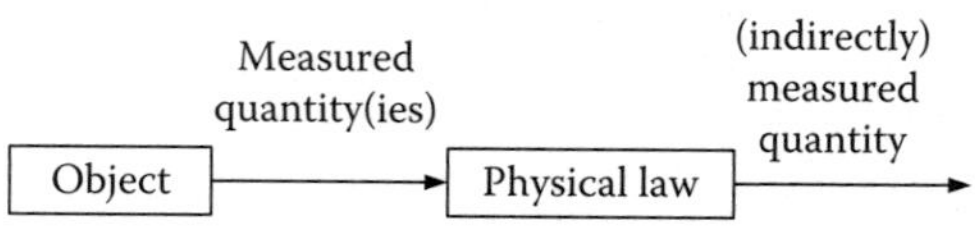


*Figure 1.2* Basic scheme for the indirect measurement of a quantity.

In the first case, derived measurements are essentially reduced to fundamental ones and do not have an independent foundation. In the second, quantities are considered as a part of a system and the focus is shifted toward the performance of the overall system rather than on the individual properties. This concept of quantities as a part of a system was clearly affirmed, in about the same period, with the constitution of the Metre Convention.

## 1.3 The constitution of the international system of metrology

The need for reference standards for measurement in trade, agriculture, and construction has been recognized by mankind from ancient times. Metrological activities have been developed on a regional basis, following the evolution of the geopolitical scenario, up to relatively recent times. Only in the nineteenth century has international coordination been achieved, as a consequence of a process that started near the end of the previous century. At the time of the French Revolution, the *decimal metric system* was instituted and two platinum standards representing the meter and the kilogram were deposed in the *Archives de la République* in Paris (1799). This rationalization of the system of units may perhaps have been explained by the concurrence of a few factors. At that time modern science had been firmly established and the need of accurate measurements for its development had been clearly recognized. Philosophers of the Enlightenment were in search of a rational foundation of knowledge, which has a natural counterpart in science in the search for universal reference standards, independent of place and time.

This process continued in the nineteenth century and ultimately led to the Metre Convention, a treaty that was signed in Paris in 1875 by representatives of seventeen nations. The Convention created the *Bureau International des Poids et Mesures* (BIPM), the international reference body for metrology, and established a permanent organizational structure for coordinating metrology activities. The organization includes the International Committee for Weights and Measures (CIPM), a body supported by a number (currently 10) of technical committees for providing recommendations for the development of the different fields of metrology. The CIPM reports to the General Conference on Weights and Measures (CGPM), a meeting of national delegations from the member states of the BIPM that have acceded to the Metre Convention. The CGPM makes the necessary decisions for the operation of the world metrology system and, in particular the International System of Units (SI). The work of the BIPM provides the basis for a single coherent system of measurements throughout the world, acting in many forms, from direct dissemination of units to coordination through international comparisons of national measurement standards. The Convention, modified slightly in 1921, remains the basis of international agreement on units of measurement. There are now 54 members of the BIPM, including all the major industrialized countries.

From our standpoint it is useful to stress two major advantages of such a system. First, for each quantity a unique, stable, primary reference is maintained, recognized, and accepted worldwide. Second, quantities in the system are linked by a set of relations, the currently accepted physical laws, and consequently progress in one quantity influences other quantities as well and we may say that the measurability of each quantity is founded not only on the properties of that quantity, but also on the overall system's coherence, which is continually checked, both theoretically and experimentally. The international system of metrology is treated in greater detail in Chapter 3. When the international system for metrology was constituted, a noteworthy development of measurement in psychology was taking place, as we now show.

## 1.4 The role of measurement in the birth of experimental psychology

"As an exact science psychophysics, like physics, must rest on experience and the mathematical connection of those empirical facts that demand a measure of what is experienced or, when such a measure is not available, a search for it." This is Fechner, in his *Elements of Psychophysics*, published in 1860 (Fechner, 1966); in 1879 Wundt established his famous laboratory in Leipzig, giving rise to experimental psychology as an autonomous discipline, strongly grounded in measurement. But how was measurement conceived in psychophysics?

We have seen that Helmholtz founded measurement on an analogy with counting. Campbell developed this approach by introducing, in an embryonic form, the notion of measurement scale and explicating the distinction between fundamental and derived quantities. The problem Fechner had to face was even more challenging, inasmuch as "unlike physical processes, which are external, public, objective, and open to direct measurement, mental processes are internal, private, subjective, and cannot be measured directly. Somehow an indirect method had to be developed," Wozniak (1999) notes.

Fechner's idea was to measure the increments of mental activity through the measurement of the increments of the energy of the physical phenomenon that causes them. But what law links them? Weber had already shown that, in several circumstances, the increment of the physical stimulus, $\delta\varphi$, needed to cause a just perceptible variation in the corresponding sensation, is proportional to the intensity of the stimulus, $\varphi$; that is,

$$\delta\varphi = k\delta, \tag{1.1}$$

where $k$ is a constant that depends upon the sensation considered. This is called Weber's law.

But what happens on the sensation side, on the internal side? Interestingly enough, to answer this question Fechner refers, as Helmholtz, to the *counting paradigm*. He looks for a zero and a unit for the evoked sensation, with a natural and convincing choice: the zero is the perception threshold, the unit is the increment of sensation corresponding to a just noticeable difference in stimulus quantity that he assumes to be invariant and independent of the value of the stimulus: simple and genial!

In this perspective, the intensity of a sensation is the sum of a number of elementary variations of sensation intensity, all equal and corresponding to just noticeable

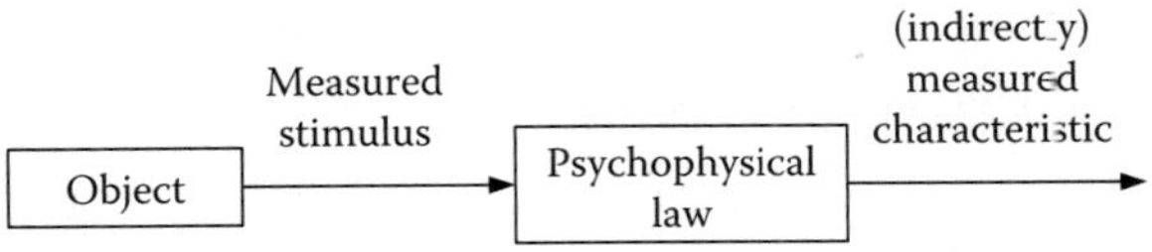


*Figure 1.3* Indirect psychophysical measurement.

differences in the stimulus (Nowell Jones, 1974). If, in turn, just noticeable differences in the stimulus follow Weber's law (1.1), a logarithmic law would follow,

$$\psi = \alpha \ln \varphi + \beta, \tag{1.2}$$

where $\psi$ is the intensity of the sensory perception and $\alpha$ and $\beta$ are constant parameters that characterize the response of an average observer to the stimulus. So it is possible to measure the intensity of a sensory perception $\psi$ indirectly by measuring the intensity of the stimulus $\varphi$ and applying the psychophysical law. This is depicted in Figure 1.3.

The similarity with the procedure for indirect physical measurement, illustrated in Figure 1.2, may be noted. Summarizing,

- What we measure is a characteristic of a physical object (or event), that has the capacity of evoking a sensory perception in individuals that has different possible degrees of intensity.
- Measurement may be performed indirectly, by measuring the intensity of the stimulus and applying the psychophysical law.
- The psychophysical law is based on Weber's law and on Fechner's hypothesis that the just noticeable differences in the stimulus intensity evoke mutually equal differences in the intensity of the sensory perception.
- The parameters of the psychophysical law refer to an average observer.

Some comments are now in order. The assumption of Weber's law, although mathematically convenient whenever applicable, is not a must. What is needed is a relation between just noticeable differences and the intensity of the stimulus, that is, the function

$$\delta\varphi = 1(\varphi) \tag{1.3}$$

which may be derived experimentally.

Fechner's hypothesis instead is crucial and it was criticized, as we show in the next section. Moreover, referring measurement to an average observer is again not a must, because methods for dealing with individual differences may be developed, as we will show at a later stage.

To sum up, thus far we have shown how in the last part of the nineteenth century a noteworthy increase in awareness of the foundations of the measurement process developed in the disciplines and in the scientific communities having an experimental basis. This ultimately led to a comparison of their views, which took place at the beginning of the twentieth century, with, unfortunately, an inauspicious result.

## 1.5 The schism: The report of the British Association for the Advancement of Science

In 1932 the British Association for the Advancement of Science (BAAS) appointed a committee including physicists and psychologists to consider and report upon the possibility of quantitative estimates of sensory events. The committee produced a final report, in 1939, some of whose conclusions are summarized here (Ferguson, Myers, & Bartlett, 1940). As we have already seen, it is possible by psychophysical experiments to obtain a curve that links just noticeable differences in a stimulus to its intensity, formula (1.3). Often this results in a smooth curve, so that it is feasible to assume that some empirical relation holds between them. On these premises, the committee agreed, but the question was if such a function fully describes the facts.

The psychologists claimed the need for some quantitative description of the intensity of the sensory perceptions involved. As we have seen, one such description may be obtained, according to Fechner, by further assuming that each just noticeable step in the intensity of the stimulus $\delta\varphi$ produces a step in sensation $\delta\psi$, and that such steps are all equal, which leads to formula (1.2).

The physicists argued that the possibility of mathematically obtaining formula (1.2) does not "prove" the measurability of the intensity of the sensation $\psi$, inasmuch as that formula is based on an assumption that cannot be verified, unless it is possible to independently measure the intensity of perception. But this is not possible, in their view, because no additive operation is definable among sensations. The main point against the measurability of the intensity of a sensation thus was ultimately the impossibility of satisfactorily defining an addition operation for it. On the other hand, the psychologists claimed that, although Fechner's position cannot be fully supported, the result of psychophysical experiments cannot, in general, be expressed only in terms of stimulus intensities (Stevens, 1936). In fact, the particular intensity changes $\delta\varphi$ that are being plotted "are obtained only by reference to the sensation they evoke, and are based on the equality or inequality of these sensation intensities."

The report of the committee had an enormous influence in the following years and we may say that it led to an essentially parallel development of measurement science in physical science on one side and in behavioral sciences on the other, with consequences up to the present day. We return soon to the conclusions of the committee, after briefly reviewing some advances in measurement that took place in the twentieth century.

## 1.6 Twentieth-century development

### *1.6.1 Development of measurement in psychology*

#### *1.6.1.1 Psychometrics*

In the beginning of the twentieth century the scope of psychological measurement broadened, and we may identify two main schools, psychophysics and psychometrics. As we have seen, psychophysics or perceptual measurement focuses on within-individual processes that can be assumed to vary very little between individuals

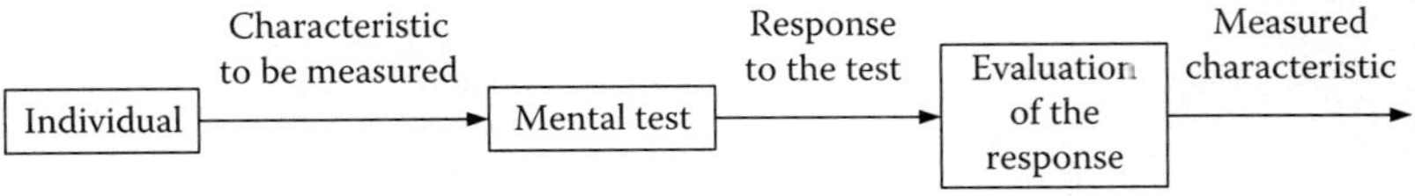


*Figure 1.4* Measurement based on a psychometric test.

(Gescheider, 1997). Thus a variation in the stimulus (outside the individual) would roughly be processed the same, or at least according to the same principles. So characteristics such as red or coffee odor are essentially perceived in the same way by individuals.

Psychometrics instead focuses on measuring "host factors," that is, concepts that are unique to an individual, such as trait, and where interindividual differences would typically exist (Lord & Novick, 1968). Examples are personality, emotions, mood, and attitudes. Thus psychophysics aims at measuring attributes of stimuli, which vary with "invariant persons," whereas psychometrics aims at measuring attributes of persons, which vary with "invariant stimuli." Here the stimuli are test items.

As we have already illustrated in Figure 1.3, psychophysics deals with the measurement of characteristics of objects, as perceived by humans. In order to do this, a psychophysical law is used, referred to a standard observer: the sensation evoked by the characteristic under investigation may be indirectly measured by measuring the stimulus and applying the psychophysical law to it. Individual differences are considered as an inherent uncertainty source, or noise, in such measurements.

An alternative approach has been pursued in psychometrics, where the characteristics of individuals are of interest. They are measured by the responses they provide to mental tests, which play the role of measuring instruments. On the basis of such responses, the psychological variables of interest may be measured. This is depicted in Figure 1.4. Similar to these are, to some extent, measurements in sociology and economics, where often preferences are assessed and the use of questionnaires is typical.

### *1.6.1.2 Stanley S. Stevens: The direct measurement of sensory events*

Let us now return to the report of the British Association. As we have noted, two main points were raised against the measurability of sensory events, the impossibility of directly measuring perceived intensity and the need for additivity as a necessary property for measurement in general. An answer to both points came from the contribution of Stevens.

For the first point, the possibility of directly evaluating the intensity of a sensation, he introduces new types of measurement (or scaling) methods, in which magnitude or ratio of sensations is estimated directly by the subjects and called *magnitude estimation* or *production* and *ratio estimation* or *production*.

> Present a line of a given length and tell the observer to call it some number, say, 10. Then present a line of some other length and say: "If the first line was 10, what would you call the second line? Use any number that seems appropriate—fractional, decimal, whole number—but try to make the number proportional

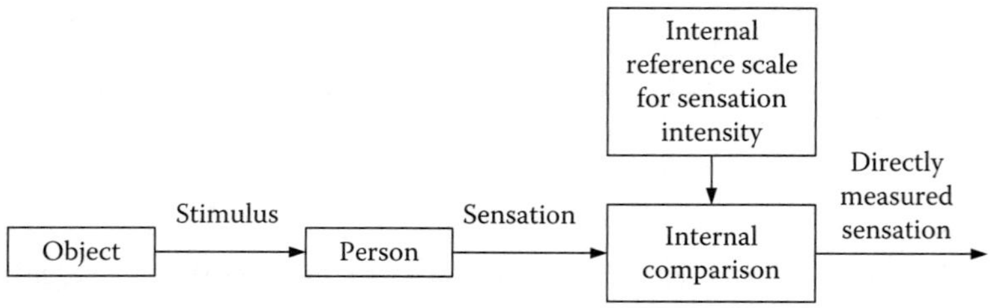


*Figure 1.5* Magnitude estimation: a person acts as a measuring system.

> to the apparent length as *you* see it." Then proceed to other lengths, in irregular order, and ask for similar estimates of apparent length. (Stevens, 1959)

This is *magnitude estimation*; in *magnitude production*, instead, the observer is asked to alter the length in order to match numbers. In *ratio estimation* the observer is asked to estimate the apparent ratio between several lengths and a standard length which is maintained constant during the experiment. Last, in *ratio production* the observer is asked to change a variable length in order to match given ratios with respect to the standard one. Note that in particular in magnitude estimation *a person acts as a measuring system* (Stevens, 1956). This is an important point, and is illustrated in Figure 1.5.

Thanks to these new methods, Stevens could check Fechner's law and actually he rejected it, proposing as a substitute the so-called *power law*,

$$\psi = \eta\varphi^{\theta}, \tag{1.4}$$

where, as usual, $\varphi$ is the physical stimulus, $\psi$ is the corresponding perceived quantity, and $\eta$ and $\theta$ are constants that depend upon the kind of sensation considered. As in Fechner's approach, the intensity of a sensation may still be measured indirectly by measuring a stimulus quantity and applying a psychophysical law, but with an important difference: here the law has not been assumed as a hypothesis about the way perception takes place, but rather it has been determined experimentally, by directly measuring both the stimuli and the resulting sensations, thanks to the new scaling methods (Stevens, 1956).

### *1.6.1.3 Stanley S. Stevens: The classification of measurement scales*

Considering the crucial point of additivity, Stevens circumvents it by taking another way.

> In the meantime, unaware that the British committee of BAAS was trying to settle the issue, some of us at Harvard were wrestling with similar problems… . What I gained from these discussions was a conviction that *a more general theory of measurement was needed*, and that the definition of measurement should not be limited to one restricted class of empirical operations.

*Table 1.1* Classification of measurement scales, according to Stevens

| *Scale* | *Basic empirical operations* | *Mathematical group structure* | *Examples* |
|---|---|---|---|
| Nominal | Determination of equality | Permutation group $m'(a) = f[m(a)]$ where $f$ is any one-to-one transformation | Perception thresholds<br>Detection of defects (for example welding defects in welded structures)<br>Pattern recognition techniques |
| Ordinal | Determination of greater or less | Isotonic group $m'(a) = f[m(a)]$ where $f$ is any increasing monotonic function | Hardness of minerals<br>Earthquake intensity<br>Wind intensity<br>Grades of leather, lumber, wool |
| Interval | Determination of the equality of intervals or of differences | Linear or affine group $m'(a) = \alpha m(a) + \beta$ with $\alpha > 0$ | Temperature (Fahrenheit or Celsius)<br>Position<br>Time (calendar) |
| Ratio | Determination of the equality of ratios | Similarity group $m'(a) = \alpha m(a)$ with $\alpha > 0$ | Length, mass, density, time intervals<br>Temperature (kelvin)<br>Loudness (sone)<br>Brightness (bril) |

*Note:* Examples have been partially changed from the original.

> The best way out seemed to approach the problem from another point of view, namely, that of *invariance*, and to classify scales of measurement in terms of the group of transformations that leave the scale form invariant. . . . A fourfold classification of scales based on this notion was worked out sometime around 1939 and was presented to the International Congress for the Unity of Science in 1941. World War II then came along, and publication was delayed until 1946. (Stevens, 1959)

This famous fourfold classification of measurement scales is summarized in Table 1.1 (Stevens, 1946).

Nominal scales are related to classification operations and numbers serve only to distinguish one class of objects from another. Any one-to-one substitution is permissible, because identification is still possible. Ordinal scales permit a rank ordering of objects and remain invariant under monotonic increasing transformations. Interval scales entail a constant unit of measurement; that is, they introduce a metric, and so permit the calculation of differences between any two values. They remain invariant under linear transformations. Ratio scales also feature constant units of measurement, but, in addition, they allow the ratio of two values to be evaluated, because an absolute zero exists. They are invariant under any simply multiplicative transformation. Note that equality of ratios here plays the role of an empirical relation, substituting empirical sum in measurements on ratio scales.

Summarizing, Stevens shows ways for overcoming the severe limitation in measurability appearing in the BAAS committee report, based on increasing the number of allowable measurement scales, through an innovative approach to their classification based on an invariance principle, and on considering ratio equality as an empirical relation.

With Stevens's contributions we have reached the second half of the twentieth century. At that time a considerable body of results had been obtained in measurement theory and there was a need for systematization, which was achieved with the representational theory of measurement. But prior to that we have to take a look at the progress of the international system of metrology.

## 1.7 Measuring the human response to physical stimuli: The candela in the SI

The Metre Convention, established in 1875, was revised in 1921, extending the scope and responsibilities of the BIPM, originally concerned with mechanical quantities (length, mass, and time) to other fields in physics. Then the Consultative Committee for Electricity (CCE, now CCEM) was created (1927) and a four-dimensional system based on the meter, kilogram, second, and ampere, the MKSA system, was adopted (1946). The number of base quantities was then extended to six, with the introduction of the kelvin and the candela, respectively, for thermodynamic temperature and luminous intensity (1954).

The name International System of Units, with the abbreviation SI, was given to the system in 1960. Lastly, in 1971, the current version of the SI was completed by adding the mole as the base unit for amount of substance, bringing the total number of base units to seven (BIPM, 2006).

For our purposes, the candela deserves special interest. Matters concerning photometry are treated, in particular, by the Consultative Committee for Photometry and Radiometry of the BIPM. In a monograph on the *Principles governing photometry* (BIPM, 1983), the special character of photometric quantities is pointed out by noting that they

> must take into account both the purely physical characteristics of the radiant power stimulating the visual system and the spectral responsivity of the latter. The subjective nature of the second of these two factors sets photometric quantities apart from purely physical quantities.

This is a very important statement, because it makes clear that it makes sense, and actually it is very useful, to measure quantities that are not "purely physical," but rather have a "subjective nature," in that they measure the human response to some external stimuli. Basically, the measurement of luminous intensity may be done by spectrophotometers, which are instruments that first detect the radiant power by sensors and then process the resulting signal by applying a spectral weighting that accounts for the spectral responsivity of an average observer. Such weighting was determined by experiments of intensity matching by panels of subjects:

> The matching of brightness is the fundamental operation of photometry. In direct visual photometry, the visual stimuli provided by two juxtaposed uniform light patches of similar shape and angular area in the observer field of view are adjusted so that the patches appear equally bright. (Wyszecki, 1982)

Therefore the ultimate foundation for the measurement of luminous intensity includes the results of panel-testing experiments. The path for introducing quantities related to perception was thus opened then, in 1954, with the introduction of the candela, although the cultural consequences of that event perhaps have not yet been fully recognized. Luminous intensity has been the outrider for what we now call "physiological quantities," to which we return at a later stage. By now it is important to note further that measurements in the field of biology, health, and safety have thus far become more and more important. Interestingly enough, in the 21st General Conference on Weights and Measures (GCPM) in 1999, it is recommended that

> those responsible for studies of Earth resources, the environment, human well-being and related issues ensure that measurements made within their programmes are in terms of well-characterised SI units so that they are reliable in the long term, are comparable worldwide and are linked to other areas of science and technology through the world's measurement system established and maintained under the Metre Convention. (BIPM, 1999)

To sum up, in the midst of the twentieth century the international system of metrology took a major step forward with the constitution of the SI, with the subsequent inclusion in the fundamental quantities of a unit, the candela, that takes account of the human perception of a physical stimulus. Increasing attention to quantities of this kind has emerged, and they have been recognized as treatable with the paradigm of derived measurement that we have discussed in the previous section. The time was right for attempting a systematization of the theory of measurement.

### 1.7.1 *An attempt at systematization: The representational theory of measurement*

A remarkable systematization of the formal theory of measurement was achieved by the representational theory (Krantz, Luce, Suppes, & Tversky, 1971; Roberts, 1979/2009; Suppes, Krantz, Luce, & Tversky, 1989; Luce, Krantz, Suppes, & Tversky, 1990), which combines the viewpoints of Campbell and Stevens, and are seen as complementary rather than opposing. The main idea, traceable, as we have seen, to Helmoltz, is that the numbers we obtain through measurement represent empirical relations. This holds true for fundamental physical measurements, as intended by Campbell, here called extensive, but also for other, weaker, scales, as envisaged by Stevens. Consequently the classification of scales proposed by Stevens may be retained and each scale is now characterized by a *representation theorem* and a *uniqueness theorem*.

A representation theorem, for a given scale, states in which way, for that scale, empirical relations are mapped into corresponding numerical ones. For example, in an ordinal scale, it reads

$$a \succcurlyeq b \Leftrightarrow m(a) \geq m(b), \tag{1.5}$$

that is, an empirical order between two objects, $a \succcurlyeq b$, holds if and only if the corresponding numerical order holds between their measures, $m(a) \geq m(b)$. Consider the notation: the symbol $\succcurlyeq$ denotes an empirical relation between two objects, whereas the symbol $\geq$ denotes a similar relation for the corresponding measures, which are numbers. This careful distinction between empirical relations and numerical ones is typical of the representational theory and requires a proper notation.

The uniqueness theorem says what transformations may be safely applied to the scale without altering the meaning of the measurement: for example, in the ordinal scale case monotonic increasing transformations may be applied, because they are order preserving. Through this theorem the meaningfulness of statements concerning measurement may be addressed: we may say that a statement concerning the results of measurement on a given scale is meaningful if its truth is unaffected by admissible transformations on that scale.

A summary of the representation framework is presented in Table 1.2, which is provided here just to give an overview of some of the main results of the representational

*Table 1.2* Summary of the main scales for fundamental measurement, as considered in the representational theory

| *Empirical structure* | *Empirical relations* | *Scale type* | *Representation* | *Admissible transformations* |
|---|---|---|---|---|
| Nominal | Equivalence among elements in each class | Nominal | $a \sim b \Leftrightarrow m(a) = m(b)$ | Bi-univocal |
| Order | Weak order among the objects | Ordinal | $a \succcurlyeq b \Leftrightarrow m(a) \geq m(b)$ | Monotonic increases |
| Difference | As above plus weak order among intervals | Interval | $\Delta_{ab} \succcurlyeq \Delta_{cd} \Leftrightarrow$ $m(a) - m(b) \geq m(c) - m(d)$ | Linear positive $m' = \alpha m + b$ $\alpha > 0$ |
| Extensive | As above plus a concatenation operation | Ratio | $a \sim b \circ c \Leftrightarrow$ $m(a) = m(b) + m(c)$ | Similarity $m' = \alpha m$ $\alpha > 0$ |

*Note:* Symbols ~, ≻, ≽, ∘ denote relations or operations among objects, whereas =, >, ≥, + denote similar relations or operations among numbers. In particular, "~" means "equivalent to", "≻" "greater than", "≽" "greater than or equivalent to, and "∘" denotes empirical addition.

approach. We do not go into details now; the representational approach is probed further in Chapter 4, with a special focus on uniqueness, and is also discussed in Chapter 5, where the formalism is reviewed and a probabilistic reformulation provided.

The representational theory has been developed mainly in the field of behavioral sciences (Iverson & Luce, 1998) but has been brought to the attention of physicists and engineers since the 1970s, mainly by Finkelstein, who has supported its feasibility for all kinds of measurements. His definition of measurement as "a process of empirical, objective assignment of symbols to attribute of objects and events of the real world, in such a way as to represent them or to describe them" (1982) is famous. This theory also received, afterwards, contributions from that community (Finkelstein, 2005; Muravyov & Savolainen, 2001; Rossi, 2007) and it actually constitutes an excellent starting point for a unified theory of measurement.

## 1.8 Preparing the future

It is now time for briefly reviewing the current state of the art and for indicating possible development lines.

### *1.8.1 Trends in metrology*

In the last part of the twentieth century some very important issues emerged in metrology. The need of accompanying measurement results with a statement on their uncertainty was recognized as a means of fully providing measurement information. A working group was appointed to search for an internationally agreed way of expressing uncertainty and to prepare guidelines. After a long discussion, a noteworthy proposal was produced, the *Guide for Expression of Uncertainty in Measurement* (GUM), published in 1993 (BIPM, 2008a). This event has pushed parallel and successive research efforts, both on the theoretical and on the application side.

At the same time another important initiative was carried out concerning the revision of the language in metrology, which yielded the publication of the international vocabulary of basic and general terms in metrology (1984), now in its third edition (BIPM, 2008b). All the revisions have implied a profound reconsideration of the matter, which demonstrates the criticality of this issue.

Third, the cooperation among members of the BIPM has been reinforced and made more effective with the institution of a *Mutual Recognition Agreement* (CIPM MRA) (BIPM, 2008c), which specifies the organizational and technical requirements for the mutual recognition of measurements performed by national metrological institutes (NMIs). A major tool for such recognition is *key comparisons*. In some cases, comparisons are performed directly against an international reference facility at the BIPM. In others a stable traveling standard is circulated among several NMIs, which are asked to provide a measurement value for it, accompanied by an uncertainty statement. An international committee of NMI experts in the field evaluates the resulting data and provides practical information on the degree of comparability of the individual results. Similar exercises, called intercomparisons, are performed among laboratories at lower levels of the metrological structure and they are very effective for guaranteeing the performance of the overall system of metrology. Their use could perhaps be extended to measurement in behavioral sciences also, as we mention at a later stage. The CIPM MRA agreement further confirms the benefit of making a system of measurement activities performed in the world (BIPM, 2003). Such a system may perhaps undergo a noteworthy reorganization in a few years, inasmuch as there is a proposal to revise the definition of the base quantities through the natural constants that link them (Mills et al., 2006; Wallard, 2009, 2011). There is no room here for discussing this topic in detail; we simply note that the system of metrology has an evolutionary nature, and with this continuous process of revision it contributes significantly to the overall progress of science and technology.

In the core of this system, a new paradigm has recently emerged, *soft metrology*, defined as "measurement techniques and models which enable the objective quantification of properties which are determined by human perception," where "the human response may be in any of the five senses: sight, smell, sound, taste and touch" (Pointer, 2003). A unique opportunity for pursuing studies in this area has also emerged meantime.

### *1.8.2 The "measuring the impossible" environment*

The measurement of quantities related to human perception has recently received important support by a European Call, named Measuring the Impossible (MtI), as a part of the New and Emerging Science and Technology (NEST) programme. NEST aims at supporting unconventional and visionary research with the potential to open new fields for science and technology, as well as research on potential problems uncovered by science.

Motivations under the MtI Call include *scientific arguments*, "many phenomena of significant interest to contemporary science are intrinsically multidimensional and multidisciplinary, with strong cross-over between physical, biological, and social sciences," *economic aspects*, "products and services appeal to consumers according to parameters of quality, beauty, comfort, etc., which are mediated by human perception," and *social reasons*, "public authorities, and quasi public bodies such as hospitals, provide citizens with support and services whose performance is measured according to parameters of life quality, security or wellbeing" (European Commission, 2007). The focus is on "measurements which are holistic and multi-dimensional in nature, and which involve complex issues of interpretation, and/or mediation by human perception."

Several projects have been launched in this perspective and a need for coordinated action has been envisaged, which has given rise to an action called MINET, Measuring the Impossible Network. MINET is the result of a new way of approaching the problems that we have so far discussed. It starts from the recognition of the interdisciplinary character of measurement involving persons and identifies outcomes from the consideration that the interdisciplinary nature of the MtI raises new challenges. The MINET activity has included the organization of workshops, think tank events, and an international course, held in Genova, Italy, in June 2008, which was attended by 70 people from 14 different countries. This course has given rise to this book. This is where we are now: it is thus time to briefly review some current areas of research and to address future needs.

## 1.9 Current research issues and future needs

Research issues central to measurement with persons may be grouped in three main categories,

- Instrumentation and methods
- Foundation and theory
- Implementation areas and applications

### *1.9.1 Instrumentation and methods*

*Instrumentation-oriented* research concerns both the measurement of physical events (the stimuli) that give rise to a sensory response and the physiological (or behavioral) responses to internal/external stimuli. It would also include perception and interpretation processes and the development of sensors that mimic, to some extent, human perception. Since the time of the "schism" in the 1940s, progress in these areas has been enormous; concerning, for example, the measurement of sound, we now have highly accurate measurement microphones and binaural recording devices that make it possible to measure the acoustic stimuli as they appear at the input to the auditory system. We also have sophisticated binaural reproduction devices with processors and algorithms for the required signal processing. Sound perception is treated in Chapter 11 in this book. In the case of sight, we can measure not only luminous intensity and color, but also parameters of the interaction between light and matter, as well as properties of surfaces, such as texture that also involve sophisticated signal processing. Visual perception is treated in Chapter 13 and the skin senses in Chapter 12.

Concerning the measurement of physiological processes, novel techniques are available, especially in the field of brain imaging (Bronzino, 1995). These techniques developed rapidly because of their great value in neurophysiology/neuroscience and are treated amply in Chapter 14. As we have mentioned, there is increasing interest in exploring physiological quantities, that is, quantities caused by physiological responses in the human body, and their compatibility with the international system of metrology (Nelson & Ruby, 1993). A workshop on this very topic was organized in November 2009, by the BIPM, dealing with optical radiation, radio waves and microwaves, ionizing radiation, acoustics, magnetic fields, and other international standard measures and units applied, for example, in documents by the World Health Organization.

In a broader vision of human response, we may include behavioral aspects also. In this regard, image-based measurements play a key role; they are essential, for example, for studying emotions or body language, which are treated in Chapter 15. Emotional responses may also be assessed by physiologically oriented measurements with instruments. Galvanic skin response, for example, measures detectable changes in skin conductance, induced by the sympathetic nervous system due to stress or emotions. Although often replaced by brain imaging, this relatively old method is still profitably used, because of its simplicity and low cost. Another approach to emotion is to measure the activation of critical facial muscles by electromyography (Dimberg, 1990). Moreover, highly valuable information on the complex mechanism of visual perception may be gained by the tracking of saccadic eye movements: current advances in this area have revealed space–time gaps that seem to be interpretable via relativistic-like principles.

Sensors that mimic human perception include, for example, the electronic nose. In current research aiming at directly sensing the quality of indoor air, such a device has been built according to a perceptual odor space determined empirically for materials emissions. It is multidimensional and the interdistances between odor qualities were calibrated with the aid of a set of odor references that fulfills reliability requirements. Other examples are tactile sensors, that have an increasing ability to "perceive" surface texture, or the visual sensors called artificial retinas. Advanced robotics and clinical applications are expected for these sensors. One example is the artificial arm equipped with tactile sensors which make it possible to appreciate the aesthetics of sculptures.

In fact, as we have explicitly noted for the electronic nose, all these instrumentation-related possibilities should not make us forget that the screening and testing of participants as measuring instruments are absolutely necessary for reliable and valid psychological measurement. Many reliable *methods of measurement* are available, ranging from the traditional methods of psychophysics (the method of limits, of average error, and of constant stimuli, which were developed by G. T. Fechner for determining absolute thresholds of detection and just noticeable differences or, in general, equalities or inequalities among sensations) through the basic methods of direct scaling introduced by S. S. Stevens (magnitude or ratio estimation and production), to the more advanced approaches, such as the master scaling (Berglund & Harju, 2003). Psychophysical measurements are treated in Chapter 2. Psychometrics is another school of measurement in psychology, as we have briefly mentioned, that uses standardized tests for collecting data, that is, in the form of questionnaires, interviews, or performance tasks.

Thurstonian scaling (Thurstone, 1927) is somewhat intermediate between psychophysics and psychometrics and is sometimes called "indirect scaling" as opposed to Stevens's direct scaling. From a psychophysical perspective, this approach is based on the assumption that a single value of an external stimulus will evoke perceptions that are mapped on an inner psychological continuum, giving rise to a probability distribution, usually assumed to be Gaussian. So it is possible to establish a precise relation between distances on such a continuum and the probability of order relations. Accordingly, it is possible to infer, from a pair-comparison test, a metric scaling. Actually, these inner representations are not necessarily related to an external stimulus and this is why this approach may also be used in psychometrics: indeed, it was first proposed for measuring attitude. A remarkable model for psychometric tests is provided by the item response theory, in which the probability of the correct response to a test item is a function of person and item parameters.

To summarize, many methods are available for gathering information from the real world, whether outer or inner, and we must focus on how best to use such information. This is where measurement theory comes into play.

### *1.9.2 Foundations and theory*

Several foundational and theoretical issues are, in our opinion, of prime interest in this area, including

- The language
- The concepts of measurement scale and of measuring system (or instrument)
- The logic (deterministic, probabilistic, fuzzy, etc.)
- The issue of measurability
- Multidimensionality and mathematical modeling

*Language* has been a main issue in twentieth-century scientific and philosophical debate. In the metrology community, a noteworthy revision of linguistic terms has been undertaken, starting with the publication of the international vocabulary of basic and general terms in metrology (1984), now in its third edition (BIPM, 2008b). It is interesting to note the evolution of such editions, because the trend has been to include further disciplinary areas. It may be envisaged that in the near future, measurement with persons may play a role there. Moreover, in the workshops and think tank events organized by MINET, the issue of language/vocabulary soon emerged. It is natural that this will be a challenge in any multidisciplinary environment. Yet, in any revision of terms, a revision of concepts and theories must also be considered, that indeed will be beneficial for the entire world of measurement (Rossi, 2009a).

Any theory of measurement should deal, at least, with two main topics, the *measurement scale* and the *measurement process*. As we have seen, the notion of scale is central to representational theory, and it should be given more consideration in physical measurement too. Although nowadays we know much about scales, further research is still needed for ensuring that this concept is really common to measurement in physical, psychological, and social sciences. This includes, for example, a probabilistic formulation (Schweizer & Skal, 1983; Rossi, 2006), a better understanding of the notion of scale in the case of derived quantities, and a better systematization of the foundations for various psychological methods of measurement. The probabilistic approach is treated in Chapter 5 and the fuzzy one in Chapter 10.

The concept of *measurement process* has a strange history. It is closely related to the notion of *measuring system*, or instrument. Although scientific instruments have been the key to developing modern science since the time of Galileo, and they are a key topic in university courses on measurement (Bentley, 2005), it is interesting to realize that instruments were ignored in the research on the foundation of measurement. Only recently was the theoretical role of the measuring system outlined. In particular, it is important to consider whether this is important only for physical measurement or for psychological measurement, too.

The question of the *logic* is transversal to all the above. If uncertainty is recognized as an essential aspect in measurement, a probabilistic or a fuzzy logic may be best suited (De Coensel, Botteldooren, Debacq, Nilsson, & Berglund, 2008). Systematic studies in these latter perspectives are still in their infancy.

*Measurability* has recently been discussed and proposals, mainly based on the representational approach, have been presented (Finkelstein 2005, 2008; Rossi, 2007). This is clearly a key point requiring careful discussion together with *mise en pratique* issues.

As outlined in the MtI Call, *multidimensionality* is often involved in the processes of human perception and interpretation. A shift from unidimensional to multidimensional measurements will result in significant changes. In a unidimensional scale, the key property is order, whereas in a multidimensional space, the key property is distance (or content). Moreover, in the latter case the problem of dimensionality reduction becomes most important. In future work, it would be beneficial to proceed with foundational search in parallel with mathematical and numerical developments of models and methods (Muravyov & Savolainen, 2001). Multidimensionality is treated in Chapters 6–9, from various standpoints.

Human perception and interpretation of, say, the living or working environment, may be understood through the mediation of *modeling*. Modeling of complex perceptual environments requires a combination of physical and perceptual measures. An example of modeling is presented in Chapter 8.

### *1.9.3 Implementation areas and applications*

Measurements related to human perception and interpretation have a wide range of actual and potential applications (European Commission, 2007; Rossi, 2009b; Rossi & Berglund, 2009). Here we briefly mention the areas of perceived quality (of products and services), environment, ergonomics, safety, security, and clinics. The role of measurement in decision making is addressed in Chapter 16.

In the first part of the last century, the impact of mass production was so high that qualitative aspects of goods were somewhat neglected. Today, the shortage of energy sources and the concern for pollution may cause an increasing request for durable, high-quality goods. Thus, *perceived quality*, which results from perception and interpretation of sensory input, may play a key role in industrial competition. Examples of products include food, materials, and simple and complex devices. A good cup of coffee, for example, is appreciated on the basis of a combination of taste, smell, sight, and touch. Common materials of daily use include fabric, paper, wood, and stone. For these, the feeling of naturalness is important: in this regard, as already mentioned, research is ongoing for relating naturalness with a combination of visual and tactile inputs (Goodman et al., 2008). Domestic electric appliances are appreciated not just on the basis of their performance, but also, perhaps mainly, because of the sound quality they produce as well as their visual appearance. Color photocopiers seem to be evaluated mainly on the basis of pleasantness instead of fidelity; in the case of single colors, pleasantness seems mainly to depend on hue, lightness, and chroma, whereas for combinations of colors, predictions are more difficult. The next generation of touch screens on mobile devices may provide some touch feedback, that is, simulating texture by varying friction factor through controlled ultrasonic oscillation. Last, for many years, car producers have been aware of how interior car noise, door-closure sound, and even interior smell will affect a customer's decision to buy a new car.

The last example is particular significant because in the last, say, 20 years, perceived quality has been the main (or even the only) motivation for supporting research in the product development area, at least at the European Community level. Yet, we believe that even if this remains an important application area, as we have claimed, there are other emerging areas, perhaps even more valuable in a strategic perspective.

Outdoor and indoor *environments* are going to be of major concern in the years to come. Outdoors, visual, olfactory, and auditory perception provide the basis for quality evaluation. Research projects concerned with the characterization of landscapes and soundscapes (i.e., a combination of sounds that results from an immersive environment) may be mentioned, as well as measurement campaigns for reducing loudness or odor intensity of fertilizers in the surroundings of industrial plants. This study area, called "environmental psychophysics," faces challenges of characterizing exposures in a multisensory way, varying over time, and often obscured by background conditions, that requires carefully designed and controlled measurement procedures (Berglund, 1991). Indoor environment is also of great importance, because people spend about 90% of their time indoors, either at work, at home, or when commuting between work and home. The quality of the indoor environment depends upon the quality of its subsystems: air quality, soundscapes, visual–tactual surfaces, and their integration. Perceptual studies and measurements must thus be combined with sophisticated modeling of complex systems.

The indoor environment provides an immediate link to *ergonomics*. Although originally intended to deal with work systems only, ergonomics has now a new definition by the International Ergonomics Association:

> The scientific discipline concerned with the understanding of the interactions among human and other elements of a system, and the profession that applies theory, principles, data, and methods to design in order to optimize human well-being and overall system performance.

It is now concerned with human activities in general, including work, study, recreation, or rest. The relationship between human beings and their environment, including machines and devices, is experienced through the senses and perceptual measurements are key ways for obtaining valuable scientific and professional data. A typical ergonomic concern is the measurement of comfort. In transportation systems discomfort is often associated with noise and vibration exposures in which case perception plays a central role. Epidemiological or quasi-experimental studies in their various forms rely on measurement with persons as their main tool.

Ergonomics aims at ensuring a good quality of life for operators and, on the other hand, a best performance of the system concerned. Consider the case of a driver: ensuring that he or she is working in optimal conditions is possibly the best means of guaranteeing the *safety* of the people carried. Consider also the case of a watchman: here his or her performance affects *security*.

Security is another important application area. The case of face recognition for the identification of suspected persons may be briefly considered. So far, several approaches have been implemented for the automation of this task: comparing a picture of a suspect with a database of criminals may be too heavy a task for a human being. At present, approaches related to the psychology of face recognition seem to be promising (Wenger & Townsend, 2001). They are related to multidimensional measurements and to perceptual models and are treated in Chapter 7. Forensic science is a closely related field; a major problem there is the reliability of eyewitness testimony, not because of any wish to lie, but to failures in memory. There are ongoing studies in perception and memory formation that may result in practical methods for assessing the reliability of eyewitnesses.

*Clinical* applications are also important. The measurement of the intensity of pain may help to optimize treatments (Berglund & Harju, 2003); changes in sensorial sensitivity may be used in diagnostics (e.g., decreased smell sensitivity as an early warning symptom for Alzheimer's disease) or for the monitoring of rehabilitation processes. Last, humanoid robotics aims at developing machines that resemble, to some extent, some aspect of human behavior. They must be equipped with sophisticated sensor interfaces that mimic certain aspects of human perception and may be used in rehabilitation and special assistance programs.

## 1.10 Final remarks

We are now at the end of this short journey along the development of measurement across the physical and behavioral sciences. We have paid special attention to the schism of the 1930s that impeded coordinated progress in the various disciplines involved. We have tried and explicated the terms of the dispute in some detail and we have shown how the successive development of measurement science, in its various aspects, has essentially contradicted the conclusions of the BAAS report on the impossibility of finding a common ground for investigation. Contact points between measurement in physics and in psychology are now more substantial than differences, in our opinion, and there are signs of initiatives to rebuild the bridge between the disciplines.

The case of physiological quantities is emblematic: the ultimate foundation for the measurement of luminous intensity, for example, is summarized in a set of experimental curves that basically express the perceptual response of persons to some aspects of light, as collected, checked, and finally accepted, in a thorough experiment carried out at the beginning of the last century (BIPM, 2009).

We have also seen that sound scientific, social, and economic reasons push now for a concerted effort by the scientific community to face the challenge of measurement with persons. We are now at the beginning of a path that will require proper steps. We try to figure out three of them (Rossi & Berglund, 2011).

The first step may somehow be the hardest; it requires some change in the conventional attitudes of both parties. Physicists and engineers should perhaps be more open to accept that measurement may also be performed through the human perception and interpretation, although, obviously, in properly designed and conducted experiments. This may contrast somewhat with the traditional education of many that often interprets the requisite of "objectivity" as absence of human intervention, rather than as collective (i.e., intersubjective) agreement on methods and procedures. On the other hand, psychologists and behavioral scientists should perhaps develop a greater sensitivity to the benefit of an international organization supporting the measurement of, at least, some key perceptual quantities, such as, for example, loudness or odor intensity. Some of the quality-control procedures of the international system of metrology, such as intercomparisons, could perhaps be applied, after proper adaptation, to the qualification of methods for measuring perceptual quantities.

Another major step would consist in making a joint effort to develop a common theory for measurement. This would also greatly help in achieving a common language: once common ideas are developed, the words for phrasing them will be found as well.

Last, the third step (logically, not necessarily temporally) would be to work together on common projects. An excellent opportunity in this regard has been provided by the MtI Call and in particular by the associated MINET Action. This book is a result of such a collaboration and it is hoped that it will inaugurate a new era for this subject. A large band of scholars and scientists from physical, psychological, biological, and social sciences have accepted the challenge of working together to reach a common understanding of measurement theory and methods. The aim is to provide, seemingly, the first book ever issued covering the topic of measurement with persons through a multi- and interdisciplinary approach. The complementary aspects of general theory, measurement methods, instrumentation, and modeling are treated together by scientists in the related fields of psychophysics and general psychology, measurement theory, metrology, and instrumentation, neurophysiology, engineering, biology, and chemistry.

The book is organized in two parts. In the first, generic theoretical and methodological issues are treated, including the conceptual basis of measurement in the various fields involved, the development of formal, representational, and probabilistic theories, the approach to experimentation and the theories, models, and methods for multidimensional problems. In the second, several implementation areas are presented, including sound, visual, skin, and odor perception, functional brain imagining, body language and emotions, and, finally, the use of measurements in decision making.

## References

Bentley, J. P. (2005). *Principles of measurement systems* (4th ed.). Harlow, Essex, UK: Pearson Education.

Berglund, B., (1991). Quality assurance in environmental psychophysics. In S. J. Bolanowski, & G. A. Gescheider (Eds.), *Ratio scaling of psychological magnitudes*. Hillsdale, NJ: Erlbaum.

Berglund, B., & Harju, E. (2003). Master scaling of perceived intensity of touch, cold and warmth. *European Journal of Pain*, *7*, 323–334.

BIPM. (1983). *Principles governing photometry*. Luisant: Imprimerie Durand.

BIPM. (2001). *Proceedings of the 21st General Conference on Weights and Measures*, 11–15 October.

BIPM. (2003). *Guidelines to CIPM key comparisons*.

BIPM. (2006). *The International System of Units* (8th ed.). Paris: STEDI.

BIPM. (2008a). *Evaluation of measurement data—Guide to the expression of uncertainty in measurement.* (JCGM 100:2008).

BIPM. (2008b). *International vocabulary of metrology—Basic and general terms (VIM).* (JCGM 200:2008).

BIPM. (2008c). *Mutual recognition.* Paris: STEDI.

BIPM. (2009). BIPM Workshop on Physiological Quantities and SI Units. Online. Available HTTP: http://www.bipm.org/en/events/physiological_quantities/ (accessed 14 April 2011)

BIPM. (2010). The new SI. Online. Available HTTP: http://www.bipm.org/en/si/new_si/ (accessed 14 April 2011)

Bronzino, J. D. (Ed.). (1995). *The biomedical engineering handbook.* Boca Raton, FL: CRC & IEEE Press.

Campbell, N. R. (1957). *Foundations of science.* New York: Dover. (Original work, *Physics—The elements,* published 1920)

De Coensel, B., Botteldooren, D., Debacq, K., Nilsson, M. E., & Berglund, B. (2008). Clustering outdoor soundscapes using fuzzy ants. Paper presented at the *2008 IEEE World Congress on Computational Intelligence, WCCI 2008*, Hong Kong.

Dimberg, U. (1990). Facial electromyography and emotional reactions. *Psychophysiology*, *27,* 481–494.

European Commission. (2007). *Measuring the impossible.* (EUR 22424). European Communities.

Fechner, G. T. (1966). *Elements of psychophysics* (Vol. I). New York: Holt, Rinehart and Winston. (Original work published 1860)

Ferguson, A., Myers, C. S., & Bartlett, R. J. (1940). Quantitative estimation of sensory events—Final BAAS Report. *Advances of Science*, *2*, 331–349.

Finkelstein, L. (1982). Theory and philosophy of measurement. In P. H. Sydenham (Ed.), *Handbook of measurement science* (Vol. 1, pp. 1–30). Chichester, UK: Wiley.

Finkelstein, L. (2005). Problems of measurement in soft systems. *Measurement, 38*, 267–274.

Finkelstein, L. (2008, September). Problems of widely-defined measurement. Paper presented at the *12th IMEKO TC1 and TC7 Symposium on Man, Science and Measurement*, Annecy, France.

Gescheider, G. A. (1997). *Psychophysics: the fundamentals* (3rd ed.). London: Erlbaum.

Goodman, T., Montgomery, R., Bialek, A., Forbes, A., Rides, M., Whitaker, T. A., Overvliet, K., McGlone, F., & van der Heijden, G. (2008, September). The measurement of naturalness. Paper presented at the *12th IMEKO TC1 and TC7 Symposium on Man, Science and Measurement,* Annecy, France.

Helmholtz, H. (1971). An epistemological analysis of counting and measurement. In R. Karl (Ed. and Trans.), *Selected writing of Hermann Helmholtz.* Middletown, CT: Wesleyan University Press. (Original work published 1887)

Iverson, G., & Luce, R. D. (1998). The representational measurement approach to psychophysical and judgmental problems. In M. H. Birnbaum (Ed.), *Measurement, judgment, and decision making* (pp. 1–79). New York: Academic Press.

Krantz, D. H., Luce, R. D., Suppes, P., & Tversky, A. (1971). *Foundations of measurement* (Vol. 1). New York: Academic Press.

Lord F. M., & Novick, M. R. (1968). *Statistical theories of mental test scores.* Reading, MA: Addison-Wesley.

Luce, R. D., Krantz, D. H., Suppes, P., & Tversky, A. (1990). *Foundations of measurement—Representation, axiomatization and invariance.* New York: Academic Press.

Mills, J. M., Mohr, P. J., Quinn, T. J., Taylor, B. N., & Williams, E. R. (2006). Redefinition of the kilogram, ampere, kelvin and mole: A proposed approach to implementing CIPM recommendation 1 (CI-2005). *Metrologia, 43,* 227–246.

Muravyov S., & Savolainen, V. (2001). Special interpretation of formal measurement scales for the case of multiple heterogeneous properties. *Measurement, 29,* 209–224.

Nelson, R. A., & Ruby, L. (1993). Physiological units in the SI. *Metrologia, 30,* 55–60.

Nowell Jones, F. (1974). History of psychophysics and judgement. In E. C. Carterette, & M. P. Friedman (Eds.), *Handbook of perception* (Vol. 2). New York: Academic Press.

Pointer, M. R. (2003). *New directions—Soft metrology requirements for support from mathematics statistics and software* (NPL Report CMSC 20/03).

Roberts, F. S. (1979). *Measurement theory, with applications to decision-making, utility and the social sciences.* Reading, MA: Addison-Wesley. Digital Reprinting (2009). Cambridge, UK: Cambridge University Press.

Rossi, G. B. (2006). A probabilistic theory of measurement. *Measurement, 39,* 34–50.

Rossi, G. B. (2007). Measurability. *Measurement, 40,* 545–562.

Rossi G. B. (2009a). Cross-disciplinary concepts and terms in measurement. *Measurement, 42,* 1288–1296.

Rossi, G. B. (2009b) Measurement of quantities related to human perception. In F. Pavese et al. (Eds.), *Advanced mathematical and computational tools in metrology and testing (AMCTM VIII)* (pp. 279–290). Singapore: World Scientific.

Rossi, G. B., & Berglund, B. (2009, September). Measurement related to human perception and interpretation—State of the art and challenges. Paper presented at the *XIX IMEKO World Congress*, Lisbon.

Rossi, G. B., & Berglund, B. (2011). Measurement involving human perception and interpretation. *Measurement, 44,* 815–822.

Schweizer, B., & Sklar, A. (1983). *Probabilistic metric spaces.* New York: North Holland.

Stevens, S. S. (1936). A scale for the measurement of psychological magnitude, loudness. *Psychological Review, 43,* 405–416.

Stevens, S. S. (1946). On the theory of scales and measurement. *Science, 103,* 677–680.

Stevens, S. S. (1956). The direct estimation of sensory magnitudes: Loudness. *American Journal of Psychology, 69,* 1–25.

Stevens, S. S. (1959). Measurement, psychophysics and utility. In C. W. Churchman, & P. Ratoosh (Eds.), *Basic concepts of measurements* (pp.1–49). Cambridge, UK: Cambridge University Press.

Suppes, P., Krantz, D. H., Luce, R. D., & Tversky, A. (1989). *Foundations of measurement—Geometrical, threshold and probabilistic representations.* New York: Academic Press.

Thurstone, L. L. (1927). A law of comparative judgements. *Psychological Review, 34,* 273–286.

Wallard, A. (2009, September). World metrology—The next ten years. Invited paper presented at the *XIX IMEKO World Congress*, Lisbon.

Wallard, A. (2011). News from the BIPM—2010. *Metrologia, 48,* 59–67.

Wenger, M. J., & Townsend, J. T. (Eds.). (2001). *Computational, geometric and process issues in facial cognition: Progress and challenges.* Hillsdale, NJ: Erlbaum.

Wozniak, R. H. (1999). *Classics in psychology, 1855–1914: Historical essays.* Bristol, UK: Thoemmes Press.

Wyszecki, G. (1982). *Color science.* New York: John Wiley & Sons.

# 2 Measurement in psychology

*Birgitta Berglund*

Department of Psychology
Stockholm University
and
Institute of Environmental Medicine, Karolinska Institutet
Stockholm, Sweden

## 2.1 Introduction

In psychology, there are two main schools of metrology: psychophysics and psychometrics. The former is grounded in physics and the latter in statistics, but both presume that attributes of psychological experience may be viewed as quantities, which, in turn, may be represented by numbers. In practice, psychophysics has utilized the assumption of a "standard observer." This would mean that single individuals are in principle viewed as measuring instruments (persons) that may be used for measuring certain perceptual/evaluative features of the environment or of other persons (e.g., detection, discrimination, perceived intensity, pleasantness, naturalness, friendliness, and so on; "measurement *with* person(s)"). In practice, psychometrics has utilized the idea of a "standard stimulus." Stimuli or sets of test items are in principle viewed as a measuring instrument (psychological test) that may be used for measuring mainly mental processes of single and unique individuals (e.g., emotions, personality, political attitudes, psychomotor skills, etc.; "measurement *of* person(s)").

Whereas the main focus of psychometrics has been to measure interindividual differences in psychological processes, psychophysics has focused on utilizing similarities in sensory functions for measuring perception, interpretation, and evaluation of complex phenomena. Early applications of psychophysics were primarily concerned with interindividual differences in sensory functions, for example, diagnosing specific color blindness and fitting eyeglasses or determining the degree of hearing loss and fitting hearing aids or diagnosing chronic pain conditions.

Metrology schools grounded in theories of psychophysics have also developed in other fields of science, including neuroscience, ergonomics, sensory analysis, robotics, acoustics, optics, and aesthetics. Similar to psychometrics, statistically based metrology schools are found in biometrics, chemometrics, political science, sensory analysis, sociology, epidemiology, mathematical psychology, assessment designers, marketing, and education, among others. This chapter introduces the main psychophysical measurement techniques, which the author and many others have found useful in application areas inside and outside psychology. Although measurement with persons and measurement of persons require well-designed experiments, the issues of experimental design are not discussed here, nor is the methodological research on the methods themselves (for introductions, see, e.g., Cook & Campbell, 1979 and Gescheider, 1997, respectively).

## 2.2 Perceptual, hedonic, and multisensory constructs

Psychophysics provides many methods and complementary techniques for measuring human sensory perception such as *perceived intensity* and *perceived quality*. The different methods and techniques are linked to certain kinds of constructs to be measured. It is important to keep perceptual (or physical) constructs separate because they refer to different kinds of abilities of our sensory–perceptual systems. Hedonic and multisensory constructs are also measured with the same techniques.

Basic *perceptual constructs* are linked to how human sensory systems are functioning or what they can do in terms of measurement. Because the methods for measuring perception deliver information specific to a sensory modality, the examples shown here are primarily from human olfaction. These are odor detection (or absolute odor threshold), odor-quality identification (or recognition), odor-intensity discrimination, odor-quality discrimination, odor-intensity quantification, and odor-quality classification, mapping, or labeling (data collection concerning categorization, similarities/dissimilarities, and odor-quality profiling, respectively). Some of these constructs require one-point measurements (absolute odor threshold); others measure quantity (odor intensity) or categorize and map odors (odor quality).

The *hedonic constructs* are also basic and include how human emotions affect and are integrated in sensory–perceptual processes. Examples are likes/dislikes, pleasantness/unpleasantness, preferences, and similar kinds of "emotional-evaluative" attributes (beautiful, tasty, joyful, etc.). Hedonic constructs are of course grounded in sensory–emotional coprocessing acquired through perceptual learning, and feelings would be as immediate as the sensory perceptions. Hedonic evaluations involve perception and cognition, learning, memory, and last but not least, *emotions*. One way of understanding a hedonic construct is to view emotions as being attributed to objects or events perceived with the aid of sensory systems. To exemplify, red is a perception, like odor, whereas favoring a red color of a particular carpet or an odor of a particular perfume is a matter of personal preference (= hedonic evaluation). We would all agree that we see red, but all will not agree that red is a beautiful color. The same is true for perfumes or air deodorants or indeed indoor air qualities. It follows that there are large interindividual differences in measurements of hedonic constructs as compared to sensory–perceptual constructs.

A third set of constructs is the *multisensory–perceptual* constructs, such as the perception of indoor air quality. Obviously, this is a more complex construct than odor quality, which originates in one sensory modality. Perceived air quality involves many kinds of sensory perceptions apart from odor [here given within brackets] and all these are interpreted and evaluated. The physical or chemical inputs [perceptions] are temperature [warmth or cold], air movement [cooling, warming, active touch], humidity [dryness, wetness], and irritants [sensory irritation, pain]. Nearly all odorous substances in indoor air have the potential to produce sensory irritation (e.g., Kobal & Hummel, 1991), but at much higher concentrations than is common in indoor or outdoor air. There has been renewed scientific interest in multisensory perception (e.g., Culvert, Spence, & Stein, 2004). Multisensory perceptual interpretations and evaluations should be recognized as measuring abilities unique to human beings.

## 2.3 Measurement with persons require experiments or other study designs

Measurement of perceptual, hedonic, and multisensory constructs (each assumed to be one-dimensional), is conducted with persons as the main measuring instrument. This means that a group of persons has to be selected who individually or as a panel constitute the measuring instrument of the perceptual, hedonic, or multisensory evaluations. Similarly, a sample of stimuli has to be provided, which specific physical–chemical properties have also to be defined as relevant and measured separately. Depending on what kind of study is to be conducted, either well-controlled stimuli (odorous substances, material emissions) are provided in a psychophysical experiment with persons in a laboratory or natural stimuli (indoor air) are provided in a quasi-experiment with visitors of buildings (field study). In the latter case, the environment (location, time of the day, ventilation rate, temperature, humidity, etc.) is well controlled and measured in parallel with the visitors' perceptual, hedonic, and multisensory measurements (alternatively, residents or occupants may constitute a panel). Often in psychological research, the concept of measurement is replaced by more imprecise words such as assessment and evaluation.

As illustrated in Figure 2.1, the method selected for measuring perceptions with the aid of individuals or panels is but one of the necessary components for the psychophysical experiment or the quasi-experiment in field situations. The quality of the olfactometer, the sample of stimuli and the panel (sample of persons) are all very important ingredients as are the instructions, experimental procedure, and types of data treatments planned in order to construct the scales from the sets of collected data (e.g., assumptions on the form of psychophysical function and type of distribution models applied for uncertainty). The kinds of scale delivered by the panel (nominal, ordinal, interval, or ratio) are vital to subsequent statistical or mathematical modeling of perceptual/hedonic or psychophysical data (e.g., S. S. Stevens, 1946).

Measurement in psychology has developed in parallel with the development within the general philosophy of science and measurement in physics. Impressive knowledge is found in Torgerson (1958), Lord and Novick (1968), Baird and Noma (1978), Roberts (1979), Falmagne (1985), and Gescheider (1997).

## 2.4 Psychophysical methods

### *2.4.1 What is measured?*

The psychophysical experiment may be used for measuring various functions of human *sensory perception*. Basic aspects are:

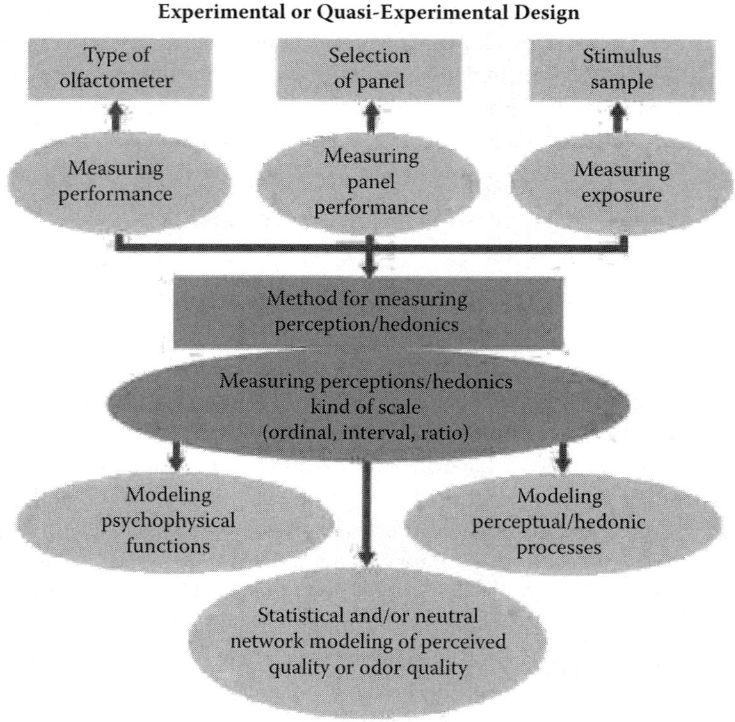


*Figure 2.1* Illustration of relevant components of experiments or quasi-experiments designed for perceptual, hedonic, or multisensory measurements with persons as measuring instruments.

1. *Identification:* Mere detection or recognition (presence of physical quantity)
2. *Discrimination:* Minimal change in perceived intensity (certain physical quantity)
3. *Perceived Intensity:* One-dimensional scaling of a quantity (perceptual quantity)
4. *Perceived Quality:* Sorting, clustering, or multidimensional scaling (mapping qualities)

Identification, discrimination, and perceived intensity are all possible to measure with psychophysical methods. Strictly, this would mean measuring perceptual constructs in terms of a physical quantity. Identification is a one-point physical measurement (threshold), whereas discrimination is a two-point physical measurement (minimal distance). The psychophysical method for measuring perceived intensity is the equal-intensity matching of two different qualities (of the same or different sensory modalities) at different intensity levels. Also perceived quality has been measured psychophysically. For example, the color triangle was originally constructed with the psychophysical method of perceived-quality discrimination combined with wavelengths representing perceived qualities (=colors). The psychophysical methods described above all measure a perceptual construct on a physical scale. For example, the method of equal-intensity matching would provide equal-loudness functions with different slopes for tones of different frequencies. Even if several different tones were matched to the same 1,000-Hz tone, it would not be appropriate to infer that a certain dB-increase of several tones actually corresponds to an invariant increase in loudness ("perceived intensity" of sound).

Sections 2.4.2, 2.4.4, and 2.4.6 present psychophysical methods of measurement, which all measure various aspects of perceptions in terms of a physical quantity and unit.

### 2.4.2 Detection or recognition

To measure perceptual detections is a psychophysical problem. A prerequisite is that people are put into situations, typically experiments (olfactometer and clean-air booth) but also field studies, where they may be stimulated and become aware that, for example, an olfactory stimulus is present. There are two principal detection theories: the "traditional" absolute threshold theory (e.g., Engen, 1971) and the signal detection theory (SDT, e.g., Green & Swets, 1962). Notably, the three basic methods for measuring the *absolute detection threshold* were originally contributed by Gustav Theodor Fechner himself. Signal detection theory grew out of the development of information theory in mathematical statistics and from work on electronic communications.

Odor detection experiments require an advanced *precision* olfactometer by which small steps of low concentrations can be produced repeatedly and presented to humans in well-controlled samples for inhalations (Berglund, Berglund, & Lindvall, 1986). In general, it has been found that the absolute detection threshold, which is expressed as a concentration or dilution value, varies widely with chemical substances (Devos, Patte, Rouault, Laffort, & van Gemert, 1990). It also varies with the method selected for determining the threshold. The method of limits usually gives lower thresholds than the method of constant stimulus. Recognition thresholds (including identification of odor quality) are generally higher than the mere detection thresholds of "something" unidentified.

The absolute odor threshold is a measure of one person's sensitivity to an odorous substance. As in other senses, for instance, vision and hearing, the interindividual differences in olfactory sensitivity may also be large. Typically, threshold distributions for different individuals are positively skewed even if expressed in log scale of concentration (Figure 2.2). It is not known if the absolute odor thresholds for a larger set of odorous substances would rank the same for different persons believed to be normosmics. In epidemiology, the method of limits is sometimes used for determining the effective dose 50 ($ED_{50}$) for a population of people or animals, for instance, for testing the impacts of drugs or odorous air pollutants (e.g., WHO, 1989, formaldehyde). The persons or animals are then assumed to be interchangeable (invariant detector) and a Gaussian distribution of individual thresholds is typically postulated. $ED_{50}$ is inappropriate to use for small samples of people because it relies on statistically representative random samples of a target population.

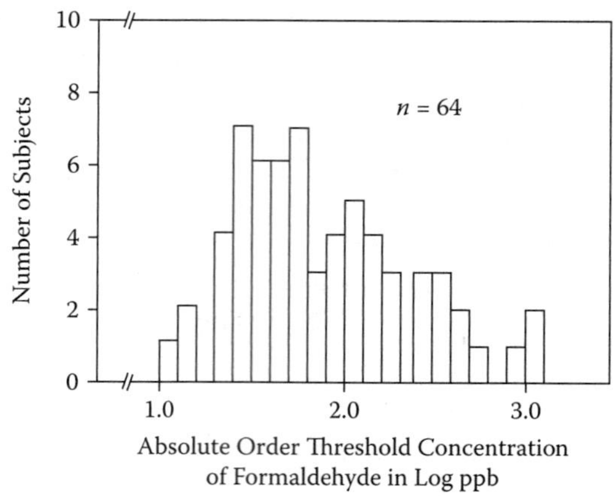


*Figure 2.2* Absolute odor thresholds of formaldehyde determined by the method of limits for each of 64 persons. The distribution of individual thresholds is given in a logarithmic scale of concentration in ppb. Reprinted from Ahlström et al. (1986).

### *2.4.2.1 The method of limits*

The method of limits measures just noticeable difference (JND) or minimal change and can be characterized as serial exploration. It is the most direct method for locating the threshold. The task of the observer is to detect the presence of a stimulus (odorous substance) in a series of small concentration (or dilution) steps (ca. 18–20) in an ascending and descending presentation order. The "one-point" of the momentary absolute threshold can be estimated directly from each series according to a predefined rule, for example, in ascending series two detections in a row and in descending series two nondetections in a row. The starting concentration should be irregularly varied between trials. The method gives a fairly quick measurement of the *individual absolute threshold* calculated as the mean of the response distribution measured in concentration (or dilution) values from each trial. The standard deviation or standard error is typically used as the uncertainty measure.

Figure 2.2 shows a distribution of individual absolute thresholds for formaldehyde odor determined by the method of limits. Even in a logarithmic scale of concentration, the absolute threshold distribution for a group of persons is typically positively skewed (Ahlström, Berglund, Berglund, Lindvall, 1986). Figure 2.2 therefore also shows the $ED_{50}$ measure for determining the absolute threshold for a group of 64 persons (effective dose for 50% of the 64 persons). This is not an optimal population estimate of the formaldehyde absolute threshold because the distribution is not symmetrical or normal and the sample is too small and consists of voluntary observers.

### *2.4.2.2 The methods of adjustment*

The method of adjustment measures the average error and the "reproduction," and it can be characterized as the equation method. The observer himself typically adjusts the concentration value of a stimulus (odorous substance), which can be varied continuously, and repeatedly sets it to a value that he judges to be the lowest that he can detect; the average of these settings is taken to be the individual absolute odor threshold. The different starting concentrations, both below and above the expected threshold, are presented in irregular order by the experimenter. Similar to the method of limits, the stimulus concentration is systematically increased or decreased until a change in response occurs (odor or no odor detections). The difference is that the observer adjusts the concentration continuously in the method of adjustment, whereas the experimenter changes the concentration in predetermined invariant distinct steps in the method of limits.

The method of adjustment gives a measurement of the individual absolute threshold calculated as the mean of the response distribution measured in concentration (or dilution) values from each trial. The standard deviation or standard error is typically used as the uncertainty measure. The method of adjustment is not well suited for determining odor thresholds because of the difficulties of changing odor concentrations continuously by an olfactometer.

### *2.4.2.3 The method of constant stimuli*

The method of constant stimuli is used to determine right and wrong cases and can be characterized as the frequency method. A series of concentration steps are chosen, similarly to the method of limits. However, instead of presenting the concentration steps in systematic order, they are now presented repeatedly in random order. The observer's task is simple. She should respond "Yes" if an odor is present or "No" if the odor is not present. A forced choice procedure (which does not allow "doubtful") is usually used. Two kinds of recommended procedures are in common use: (a) random presentation of the concentrations together with blanks (clean air), and (b) random presentation of the concentrations in one of two, three, or four marked time intervals; the other intervals are then blanks (clean air).

In the first case, chance performance (guessing) is determined for the blanks (ca. 33% of all presentations) and used for estimating the actual detection performance for each concentration. In the second case, chance performance is determined as 50% correct, 33% correct, or 25% correct for two, three, or four intervals, respectively.

In the first procedure, a psychometric curve is determined for each observer by plotting the proportion of correct detections ($Pc$) for each of the concentrations (10–18 steps) after adjusting the hit rate ($P_{Hits}$) for false alarms ($P_{FA}$). The absolute threshold ($P_c$ in Equation (2.1)),

$$P_c = \frac{P_{Hits} - P_{FA}}{1 - P_{FA}}, \qquad (2.1)$$

is determined as the concentration corresponding to the 50% probability of correct detection ($P_{50}$). The quartile range ($P_{75}$–$P_{25}$) expressed in concentration is typically used for estimating uncertainty. In the second procedure, the probability of detection above chance level is determined. The absolute threshold may then be defined as the concentration at 75% probability of detection, if 50% is chance performance.

### 2.4.3 *Signal detection theory and choice theory*

There is a theoretical mathematical system that formally deals with both decisional and sensory components in detection and discrimination tasks. In signal detection theory, the distance between the means of the absent signal (noise) and the present signal (signal plus noise) distributions (typically assumed to be Gaussian distributions) is the measure of detection. There is also a likelihood criterion set by each observer. Both positive and negative false responses can be estimated (see Table 2.1). A basic assumption is that no absolute detection threshold exists. The detections depend on how well the signal can be separated perceptually from the noise. In addition, the performance of individual observers in this perceptual "separation" task also depends on their individual likelihood criterion in responding yes or no (forced choice design is used).

Typically, the measure of sensory sensitivity selected is $d'$ of signal detection theory. It represents the distance on an excitation continuum between the means of the Gaussian distributions for the absent signal ("sensory noise") and for the present signal (signal + "sensory noise"; Green & Swets, 1962). An alternative but very similar procedure for determining *identification* (simultaneous detection and recognition) of a stimulus is Luce's choice theory (Luce, Bush, & Galanter, 1963). The signal detection theory requires high-quality equipment for rapid repetitive stimulation of odorous substances/mixtures and clean air (blanks). Berglund, Berglund, and Lindvall (1974) determined the relationship between (a) the $d'$ measure and signal strength (hydrogen sulfide concentration in mg/L), and (b) the $d'$ measure and the quantity of perceived odor intensity obtained by the method of magnitude estimation (see Section 2.4.7.3). They found that $d'$ increases as a linear function of the logarithm for stimulus concentration, that is,

$$d' = k_1 + k_2 \log S, \tag{2.2}$$

where $S$ is the physical concentration, $d'$ is the index of detectability, and $k_1$ and $k_2$ are constants. In addition, they showed empirically that the logarithm of perceived intensity ($\log R$) increases as a linear function of the $d'$ measure; that is,

$$\log R = c_1 + c_2 d', \tag{2.3}$$

*Table 2.1* Outcome frequencies in a forced-choice signal detection experiment

| | *Response* | |
|---|---|---|
| *Signal* | *Yes* | *No* |
| Present | Hit | Miss |
| Absent | False alarm | Correct rejection |

where $R$ is perceived odor intensity, $d'$ the index of detectability of odor, and $c_1$ and $c_2$ are constants. The combination of Equations (2.2) and (2.3) shows that the perceived odor intensity ($R$) increases as a power function of stimulus concentration ($S$); that is,

$$\log R = a + n \log S \tag{2.4}$$

or in linear scales, a power function with a multiplicative constant and an exponent $n$ (see Equation (2.7)).

The practical use of the detection technique is limited because the method assumes error variation in the subject's judgments. The signal has to be so weak that it is to some extent confused with the noise, without at the same time causing the experiment to become unreasonably large. The detection measure $d'$ is well suited for descriptions of rapid concentration changes at extremely low odor levels. Compared to absolute threshold measurements, $d'$ determinations appear to be superior from a theoretical point of view, as they are independent of variations in the response criterion of the subject, due to altered guessing tendencies, carelessness, lack of motivation, or the effect of expectations.

### *2.4.4 Intensity discrimination*

In determining *discrimination* or the *difference threshold* for intensive continua, the same general psychophysical procedure is followed as for the absolute detection threshold. The principal difference is that on each trial, two stimuli are presented for comparison, as contrasted to one stimulus in the typical absolute threshold procedure. Several series of ascending and descending concentrations are run and the average concentration differences of one standard concentration are calculated. In the experiment, the time order or position of the standard is typically varied randomly, as is the starting concentration of the comparison stimulus in each series. As for the absolute threshold, versions of the method of limits, method of adjustments, and method of constant stimulus are all also used for determining the minimal-intensity discrimination at different concentration levels (= standard stimulus) of the same odorous substance.

#### *2.4.4.1 Method of limits*

Observers are presented with pairs of stimuli; one is the invariant standard stimulus and the other the variable comparison stimulus. Instead of detection or not, the observers are now asked to respond which of the pair is "larger," "smaller," or "similar." In the most common version, the forced choice procedure, only the response alternatives "larger" or "smaller" are used. In the method of limits, the comparison stimulus is changed systematically in very small steps in a series of increasing or decreasing concentrations of an odorous substance (or diluted emission). The standard stimulus concentration is selected to be in the middle of these series. The data are the concentration values of the comparison stimulus where the observer shifts from one of the response categories to another. Statistically, the point of subjective equality (PSE) and the variability of the comparison concentrations are used to calculate the difference limen (see Section 2.4.3.3) at different standard concentrations.

### 2.4.4.2 *Method of adjustment*

Observers themselves adjust the value of a comparison stimulus, which can be varied continuously or in very small steps, and the task is to set it to the same perceived intensity as the standard stimulus concentration. This is made repeatedly, and the central tendency and variability of the settings are computed. The average setting is a direct indication of the point of subjective equality and the variability can be used to calculate the difference limen ($\Delta I$). This method is not well suited for investigating the difference limen for odor intensity because of the need for continuous variation of concentration by the participant.

### 2.4.4.3 *Method of constant stimuli*

For the difference limen ($\Delta I$), each of several fixed, discrete values of a comparison stimulus is compared with the standard stimulus many, many times, and the relative frequency of the different responses, for example, "smaller" or "larger" are counted for each of these fixed values (= the standard). If only two response categories are used, the observer will be right half of the time by just guessing, and his or her difference limen is therefore usually defined as the increment or decrement that was correctly judged 75% of the time (= probability in between 50% and 100%); The 50% stands for chance performance. If three response categories are used (adding "equal"), the method of constant stimuli becomes very similar to the method of limits.

## 2.4.5 Weber's law and Fechner's JND scale

The well-known Weber's law describes the relationship between the difference limen or difference threshold ($\Delta I$) and the magnitude of the standard ($I$):

$$\Delta I = kI\,. \tag{2.5}$$

Weber's law, which was proposed in 1834, is well grounded in psychophysical experiments, mainly on weights. Fechner (1860), who believed it impossible to measure sensation directly, acknowledged Weber's law and postulated that if the *units of sensation* were all of equal size, then it would be possible to count them up and thus measure sensation indirectly. He himself, and others before him, had noted that in order for a change in a stimulus to become just noticeable, a fixed percentage must be added: the *just noticeable difference* (abbreviated as JND).

In accordance with Weber's law, Fechner's law states that the magnitude of sensation or response varies directly with the logarithm of the stimulus magnitude (for the derivation please see Baird & Noma, 1978; Falmagne, 1985),

$$S = \left(\frac{1}{k}\right) \cdot \ln\left(\frac{I}{I_0}\right), \tag{2.6}$$

where $S$ is the magnitude of sensation a stimulus elicits (equals number of JNDs above 0 at absolute threshold), $I/I_0$ is the physical magnitude of the stimulus (intensity [$I$] relative to the absolute threshold stimulus magnitude [$I_0$]), $1/k$ is the inverse of the Weber fraction ($k = \Delta I/I$) and ln is the natural logarithm (logarithm to the base $e$). In this equation, $S = 0$ for $I/I_0 = 1$. Fechner's contribution is recognized because he gave psychology a way of constructing sensory scales. A scale based on the JND can be obtained either by adding the individual JND steps that are obtained by actual measurement or by assuming the validity of the more convenient logarithmic type of formula. Although experimental research has shown that Weber's law does not hold for very weak or very strong stimulus intensities, the logarithmic transformation may still be satisfactory for the middle ranges, which often are of greatest interest. However, with the increased use of category scaling and magnitude estimation and the development of S. S. Stevens' kinds of measurement levels (nominal, ordinal, interval, and ratio scales), much research has been devoted to criticize Fechner's theoretically derived logarithmic function (e.g., S. S. Stevens, 1975).

### *2.4.6 Equal-intensity matching*

#### *2.4.6.1 Intramodality matching of perceived intensity*

This is a scaling procedure in which the observer adjusts the intensity of a stimulus quality until it appears to be equally intense as another stimulus quality from the same sensory modality. Thus, *intramodality matching* means that the perceived intensity of each of two (odor) qualities of one modality (olfaction) is matched to be equally intense. The result of every match is registered as a concentration value for each of the corresponding two odorous substances. Intramodality matching is in principle the same as the method of adjustment when used for determining odor discrimination at different concentration levels (variance is then, however, of intent not level). The most famous example of intramodality matching is the equal-loudness curves determined for different frequencies of sound in which the 1,000 Hz tone was used as the comparison and all the other frequencies as standard tones one by one. These data resulted in the A-filter built into standard sound level meters for measuring the A-weighted equivalent continuous sound level in dB LAeq.

To speed up data collection with subjects, an odor intensity matching procedure grounded in successive approximations was combined with a high-flow dynamic olfactometer (Svensson & Szczygiel, 1974). The observers' task is only to answer which is more intense, a reference or a matching stimulus. New matching stimulus concentrations are given according to an algorithm that bisects intervals up or down in successive trials. This method is well suited for testing consumer products for odor quality, for example, biological toilets or kitchen fans. This is but one example of a development of the matching procedure.

#### *2.4.6.2 Cross-modality matching of perceived intensity*

This is a scaling procedure in which the observer adjusts the intensity of a stimulus until it appears to be equally intense as another stimulus from a different sensory modality. Thus, in cross-modality matching, observers are asked to adjust levels of one sensory modality to match various levels of another modality (e.g., S. S. Stevens, 1975). For other aspects of the matching procedure, see intramodality matching in Section 2.4.6.1.

#### *2.4.6.3 Equal-intensity matching to a number scale of references*

Kasche (2005) presented an intramodality matching method for measuring the odor intensity of materials emissions. The proposal is first to construct an equal interval scale of perceived odor intensity of a reference substance grounded in seven concentrations of acetone. Thus each of the seven perceived odor intensities of acetone is first assigned fixed numbers (the same for all observers) to represent the psychophysical function of odor intensity as a function of acetone concentration (based on Fechnerian integration, a logarithmic function is considered). The odor intensities of the target material emissions are then scaled by assigning a number: one of the fixed numbers or any number in between these reference odor intensities. As a result, the perceived intensity of the target odor is then either expressed as a scale value of the reference odor intensity or as a reference (acetone) concentration value. In this procedure, it is assumed that no interindividual differences exist in perceived odor intensity of the acetone reference. A *well-trained panel* is therefore used to achieve a common use of the postulated number scale of perceived odor intensity. Any scale variance is viewed as uncertainty in estimating the perceived intensity of the target emission.

### ***2.4.7 Quantification: Direct scaling methods***

Apart from equal matching of perceived intensities, measured in physical quantities, there are two kinds of quantification methods: the direct scaling methods presented in this section (2.4.7), and the indirect scaling methods presented in Section 2.4.8. The most accepted direct scaling method is the *method of ranking.* It produces an ordinal scale and therefore is not further considered, because it is problematic to compare such scale values obtained in different experiments unless a set of identical stimulus quantities is introduced, which would represent a reference rank order.

#### *2.4.7.1 Category scaling*

Category scaling is a method in which odor intensities are "sorted" in a predetermined number of categories on the basis of their perceived intensity. In a 5-category scale, typically, the lowest Category 1 is used for the least intense of the stimuli (or the blank), and the highest Category 5 for the most intense of the stimuli (which at most may be "overpowering" in its perceived odor intensity, Figure 2.3, left). In the original form of category scaling, the observer was instructed to distribute the

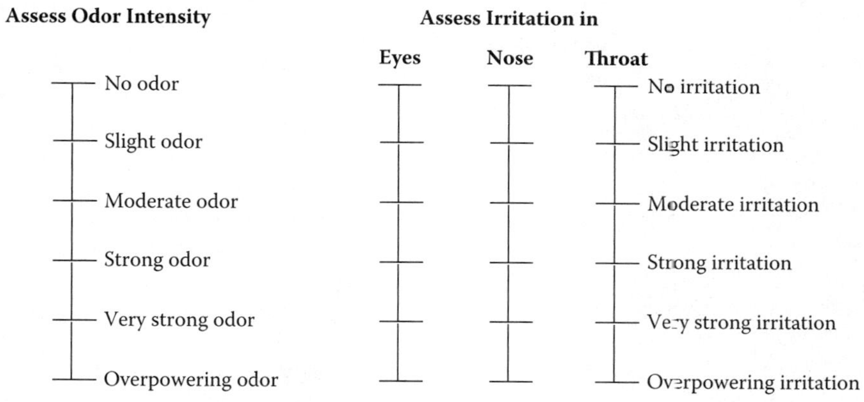


*Figure 2.3* Category scales for evaluating perceived odor intensity (left) and sensory-irritation intensity in the eyes, nose, or throat (right). Reprinted from Knudsen et al. (2003).

remaining stimuli in the other categories (e.g., Categories 2–4 of the 5-category scale) in such a way that the intervals between the category boundaries would be perceptually equal. Thus, the difference in the perceived quantity between the lower and the higher boundaries of Category 1 should be the same as that for Category 2, and so on. In other words, all categories should be the same. Thus, it is utterly important to instruct the observers to keep the principle of "equal-interval" scaling. If they do not adhere to this principle, rank ordering is potentially obtained.

In most category scales in use, the categories are given verbal labels instead of numbers (e.g., see Figure 2.3, "no," "slight," " moderate," "strong," "very strong," and "overpowering" odor intensity or irritation intensity, as used by Knudsen, Nielsen, Clausen, Wilkins, & Wolkoff, 2003). This has raised the question of whether it is possible to find verbal labels or so-called "multipliers" that would represent category distances. For example, are the perceived interdistances between "no" and "slight" irritation in the eyes the same as between "strong" and "very strong" irritation in the eyes or would "very strong" irritation in the eyes represent the same quantity as very strong irritation in the throat? Jones and Thurstone (1955), Cliff (1959), and G. Borg (1998) have shown that the way of phrasing the question and the selected verbal category labels may both be interpreted differently by different observers.

By only defining the endpoints verbally, a "2-point category scale" has been used for quantification: such a scale is called a *visual analogue scale* (VAS). The idea is that the observer should put a mark on the line of this scale, where two-endpoint categories delimit the analogue scale. The mark would directly correspond to a quantity in relation to either endpoint. An example of such a scale is the bipolar acceptability and unacceptability scale (see Figure 2.4), used in indoor air quality investigations (e.g., Knudsen, Clausen, Wilkins, & Wolkoff, 2007).

The acceptability scale is normally accompanied by the question, "Imagine that you, during your daily work, would be exposed to the air in this diffuser/room. How acceptable is the air quality?" The Danish indoor climate labeling system

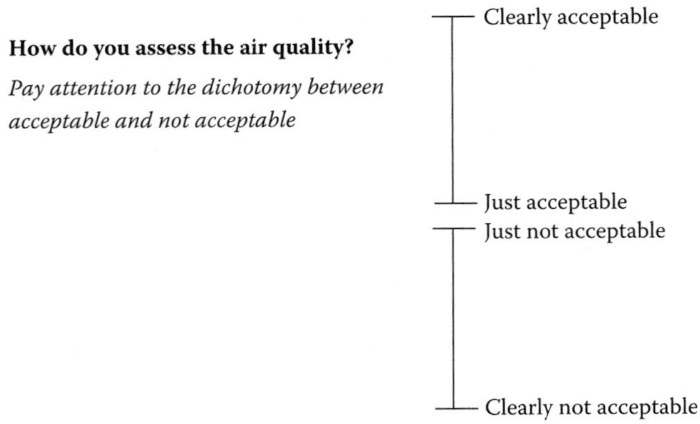


*Figure 2.4* Pair of visual analogue scales (VAS) for assessing indoor air quality on a bipolar acceptability scale, that is, as regards degree of acceptable and degree of not acceptable. Reprinted from Knudsen et al. (2007).

for materials emissions uses category scaling to distinguish between accepted and rejected construction products.

### *2.4.7.2 Borg's category-ratio scale*

Borg's category-ratio scale was developed with the purpose of adjusting interdistances between categories of the category scale such that the intervals approached a ratio scale as obtained by magnitude estimation (see Section 2.4.7.3). Another purpose was to give labels to quantities at appropriate interdistances on the category-ratio scale, thus answering questions such as how much "weaker" is "extremely weak" in relation to "very weak." In brief, the Borg's category-ratio scales (CR10© and CR100©; the number refers to the maximum level of the scale; see Figure 2.5) were intended to mimic scales obtained in absolute magnitude estimation ("numerous matching," Section 2.4.7.4) and also to give meaning to level (G. Borg, 1998).

Borg's category-ratio scaling has been applied in different areas for scaling intensive variables in perceived exertion, pain, loudness, taste, odor, and color perception. The CR10 and CR100 scales are widely used in various applications around the world, such as for perceived exertion in health, sport, disease, and rehabilitation. For safety reasons in olfaction, the method presents a problem in that maximum exposure may not be produced for many odorous and toxic substances or environmental emissions.

Borg argued that all biological systems have their boundaries, from a minimal to a maximal capacity. According to Borg's range model, the total natural, perceptual, dynamic range from zero (or minimal intensity) to a maximal or near maximal intensity should be perceptually approximately the same for most individuals. As a consequence any perceived level of intensity can be evaluated in relation to its position in the individual range, and the response for any stimulus intensity can be compared across individuals even when the physical dynamic range varies (see G. Borg, 1998).

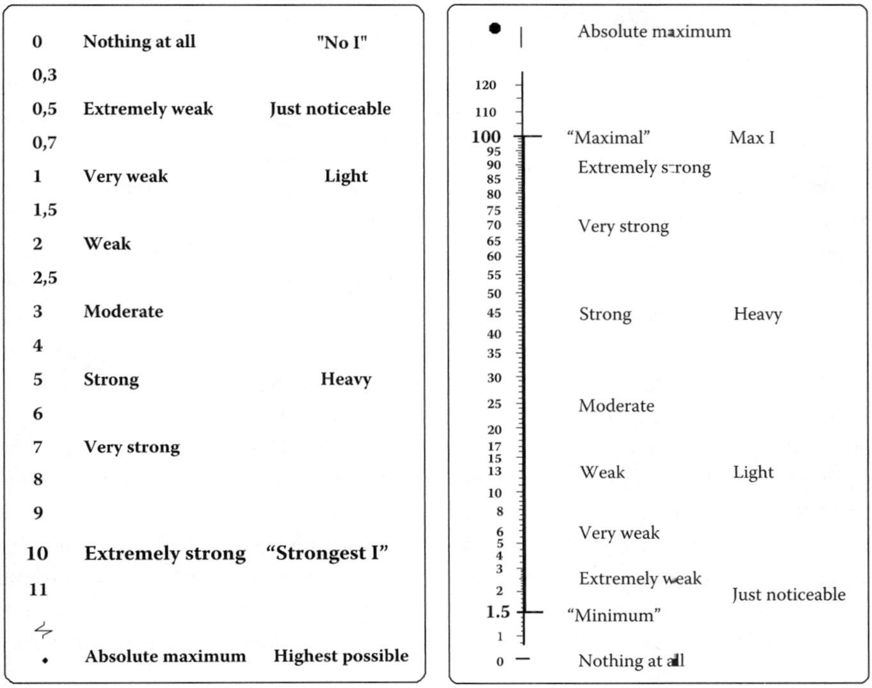


*Figure 2.5* The Borg CR10 (© G. Borg, 1998) and CR100 (© G. Borg & E. Borg, 2001) scales.

Eisler (1965) supports this idea. For perceived exertion, the CR10 and CR100 scales have been successfully validated against physiological correlates such as heart rate and blood lactate.

### *2.4.7.3 Magnitude estimation and magnitude production*

*Magnitude estimation* is a direct scaling method. It is a procedure in which observers are asked to assess directly the intensity of a perception or the quantity of any psychological variable (S. S. Stevens, 1975). In the early versions, a standard was placed in the middle of the stimulus range and called 10 (or 100). Later subjects were simply instructed to assign numbers to a series of perceived magnitudes of the presented stimulus (e.g., intensity or pleasantness). This latter procedure is called *free-number magnitude estimation* or free-number matching (cf. Zwislocki's absolute magnitude estimation in Zwislocki and Goodman, 1980; see Section 2.4.7.4).

An early version of magnitude estimation was also called the method of ratio estimation in which the more constrained "multiplying" and "dividing" were required from the participant before she reported the magnitudes. A complete *ratio scaling method* was further developed by Ekman to involve full matrices of all stimulus magnitudes, in which all possible pairs of stimulus magnitude were compared and judged (e.g., Ekman, 1958; Ekman & Sjöberg, 1965). For many continua, perceived intensity ($\Psi$) increases with stimulus magnitude ($\Phi$) as a power function,

$$\Psi = k \cdot \Phi^n , \tag{2.7}$$

where the constant $k$ depends on the units of measurement and $n$ is the value of the exponent. The exponent has been found to differ depending on the sensory continuum and perceived qualities (S. S. Stevens & Galanter, 1957; Berglund, Berglund, Ekman, & Engen, 1971). S. S. Stevens (1975) claims that the value of the exponent is an important property of a sensory continuum. For example, the exponent for pain intensity has been reported to be as high as 3.5, whereas the exponent for loudness typically is close to 0.3 (sound intensity; 0.6 sound pressure). Compared with other senses, odorous substances exhibit a large variation in exponents of their power functions for perceived odor intensity. The reason for this is not well understood, although it is believed that simultaneous trigeminal stimulation, resulting in sensory irritation perception, may cause higher exponents than "pure" odorous substances.

*Magnitude production* is the opposite scaling procedure to magnitude estimation. Instead of assigning numbers to sensation magnitudes, subjects instead adjust a stimulus continuum (e.g., sound pressure level of a pink noise) such that the perceived intensity of the stimulus quantity matches the size of the numbers given by the experimenter.

### *2.4.7.4 Absolute magnitude estimation*

Zwislocki and coworkers (Hellman & Zwislocki, 1963; Zwislocki & Goodman, 1980; see also Gescheider, 1997) suggest that free-number magnitude estimation (Section 2.3.7.3), with a special instruction, may meet with the "absolute" demands necessary for interindividual comparisons. He named the method *absolute magnitude estimation* (AME). The main idea is that through our experience of numerousness, numbers themselves acquire a kind of "absolute" magnitude and therefore AME (or the numbers) works somewhat like a second modality similarly to the method of cross-modality matching (see Section 2.4.6.2), which has been shown to work well.

### *2.4.7.5 Magnitude matching*

J. C. Stevens and Marks (1980) introduced the method of magnitude matching. It classifies as a *joint scaling procedure* (cf. Berglund, Berglund, & Lindvall, 1978). Participants make free number magnitude estimations of sets of stimuli on a "common" numerical scale, shifting between two (or more) modalities, for example, loudness and brightness, from trial to trial. The rationale is that personal numerical "idiosyncrasies" should be cancelled out of the matching function. Participants serve as their own controls reducing variability in slope, position, and shape of the psychophysical functions. Under the strong assumption that the psychophysical function of one of the modalities is "the same" in all individuals, it is possible to assess and "calibrate" for individual differences in the other, target modality in which the same individuals are "not the same" (J. C. Stevens & Marks, 1980; Marks & Algom, 1998). This method has, for example, been used by Bartoshuk (2000) to study sensory differences in taste perception between nontasters, tasters, and supertasters. Berglund and Nordin (1992) found that the assumption of finding a modality, which is the same for all individuals, whereas another target modality is not, is not easily fulfilled. They showed that in smokers, as compared to nonsmokers, not only the odor perception was affected but also the loudness perception, a finding that rejected the invariance assumption but found support in thus far unknown findings.

### *2.4.7.6 Constrained scaling*

Compared to the method of magnitude matching (Section 2.4.7.5) and of master scaling (Section 2.4.7.7), Ward (1992) takes on a somewhat opposite view on how to treat individual differences, namely to view it as measurement behavior (West & Ward, 1994; West, Ward, & Kohsla, 2000). He emphasizes the value of "constrained" scaling by using an arbitrary scale. According to this method, participants are taught and trained in the use of a certain standard scale (cf. Section 2.4.6.3) with a specific exponent of the psychophysical power function for some chosen modality, until they are able to reproduce the chosen exponent of a particular power function with high accuracy. The same persons then use the same scale for scaling perceptual magnitudes of target stimuli.

A similar approach has also been developed by Fanger (1988) and been proposed for applications in the field of indoor air quality. The participants are trained to scale perceived odor intensity of acetone and subsequently told to use this same number scale also when scaling other quantities, such as perceived air quality in rooms (visitors' condition). Both Fanger (1988) and Kasche (2005) train observers to use a specific postulated scale, thus getting rid of between-observer variance for the *odor-intensity set of concentrations* of a reference substance. In principle, constrained scaling is often the psychophysical method also preferred in sensory analysis of food products.

### *2.4.7.7 Master scaling*

In order to keep the experimental context invariant, Berglund (1991) recommends joint scaling of references and target stimuli. Her master scaling was originally developed for the calibrated measurement of one point on a continuum of perceived intensity (the one target) with the aid of one individual. The method has been used with great success in studies of, for example, traffic noise, odorous air pollution, and in patients with chronic pain (e.g., Berglund et al., 1974; Berglund & Lindvall, 1979; Berglund & Harju, 2003; Berglund, Harju, Kosek, & Lindblom, 2002).

In master scaling, measurement of perceived odor intensity is viewed as a contextually based dynamic process. Characteristically, sensory systems are dynamic and adaptable. Each observer's magnitude estimates (Section 2.4.7.3) consist of context-dependent relative values rather than absolute levels or invariables. Between-observer variation is assumed to reflect true perceptual differences. This is not to say that an observer has no measurement error, only to say that true among-observer differences in (perceived) odor intensity exist. Master scaling means, for example, that odor intensity of a set of well-defined reference concentrations (e.g., pyridine) is scaled jointly with the target odor emission(s); hereafter the odor intensity of the target is *calibrated* to the agreed-upon master scale of the references. There are two principal goals with master scaling: (a) The experimental procedure of master scaling is used for measuring and evaluating each observer's scaling behavior with the aid of reference stimuli (scaling context); and (b) the master scale transformation is used to measure each observer's perceived intensity of target odor emissions on a calibrated (perceived) odor intensity scale. It is considered especially important to differentiate the odor-intensity variance of the references from the variance of the target, a problem inherent in any direct equal-intensity matching procedure.

The master scale transformation is as follows. The perceived odor intensity ($R$) of the references is a power function of concentration ($S$), $R = c\,S^n$, and $c$ and $n$ are multiplicative constant and exponent, respectively (see Equation (2.7)). Let this equation of the master function for the pyridine references be subscribed by $m$ and the corresponding equation for each observer's empirical odor intensities for the references be subscribed by $i$. Because the concentration measures of the *references* are the same in these two power-function equations ($S_m = S_i$), equating the two and rearranging the terms give the equation for the master scale transformation,

$$R_m = c_m \left( \frac{R_i}{c_i} \right)^{\frac{n_m}{n_i}}, \tag{2.8}$$

where $R_i$ is the empirical odor intensity of each subject's reference scale, and $R_m$ is the corresponding odor intensity transformed to the master scale. By inserting the individual empirical (perceived) odor intensity values of the *target materials emission* ($R_i$) into Equation (2.8), these can be transformed to the *unit* and *reference points of the master scale of odor intensity* ($R_m$), defined for the set of odor intensities of the pyridine concentrations.

The participants are quality assured in that they are to produce a power function for the reference concentrations. Participants are screened ad hoc on the quality of these power functions, which they produce in the scaling experiment. They are free to use the number scale they feel comfortable with, as is the case in magnitude estimation. In principle, master scaling involves a "calibration" of individual participant's perceived odor intensity scales. The uncertainty is determined for each participant with the aid of the references. A criterion of acceptable uncertainty may thus be used before averaging the empirical data. The odor intensity of the target stimuli can either be expressed in master-scale numbers or in equivalent concentration values of the reference.

### *2.4.8 Quantification: Indirect scaling methods*

Indirect scaling methods may be particularly suited for scaling psychological attributes of complex stimuli for which a relevant and common stimulus quantity is lacking. The indirect scaling methods differ from direct scaling methods in that the collected data will not carry enough information for measurement at interval or ratio scales. The judgments are at ordinal level: larger than or smaller than. To obtain measurement on a higher order scale than the ordinal scale, certain assumptions have to be introduced and applied to the collected empirical data. and it is also necessary to test the assumptions introduced (data theory; Jacoby, 1991). A potential conclusion of the measurement with indirect scaling methods may be that the assumed measuring model did not fit the data.

### *2.4.8.1 Thurstone's judgment scaling model: Pair comparisons of stimuli*

In Thurstonian scaling, the scaling of stimuli must always be done indirectly (Torgerson, 1958). Each stimulus, when presented to an observer, gives rise to a discriminatory process, which has a value on the psychological continuum (e.g., degree of annoyance). Because of momentary fluctuations in the organism, a given stimulus does not always excite the same discriminatory process, but may excite one with a higher or lower value on the continuum. The discriminatory process reflects how the organism identifies, distinguishes, or reacts to stimuli. It is postulated that the values of the discriminatory process form normal frequency distributions on the psychological continuum. The mean ($s_j$ and $s_k$) and the standard deviation ($\sigma_j$ and $\sigma_k$) of the distributions associated with two different stimuli, *j* and *k*, are their scale value and discriminatory dispersion, respectively.

*2.4.8.1.1 Law of Comparative Judgment.* The complete form of the law of comparative judgment reads (Torgerson, 1958, p. 161):

$$s_k - s_j = z_{jk}\,(\sigma_j^2 + \sigma_k^2 - 2r_{jk}\,\sigma_j\sigma_k)^{1/2}, \qquad (2.9)$$

where $z_{jk}$ is the distance from the mean expressed with the variance measure as unit. By assuming zero correlations ($r = 0$) and equal discriminatory dispersions ($\sigma_j = \sigma_k = c$), the law of comparative judgment reduces to Thurstone's Case V:

$$s_k - s_j = z_{ik}\, c\, (2)^{1/2.} \qquad (2.10)$$

If $c\ (2)^{1/2}$ is used as unit, the equation reduces to

$$s_k - s_j = z_{jk}. \qquad (2.11)$$

As an example, a group of 100 participants conducts pairwise comparisons of annoyance attributed to seven sound recordings of different kinds of aircraft overflights. Each participant is to report which of two aircraft overflights is more annoying among the 21 unique pairs. The response proportions for the 100 participants are calculated and transformed to *z*-values, which according to Case V constitute scale intervals. By adding the *z*-values of each column of the square matrix, and by selecting a zero-point of the scale, the annoyance scale is established as an interval scale.

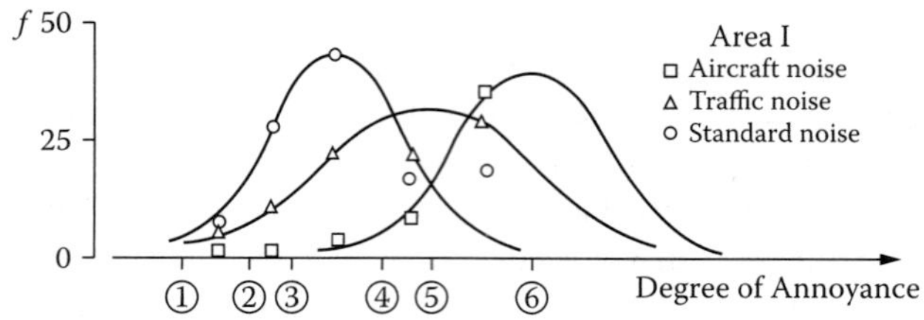


*Figure 2.6* Empirically obtained frequency distributions of annoyance with regard to three different kinds of noises. The means of the distributions represent the degree of annoyance on a calibrated interval scale. Reprinted from Berglund, Berglund, & Lindvall (1975).

*2.4.8.1.2 Law of Categorical Judgment.* In principle, this law states that the boundaries between adjacent points on a category scale behave as do the stimuli in the example above. It also assumes there is a psychological continuum of the observer that can be divided into a specific number of ordered categories. For this case different scaling models may be used depending on the type of replications in collecting the data (several trials per observer or observers viewed as replications or a mix of these two).

Berglund, Berglund, and Lindvall (1975) applied Thurstone's Case V to annoyance questionnaire data (6-point category scale) in an epidemiological study of 1,400–2,000 inhabitants in each of five areas of aircraft noise exposure. The frequency of response for each of three environmental agents was tabulated relative to the 6 points of a category scale. Frequencies were then transformed to proportions of the total number of responses, and the proportions further transformed into a normal deviate. It is from the normal deviates that the continuum of annoyance was derived on which both category boundaries and the participant's degree of annoyance to the environmental noise were scaled; in this case Gulliksen's method of least squares was used (Torgerson, 1958). Once the annoyance scale is established, locations of the boundaries for the verbal categories and the environmental agents in each area are easily determined.

The interval property of the scale means that the annoyance scales for differently exposed areas can be calibrated to a common reference point and a common unit of measurement. In Figure 2.6, the degree of annoyance for three environmental agents is provided on the same calibrated scale as obtained in the aircraft noise investigation (all five areas). The specific assumptions applied are that the variances of each response category boundary are constant and independent of the specific environmental agent. In this specific Area I, the degree of annoyance for each agent is expressed by the mean of the distributions. The means are located on an interval scale of annoyance and therefore quantitative comparisons of the agents are possible.

### 2.4.9 Combining methods

The research problem has certain requirements as to what method to use. It may be impossible to know beforehand the range of stimulus intensities to use, for example, if the odor sensitivity of smokers and nonsmokers (Berglund & Nordin, 1992) were to be tested or of patients with Alzheimer's disease (Nordin, Almkvist, Berglund, & Wahlund, 1997). In such cases, it may be favorable to introduce blanks in an experiment designed for the method of constant stimuli such that signal detection theory may be applied in the data treatment. The reason for this precaution is that the expected absolute threshold may differ a great deal among patients and individual smokers or nonsmokers.

In some cases, it may also be favorable to combine the method of constant stimuli with magnitude estimation (Berglund & Nordin, 1992). For example, first ask if the subject can perceive a smell or not (blanks may still be presented), and, if the subject says yes, then ask how intense the odor of the sniff is and get a quantity by the method of magnitude estimation.

## 2.5 Descriptor profiling and multidimensional scaling

In environmental field applications, it is not possible to present exactly the same exposure several times. For example, the annoyance of an aircraft overflight cannot be repeated with a short time interval or the odor of indoor air will not be stable for long. Alternatively, it may then be possible to ask a group of subjects to judge several aspects of their perceptions by a profiling technique. For example, several category scales could be used for measuring the sound of the overflight (e.g., loudness and/or annoyance of the maximum, the perceived duration of the overflight, etc.) or the quality of the indoor air (e.g., warmth, stuffiness, odor intensity, etc. to create a quantity profile of the qualities).

Ideally, descriptor profiles would be built from 8–10 perceptual–emotional attributes, all describing the "quality of the indoor air." A sheet with visual analogue scales for each attribute is prepared with endpoints marked 0% match and 100% match. The selection of attributes has to be piloted before the descriptor profile may be considered part of a measuring instrument for perceived air quality (or materials emissions). Alternatively, applicability of attributes to indoor air samples or materials emission may be used (Baird, Berglund, & Shams Esfandabad, 1994). It is important that careful cross-translations are made between languages of different countries.

The scale values of attribute matches (0–100% interval scale) provide a characteristic profile over attributes for each respondent. A correlation matrix may be formed from pairs of profiles, each profile characterizing the indoor air quality in parts of buildings or different buildings. Inasmuch as a profile represents one emission (one indoor air), the correlation matrix can be viewed as a matrix of "similarities" ($r^2$ = shared variance). Data treatment by PCA (principle components analysis, content model) or MDS (multidimensional scaling, distance model) would deliver a representation of the interrelations among the materials emissions or the samples of indoor air. There are methods by which interindividual differences may be treated according to specific theory (e.g., INDSCAL, see Schiffman, Reynolds, & Young, 1981). Joint space analysis (attributes and stimuli) with correspondence analysis is also a possibility (Noma, Berglund, Berglund, Johansson, & Baird, 1988; Greenacre, 1984).

## References


Ahlström, R., Berglund, B., Berglund, U., & Lindvall, T. (1986). Formaldehyde odor and its interaction with the air of a sick building. *Environment International, 12,* 289–295.

Baird, J. C., Berglund, B., & Shams Esfandabad, H. (1994). Longitudinal assessment of sensory reactions in eyes and upper airways of staff in a sick building. *Environment International, 20,* 141–160.

Baird, J. C., & Noma, E. (1978). *Fundamentals of scaling and psychophysics.* New York: Wiley.

Bartoshuk, L. (2000). Comparing sensory experiences across individuals: Recent psychophysical advances illuminate genetic variation in taste perception. *Chemical Senses, 25,* 447–460.

Berglund, B. (1991). Quality assurance in environmental psychophysics. In S. J. Bolanowski & G. A. Gescheider (Eds.), *Ratio scaling of psychological magnitudes–In honor of the memory of S. S. Stevens* (pp. 140–162). Hillsdale, NJ: Erlbaum.

Berglund, B., & Harju, E.-L. (2003). Master scaling of perceived intensity of touch, cold and warmth. *European Journal of Pain, 7,* 323–334.

Berglund, B., & Lindvall, T. (1979). Olfactory evaluation of indoor air quality. In P. O. Fanger & O. Valbjørn (Eds.), *Indoor climate. Effects on human comfort, performance, and health in residential, commercial, and light-industry buildings* (pp. 141–157). Copenhagen: Danish Building Research Institute.

Berglund, B., & Nordin, S. (1992). Detectability and perceived intensity for formaldehyde in smokers and non-smokers. *Chemical Senses, 17,* 291–306.

Berglund, B., Berglund, U., & Lindvall, T. (1974). A psychological detection method in environmental research. *Environmental Research, 7,* 342–352.

Berglund, B., Berglund, U., & Lindvall, T. (1975). Scaling of annoyance in epidemiological studies. In *Proceeding of the International Symposium Recent Advances in the Assessment of the Health Effects of Environmental Pollution,* Vol. I (pp. 119–137). Luxembourg: Commission of the European Communities.

Berglund, B., Berglund, U., & Lindvall, T. (1978). Separate and joint scaling of perceived odor intensity of n-butanol and hydrogen sulfide. *Perception & Psychophysics, 23,* 313–320.

Berglund, B., Berglund, U., & Lindvall, T. (1986). Theory and methods of odour evaluation. *Experientia, 42,* 280–287. (Odour Biology Issue)

Berglund, B., Berglund, U., Ekman, G., & Engen, T. (1971). Individual psychophysical functions for 28 odorants. *Perception & Psychophysics,* 9 (3B), 379–384.

Berglund, B., Harju, E.-L., Kosek, E., & Lindblom, U. (2002). Quantitative and qualitative perceptual analysis of cold dysesthesia and hyperalgesia in fibromyalgia. *Pain, 96,* 177–187.

Borg, G. (1998). *Borg's perceived exertion and pain scales.* Champaign, IL: Human Kinetics.

Borg, G., & Borg, E. (2001). A new generation of scaling methods: Level-anchored ratio scaling. *Psychologica, 28,*15–45.

Cliff, N. (1959). Adverbs as multipliers. *Psychological Review, 66,* 27–34.

Cook, T. S., & Campbell, D. T. (1979). *Quasi-experimentation. Design and analysis issues for field settings.* Boston: Houghton Mifflin.

Culvert, G., Spence, C., & Stein, B. E. (Eds.). (2004). *The handbook of multisensory processes.* London, Boston: Bradford Book (MIT).

Devos, M., Patte, F., Rouault, J., Laffort, P., & van Gemert, L. J. (Eds.). (1990). *Standardized human olfactory thresholds.* Oxford, UK: IRL Press.

Eisler, H. (1965). The ceiling of psychophysical power functions. *American Journal of Psychology, 78,* 506–509.

Ekman, G. (1958). Two generalized ratio scaling methods. *Journal of Psychology, 45,* 287–294.
Ekman, G., & Sjöberg, L. (1965). Scaling. *Annual Review of Psychology, 16,* 451–474.
Engen, T. (1971). Psychophysics. I. Discrimination and detection. In J. W. Kling & L. A. Riggs (Eds.), *Woodworth and Schlosberg's experimental psychology* (pp. 11–46). New York: Holt, Rinehart & Winston.
Falmagne, J.-C. (1985). *Elements of psychophysical theory.* New York: Oxford University Press.
Fanger, P.O. (1988). Introduction of the olf and the decipol units to quantify air pollution perceived by humans odors and outdoors. *Energy and Buildings, 12,* 1–6.
Fechner, G. T. (1860). *Elemente der psychophysik [Elements of psychophysics]* (Vol. 2). Leipzig: Breitkopf and Härtel.
Gescheider, G. A. (1997). *Psychophysics: The fundamentals* (3rd ed.). London: Erlbaum.
Green, D. M., & Swets, J. A. (1962). *Signal detection theory and psychophysics.* New York: Wiley.
Greenacre, M. J. (1984). *Theory and applications of correspondence analysis.* London: Academic Press.
Hellman, R., & Zwislocki, J. J. (1963). Monaural loudness function at 1000 cps and interaural summation. *Journal of the Acoustical Society of America, 35,* 856–865.
Jacoby, W. G. (1991). Data theory and dimensional analysis. London: Sage. (No. 07-078)
Jones, L. V., & Thurstone, L. L. (1955). The psychophysics of semantics: An experimental investigation. *Journal of Applied Psychology, 39,* 31–36.
Kasche, J. (2005). The new perceived intensity scale. Presentation at TU Berlin (Unpublished).
Knudsen, H. N., Clausen, P. A., Wilkins, C. K., & Wolkoff, P. (2007). Sensory and chemical evaluation of odorous emissions from building products with and without linseed oil. *Building and Environment, 42,* 4059–4067.
Knudsen, H. N., Nielsen, P. A., Clausen, P. A., Wilkins, C. K., & Wolkoff, P. (2003). Sensory evaluation of emissions from selected building products exposed to ozone. *Indoor Air, 13*(3), 223–231.
Kobal, G., & Hummel, T. (1991). Olfactory potentials in humans. In T. V. Getchell, R. Doty, L. M. Bartoshuk, & J. B. Snow, Jr. (Eds.), *Smell and taste in health and disease* (pp. 255–275). New York: Raven Press.
Lord, F. M., & Novick, M. R. (1968). *Statistical theories of mental test scores.* Reading, MA: Addison-Wesley.
Luce, R. D., Bush, R. R., & Galanter, E. (Eds.). (1963). *Handbook of mathematical psychology.* New York: Wiley.
Marks, L. E., & Algom, D. (1998). Psychophysical scaling. In M. H. Birnbaum (Ed.), *Measurement, judgment, and decision making* (pp. 81–178). Boston: Academic Press.
Noma, E., Berglund, B., Berglund, U., Johansson, I., & Baird, J. C. (1988). Joint representation of physical locations and volatile organic compounds in indoor air from a healthy and a sick building. *Atmospheric Environment, 22,* 451–460.
Nordin, S., Almkvist, O., Berglund, B., & Wahlund, L.-O. (1997). Olfactory dysfunction for pyridine and dementia progression in Alzheimer's disease. *Archives of Neurology, 54,* 993–998.
Roberts, F. S. (1979). Measurement theory with applications to decision making, utility, and the social sciences. In C.-C. Rota (Ed.), *Encyclopedia of mathematics and its applications.* Vol. 7. Reading, MA: Addison-Wesley.
Schiffman, S. S., Reynolds, M. L., & Young, R. W. (1981). *Introduction to multidimensional scaling. Theory, methods and applications.* London: Academic Press.

Stevens, J. C., & Marks, L. E. (1980). Cross-modality matching functions generated by magnitude estimation. *Perception & Psychophysics, 27,* 379–389.

Stevens, S. S. (1946). On the theory of scales of measurement. *Science, 103,* 677–680.

Stevens, S. S. (1975). *Psychophysics. Introduction to its perceptual, neural and social prospects.* New York: Wiley.

Stevens, S. S., & Galanter, E. H. (1957). Ratio scales and category scales for a dozen perceptual continua. *Journal of Experimental Psychology, 54,* 377–411.

Svensson, L. T., & Szczygiel, K. (1974). A matching method of successive approximations and its instrumentation. *Behavioral Research Methods & Instrumentation, 6*(1), 13–18.

Torgerson, W. A. (1958). *Theory and methods of scaling.* New York: Wiley.

Ward, L. M. (1992). Who knows? In G. Borg & G. Neely (Eds.), *Fechner Day 92* (pp. 217–222). Stockholm: International Society for Psychophysics.

West, R. L., & Ward, L. M. (1994). Constrained scaling. In L. M. Ward (Ed.), *Fechner Day 1994* (pp. 225–230). Vancouver: University of British Columbia.

West, R. L., Ward, L. M., & Kohsla, R. (2000). Constrained scaling: The effect of learned psychophysical scales on idiosyncratic response bias. *Perception & Psychophysics, 62,* 137–151.

WHO. (1989). *Formaldehyde. Environmental Health Criteria 89.* Geneva, Switzerland: The World Health Organization.

Zwislocki, J. J., & Goodman, D. A. (1980). Absolute scaling of sensory magnitude: A validation. *Perception & Psychophysics, 28,* 28–38.

# 3 Measurements of physical parameters in sensory science

*Teresa Goodman*

National Physical Laboratory
Teddington, United Kingdom

## 3.1 The importance of measurement

Measurement is the process of quantifying the extent or quantity of something by comparison with a fixed unit or a reference object of known size. It is the means by which we make objective comparisons between things on a consistent and reproducible basis, and provides a common language by which we can describe objects or behaviors. Measurement therefore sits at the heart of our modern technological world, supporting business, trade, industry, and science, and underpinning the regulatory framework that helps maintain and improve our quality of life, in areas as diverse as public health and safety, climate change, and sports and leisure. It is an essential part of all scientific and technological research and development, allowing us, for example, to specify the physical or chemical attributes of a substance or an object, to evaluate the activity of different parts of the brain, to quantify human perceptual responses and behaviors, to assess societal trends, or even (through the choice of an appropriate measurement method and scale) to enumerate such seemingly abstract qualities as intelligence or happiness. In the words of Lord Kelvin:

> When you can measure what you are speaking about, and express it in numbers, you know something about it; but when you cannot measure it, when you cannot express it in numbers, your knowledge is of a meagre and unsatisfactory kind: it may be the beginning of knowledge, but you have scarcely, in your thoughts, advanced to the stage of science (as quoted in American Association for the Advancement of Science).

The importance of physical measurements for applications such as manufacturing, construction, and commerce has been recognized since the beginnings of human civilization. In the time of the Egyptian pharaohs, for example, the architects responsible for building the pyramids faced the death penalty if they failed to calibrate their reference measurement standards ("cubit sticks") at each full moon. By implementing such a rigorous measurement regime, they were able to achieve construction accuracy of 0.05%. Early measures of length were generally based on human-centered references. In the case of the Royal Egyptian cubit, for example, the reference was the length of the forearm of the pharaoh ruling at that time (measured from his bent elbow to the tip of his extended middle finger) plus the width of the palm of his hand. This was then transferred to a carved granite reference stick, against which all other measuring sticks could be compared. Similarly, the references used for other basic measures, such as weight, were based on commonly available materials; for example, the Egyptians and Greeks used a wheat seed as the smallest unit of weight, a standard that was very uniform and accurate for the times.

However, despite their success, there were significant problems associated with all such measures, due to the fact that they were impossible to reproduce reliably over a long period of time, or in different locations. The death of a pharaoh in Egypt, for example, would result in a step change in the system for length measurement used in that country, and a year of drought or excessive rain could change the weight of a wheat seed. As the need for consistent and reliable measurement units increased, particularly for the purposes of trade between regions, so the systems of measurement moved to being based on internationally agreed reference artifacts, which were kept in carefully controlled conditions to ensure long-term consistency and against which all others could be compared to ensure region-to-region agreement. Even this approach had its limitations, however, inasmuch as not only could the reference artifacts change with time (even if carefully maintained) but also because the accuracy with which they could be transferred was limited by the accuracy of the measuring instrumentation used. Modern physical measurements are therefore based on a system of seven *base units*, which are all defined from first principles (with the exception of the unit of mass, the kilogram, which is still based on a single reference artifact) and from which all other physical measures can be derived. This is the so-called International System of Units (SI), which is discussed further in Section 3.2.

Of course, as already mentioned, the concept of measurement is not limited to the quantification of physical parameters, such as mass, time, or electric current, but is also used in many other areas of science, business, and industry. Often these types of measurement are directly (and obviously) linked to physical measurements. For example, measurements of activity in different regions of the brain carried out using an electroencephalography (EEG) system are based directly on measurements of the electric current (or voltage) for each of the sensors and on knowledge of the position of each sensor on the head. If the electrical measurements are made using equipment that has not been calibrated (or whose performance has not been otherwise validated), or if the sensors are incorrectly positioned, then any conclusions drawn from such EEG measurements may be invalid. In other cases, however, the link with physical measurements is less clear, but nevertheless important. For example, measures of human subjective responses, such as the level of enjoyment experienced when listening to different types of music, may be derived solely from responses to questionnaires, but increasingly this information is linked with the measurement of physical responses (e.g., heart rate or blood pressure) to provide additional information. Thus physical measurement plays an important role in all areas related to understanding human perception and interpretation or "measuring the impossible."

## 3.2 The Metre Convention and the International System of Units

The value of a quantity is generally expressed as the product of a number and a unit, where the unit is a particular example of the quantity concerned which is used as a reference, and the number is the ratio of the value of the quantity to the unit. It is possible to use any defined reference as the basis for a given measurement; all that is necessary is for the chosen reference to be available at the time the measurement is made. This, as we have seen, was the approach taken for the earliest measurements and it is sometimes still used in cases where consistency between different people making the measurements is not needed and where long-term continuity of measurement is not important. Which of us has not, for example, at some time "measured" length by comparison with our own thumb or arm length, in order to provide an approximate assessment of "size." But such measurements are by definition imprecise and difficult to communicate reliably. They are entirely unsuited for modern science, technology, industry, and commerce where, for example, components are sourced from many different suppliers, goods are traded internationally, safety needs to be demonstrated and assured, and performance specifications need to be met.

This need for consistency and reproducibility in measurement has been enshrined in an international treaty, named the Metre Convention, which was first signed in Paris in 1875 by representatives of 17 nations and established a permanent organizational structure under which member governments act in common accord on all matters relating to units of measurement. This treaty, which was modified slightly in 1921, remains the basis of international agreement on units of measurement and now has 53 member states, including all the major industrialized countries. The Metre Convention created the International Bureau of Weights and Measures (BIPM), an intergovernmental organization that operates under the authority of the General Conference on Weights and Measures (CGPM) and is supervised by the International Committee for Weights and Measures (CIPM). The task of the BIPM is to ensure worldwide unification of measurements and act as a central focus for world metrology, particularly concerning the demand for measurement standards of ever-increasing accuracy, range, and diversity, and the need to demonstrate equivalence between national measurement standards.

A key feature of the Metre Convention is the establishment of a practical system of units of measurement, known as the Système International d'Unités (International System of Units, international abbreviation SI; see Organisation Intergouvernementale de la Convention du Mètre, 2006), which has been used around the world as the preferred language of science and technology since its adoption in 1948 through a Resolution of the 9th CGPM. Under this system there are seven well-defined *base units*, which are defined by international agreement by the CGPM and which are, by convention, regarded as dimensionally independent. These base units are: the metre, the kilogram, the second, the ampere, the kelvin, the candela, and the mole (see Table 3.1). All other units within the SI are termed *derived units*, formed by combining base units according to the algebraic relations linking the corresponding quantities (which are accordingly described as *base quantities* and *derived quantities*). Thus although for simplicity some derived units have been given special names, such

*Table 3.1* Base quantities and units of the SI

| *SI base quantity* | *SI base unit* | *Unit symbol* | *Quantity symbol* | *Definition* |
|---|---|---|---|---|
| Length | Metre | m | *l*, *x*, etc. | The metre is the length of the path travelled by light in a vacuum during a time interval of 1/299,792,458 of a second. |
| Mass | Kilogram | kg | *m* | The kilogram is the unit of mass; it is equal to the mass of the international prototype of the kilogram. |
| Time, duration | Second | s | *t* | The second is the duration of 9,192,631,770 periods of the radiation corresponding to the transition between the two hyperfine levels of the ground state of the caesium 133 atom. |
| Electric current | Ampere | A | *I*, *i* | The ampere is that constant current which, if maintained in two straight parallel conductors of infinite length, of negligible circular cross-section, and placed 1 metre apart in a vacuum, would produce between these conductors a force equal to $2 \times 10^{-7}$ newton per metre of length. |
| Thermodynamic temperature | Kelvin | K | *T* | The kelvin, unit of thermodynamic temperature, is the fraction 1/273.16 of the thermodynamic temperature of the triple point of water. |
| Luminous intensity | Candela | cd | $I_v$ | The candela is the luminous intensity, in a given direction, of a source that emits monochromatic radiation of frequency $540 \times 10^{12}$ hertz and that has a radiant intensity in that direction of 1/683 watt per steradian. |

*Table 3.1 (continued)* Base quantities and units of the SI

| *SI base quantity* | *SI base unit* | *Unit symbol* | *Quantity symbol* | *Definition* |
|---|---|---|---|---|
| Amount of substance | Mole | mol | $n$ | 1. The mole is the amount of substance of a system which contains as many elementary entities as there are atoms in 0.012 kilogram of carbon 12.<br>2. When the mole is used, the elementary entities must be specified and may be atoms, molecules, ions, electrons, other particles, or specified groups of such particles.<br><br>In this definition, it is understood that unbound atoms of carbon 12, at rest and in their ground state, are referred to. |

as the hertz, volt, watt, newton, and lumen, all derived units can also be expressed as products of powers of the base units. The equations that express the derived quantities in terms of the base quantities also define the expression for the derived units in terms of the base units. For example, the derived quantity velocity is defined as the distance moved divided by the time taken, that is, as length divided by time, so the derived unit for velocity is metre per second ($m \cdot s^{-1}$). Similarly the derived quantity force, *F*, is related to the SI base quantities through the relationship:

$$F = ma = \frac{ml}{t^2}$$

where *m* is the mass, *a* is the acceleration, *l* is the distance moved, and *t* the time taken. Thus the SI unit for force is kilogram meter per second squared ($kg \cdot m \cdot s^{-2}$), which is given the special name of the newton, symbol N.

It is important to note that the SI is not static, but continues to evolve to match the world's increasingly demanding requirements for measurement. Historically the first units to be defined as base units were the metre, the kilogram, and the second, with the ampere, the kelvin, and the candela being added by a resolution of the 10th CGPM, in 1954, and the mole being agreed as a seventh base unit at the 14th CGPM in 1971, after lengthy discussions between physicists and chemists. The definition of each base unit of the SI is carefully drawn up so that it is unique and provides a sound theoretical basis upon which the most accurate and reproducible measurements can be made. The realization of the definition of a unit is the procedure by which this definition is used to establish the value and associated uncertainty of the unit. As technology has advanced, it has become both possible and necessary to change the definitions of the base units, to achieve lower uncertainties or greater consistency. For example, the unit of time, the second, was at one time considered to be the fraction 1/86,400 of the mean solar day, with the exact definition of "mean solar day" being left to the astronomers. However, measurements showed that irregularities in the rotation of the Earth made this an unsatisfactory definition, and it would certainly not be suitable for use in modern technological applications, such as global positioning systems. This need for more precise and reproducible measurements of time, coupled with advances in technology that allowed measurements of time based on the frequency of atomic oscillations, has led to the adoption of an atomic standard of time, based on a transition between two energy levels of the cesium 133 atom. The most recent change in the definition of one of the SI base units was in 1983 (at the 17th CGPM) and was related to the definition of the unit of length, the metre. Many of the changes that have been made to the definition of the units, particularly since the earliest days of the SI, reflect a desire to ensure that all the base units can be realized independently from first principles, without reference to a physical artifact; an objective which is driving current international research aimed at establishing a new definition for the kilogram (the last unit to be linked to a physical reference artifact).

In the context of measurements relating to human perception and cognition, which is a major focus of "measuring the impossible," the position of the SI with respect to units for quantities that describe biological effects is particularly important. These units are often difficult to relate to SI units because they typically involve weighting factors that may not be precisely known or defined, and which may be both energy and frequency dependent. For example, electromagnetic radiation can cause chemical changes in living or nonliving materials, but the nature and magnitude of these changes depends on the frequency (or, equivalently, the wavelength), power, and geometrical properties of the radiation. As a result it is not possible to establish a simple relationship between the SI base units and the biological response that applies for all electromagnetic radiation, or indeed even for all situations across specific limited spectral regions, such as the ultraviolet. Unique in this respect is the candela, which has been formally defined as one of the SI base units and applies to measurements of the interaction of light with the human eye in vision (so-called *photometry*). Several other photometric quantities with units derived from the candela have also been defined, such as the lumen and the lux. For all other photobiological and photochemical measurements the SI recommends that the optical radiation in question be characterized by its spectral distribution. This may then be weighted by the action spectrum (i.e., the relative spectral effectiveness of optical radiation) for the photochemical or photobiological effect considered, to give an integral value, but in this case the unit used for the integrated radiant quantity is the same as that for the underpinning spectral quantity; thus it is essential also to state the action spectrum that has been used in order to understand the meaning of the quantitative value. An example is given in Table 3.2.

Many psychophysical responses can be characterized in terms of dimensionless logarithmic ratios, most notably the response to changes in sound intensity at a given frequency. There are no specific SI units for such logarithmic ratios, but the CIPM

*Table 3.2* Calculation of photobiological quantities in radiometry

| *Wavelength, λ nm* | *Lamp spectral flux, Φ(λ) W* | *UV hazard action spectrum, $s_{uv}(\lambda)$* | *Erythemal action spectrum, $s_{er}(\lambda)$* |
|---|---|---|---|
| <200 | 0.000000 | — | — |
| 200 | 0.000000 | 0.030000 | 1.000000 |
| 205 | 0.051863 | 0.051000 | 1.000000 |
| 210 | 0.112560 | 0.075000 | 1.000000 |
| 215 | 0.236439 | 0.095000 | 1.000000 |
| 220 | 0.303842 | 0.120000 | 1.000000 |
| 225 | 0.330000 | 0.150000 | 1.000000 |
| 230 | 0.360590 | 0.190000 | 1.000000 |
| 235 | 0.441261 | 0.240000 | 1.000000 |
| 240 | 0.471595 | 0.300000 | 1.000000 |
| 245 | 0.503237 | 0.360000 | 1.000000 |
| 250 | 0.526061 | 0.430000 | 1.000000 |
| 255 | 0.555685 | 0.520000 | 1.000000 |
| 260 | 0.630966 | 0.650000 | 1.000000 |
| 265 | 0.622298 | 0.810000 | 1.000000 |
| 270 | 0.771722 | 1.000000 | 1.000000 |
| 275 | 0.835807 | 0.960000 | 1.000000 |
| 280 | 0.813363 | 0.880000 | 1.000000 |
| 285 | 0.767389 | 0.770000 | 1.000000 |
| 290 | 0.724387 | 0.640000 | 1.000000 |
| 295 | 0.729527 | 0.540000 | 1.000000 |
| 300 | 0.757817 | 0.300000 | 0.648634 |
| 305 | 0.732355 | 0.060000 | 0.219786 |
| 310 | 0.709882 | 0.015000 | 0.074473 |
| 315 | 0.713278 | 0.003000 | 0.025235 |
| 320 | 0.706919 | 0.001000 | 0.008551 |
| 325 | 0.649260 | 0.000500 | 0.002897 |
| 330 | 0.640969 | 0.000410 | 0.001413 |
| 335 | 0.630451 | 0.000340 | 0.001189 |
| 340 | 0.625314 | 0.000280 | 0.001000 |
| 345 | 0.677279 | 0.000240 | 0.000841 |
| 350 | 1.271558 | 0.000200 | 0.000708 |
| 355 | 0.707310 | 0.000160 | 0.000596 |
| 360 | 0.640000 | 0.000130 | 0.000501 |
| 365 | 0.541735 | 0.000110 | 0.000422 |
| 370 | 0.455264 | 0.000093 | 0.000355 |
| 375 | 0.300987 | 0.000077 | 0.000299 |
| 380 | 0.200462 | 0.000064 | 0.000251 |
| 385 | 0.100364 | 0.000053 | 0.000211 |

*(Continued)*

*Table 3.2 (continued)* Calculation of photobiological quantities in radiometry

| *Wavelength, λ nm* | *Lamp spectral flux, Φ(λ) W* | *UV hazard action spectrum, $s_{uv}(\lambda)$* | *Erythemal action spectrum, $s_{er}(\lambda)$* |
|---|---|---|---|
| 390 | 0.054211 | 0.000044 | 0.000178 |
| 395 | 0.000000 | 0.000036 | 0.000150 |
| 400 | 0.000000 | 0.000030 | 0.000126 |
| >400 | 0.000000 | — | — |
| Integrated value (in watts – the action spectrum used must also be quoted) | 20.904 | 6.071 | 10.525 |

*Note:* In this example the total lamp flux is 20.904 W, the UV hazard flux is 6.071 W (weighted using the UV hazard action spectrum) and the erythemal flux is 10.525 W (weighted using the erythemal action spectrum). When quoting the result, the action spectrum must be given, as well as the unit (W).

has officially accepted the units of the neper, bel, and decibel for use with the SI. The neper, Np, is used to express the values of quantities whose numerical values are based on the use of the neperian (or natural) logarithm, ln = $\log_e$. The bel and the decibel, B and dB, where 1 dB = (1/10) B, are used to express the values of logarithmic ratio quantities whose numerical values are based on the decadic logarithm, lg = $\log_{10}$. Measurements of sound intensity (or "loudness") are usually expressed in decibels, relative to a specified 0 dB reference which is typically set at the threshold of perception of an average human. The main reason for using the decibel for sound perception is that the ear is capable of detecting a very large range of sound pressures, covering a ratio in excess of a million to one. Because the power in a sound wave is proportional to the square of the pressure, the ratio of the maximum power to the minimum power is more than $10^{12}$. To deal with such a range, logarithmic units are useful: the logarithm of $10^{12}$ is 12, so the ratio of maximum power to minimum power for human auditory perception represents a difference of 120 dB. When making measurements of sound for human perception, account also has to be taken of the fact that the human ear is not equally sensitive to all sound frequencies: this process is called frequency weighting and is similar to the process used for spectral weighting of photobiological quantities.

## 3.3 Relevant physical parameters for studies in sensory science

We interact with our environment, and with objects within that environment, through our five senses; therefore the physical measurements that are most relevant for sensory science are those relating to the parameters that are sensed through our sensory transducers, such as light and surface reflectance (in the case of vision) or surface roughness and thermal effusivity (in the case of touch). These are listed in Table 3.3. However, as mentioned previously, other types of physical measurement are also of interest where they are used in instrumentation to measure human behavioral

*Table 3.3* Key physical parameters for sensory transduction

| *Sensory modality* | *Physical parameter and SI units* | *Sensory response* |
|---|---|---|
| Vision | ***Luminance*** **(candela per metre squared, $cd \cdot m^{-2}$):** light reflected from or emitted by a surface | Brightness |
| | ***Gloss*** **(dimensionless):** light reflected in specific directions relative to the incident direction | Shininess |
| | ***Chromaticity for non-self-luminous surfaces*** **(dimensionless):** spectral reflectance of surface combined with spectral irradiance of illuminating light source | Color |
| | ***Chromaticity for self-luminous surfaces*** **(dimensionless):** spectral radiance of surface | Color |
| | ***Dimensional characteristics*** **(metre, m):** length, volume, etc. | Size and shape |
| | ***Chroma, saturation, hue and other color appearance measures*** **(dimensionless):** derived from spectral reflectance and spectral radiance/irradiance measurements, defined in terms of various color measurement systems | Color appearance in the context of the visual environment |
| | ***Goniometric and spatial surface characteristics*** **(dimensionless):** spectral reflectance as a function of position and angle combined with spectral irradiance of illuminating light source as a function of position and angle | Visual texture and pattern |
| | ***Light scattering characteristics*** **(dimensionless):** spectral transmittance as a function of position, angle and thickness | Transparency, clarity, haze, translucency |
| Touch | ***Surface topography*** **(metre, m):** height of surface as a function of position | Roughness/ smoothness |
| | ***Friction*** **(Newton, N):** force experienced when moving a fingertip over the surface | Stickiness, slipperiness |
| | ***Hardness*** **(dimensionless):** resistance to indentation (measured on various defined ratio scales) | Hardness |
| | ***Tensile strength, elasticity*** **(pascal, Pa, or newton per metre squared, $N \cdot m^{-2}$):** resistance to deformation | Stretchiness, bendability, drape, compressibility |
| | ***Thermal effusivity*** **(joule per metre squared per kelvin per square root second, $J \cdot m^{-2} \cdot K^{-1} \cdot s^{-1/2}$ or watt square-root second per metre squared per kelvin, $W \cdot s^{1/2} \cdot m^{-2} \cdot K^{-1}$):** ability of a material to exchange thermal energy with its surroundings | Coldness, wetness |

*(Continued)*

*Table 3.3 (continued)* Key physical parameters for sensory transduction

| *Sensory modality* | *Physical parameter and SI units* | *Sensory response* |
|---|---|---|
| Sound | ***Acoustic pressure* (pascal, Pa, or newton per metre squared, $N \cdot m^{-2}$):** sound wave amplitude | Loudness |
| | ***Acoustic intensity* (watt per metre squared, $W \cdot m^{-2}$):** sound power per unit area | Loudness |
| | ***Acoustic frequency* (hertz, Hz):** sound wave frequency | Pitch, sharpness, tone quality, timbre |
| | ***Acoustic impedance* (decibel, dB—note this is accepted for use with SI, but is not an SI unit):** attenuation of sound waves through a medium | Muffled |
| Taste and smell | ***Chemical composition* (mole per metre cubed, $mol \cdot m^{-3}$)** | Flowery, fruity, salty, sweet, bitter, sour …. |

*Table 3.4* Key physical parameters relevant for instrumentation used to measure brain activity and physiological responses for human behavioral studies

| *Instrumentation/method* | *Physical parameters* |
|---|---|
| Electroencephalography (EEG) | Voltage (volt, V), time (second, s), length (metre, m) |
| Electromyography (EMG) | Voltage (volt, V), time (second, s) |
| Event-related potential (ERP) | Voltage (volt, V), time (second, s) |
| Functional magnetic resonance imaging (fMRI) | Magnetic field strength (ampere per metre, $A \cdot m^{-1}$), time (second, s), length (metre, m) |
| Functional near-infrared imaging (fNIR) | Optical radiant power (watt, W), time (second, s), length (metre, m) |
| Magnetoencephalography (MEG) | Magnetic field strength (ampere per metre, $A \cdot m^{-1}$), time (second, s), length (metre, m) |
| Magnetic induction tomography (MIT) | Magnetic field strength (ampere per metre, $A \cdot m^{-1}$), time (second, s), length (metre, m) |
| Positron emission tomography (PET) | Radionuclide activity (becquerel, Bq), time (second, s), length (metre, m) |
| Transcranial magnetic stimulation (TMS) | Magnetic field strength (ampere per metre, $A \cdot m^{-1}$) |
| Heart rate | Frequency (hertz, Hz) |
| Blood pressure | Pressure (pascal, Pa or newton per metre squared, $N \cdot m^{-2}$) |

responses, such as brain activity. Those physical parameters that are most relevant in this context are listed in Table 3.4.

## 3.4 Calibration, traceability, and measurement uncertainty

*Calibration* is the act of checking or adjusting (by comparison with a standard) the values shown by a measuring instrument in order to confirm their validity: that is, it is the process of assigning "correct" values to the measurement scale of an instrument. At its simplest level, therefore, calibration is merely a comparison between measurements: one a measurement of known magnitude using a device of known performance (the reference or standard) and the other using the test device whose performance is to be calibrated.

*Traceability* is the process of linking the calibration values to internationally recognized measurement standards (realized at national measurement laboratories) through an unbroken chain of calibrations. One of the simplest ways of ensuring traceability is by using an approved calibration laboratory that has been assessed by an independent accreditation body against the requirements of ISO 17025 (International Organization for Standardization, 2005). This is not the only approach (e.g., many national measurement laboratories have chosen not to have a formal accreditation against ISO 17025) but if using a nonaccredited laboratory, it is up to the user to verify that the linkage to national measurement standards can be clearly demonstrated.

*Measurement uncertainty* is defined as "a parameter, associated with the result of a measurement, that characterizes the dispersion of the values that could be reasonably attributed to the measurand" (Joint Committee on Guides in Metrology, 2008). It is usually expressed in terms of the bounds of an interval within which the correct result of the measurement may be reasonably presumed to lie. The concept of measurement uncertainty is used to recognize the fact that, as explained in Section 3.4.2 below, no measurement or test is ever performed perfectly and the imperfections in the process and the instrumentation used will give rise to error in the result. Consequently, the result of a measurement is, at best, only an approximation to the true value of the quantity being measured (the "measurand") and is only complete when the measured value is accompanied by a statement of the uncertainty of that approximation. This uncertainty evaluation must include not only the uncertainty contributions arising from the measurement process, but also (where this is a significant contribution to the overall uncertainty) the uncertainty associated with the calibration of the instrumentation used.

### 3.4.1 Terms related to measurement uncertainty

The terms repeatability, reproducibility, precision, accuracy, and error are often used incorrectly and therefore merit special discussion. Although they are all associated in some way with measurement uncertainty, they have different and very specific meanings:

- *Repeatability*: A measure of the spread in results under conditions where independent results are obtained with the same method on identical test items in the same laboratory by the same operator using the same equipment within short intervals of time. The usual way to quantify repeatability is in terms of the standard deviation of the results.
- *Reproducibility*: A measure of the closeness-of-agreement between the results of measurements of the same property on identical test items, when carried out under changed conditions of measurement (e.g., by a different operator or a different method, or at a different time). Reproducibility is

usually quantified in terms of the standard deviation of the mean result obtained from each of the independent sets of measurements.

- *Precision*: In science and metrology this refers to the closeness-of-agreement between indications or measured quantity values obtained by replicate measurements on the same or similar objects under specified conditions. It can be synonymous with repeatability or with reproducibility depending on the conditions under which the replicate measurements are made. Precision is often misused, especially in colloquial usage, to mean "accuracy," "uncertainty," "resolution," or "fineness of discrimination," and it should therefore be used with caution.
- *Measurement accuracy*: An expression of the closeness-of-agreement between the measured value and the true value. As the true value is not known, accuracy is a qualitative term only and cannot be given a numerical value. A measurement is said to be more accurate when it offers a smaller measurement error.
- *Measurement error*: This is defined as the measured quantity value minus a reference quantity value. It should not be confused with a production error or mistake. Measurement errors can take two forms:
  - *Systematic measurement error*: The component of measurement error that in replicate measurements remains constant or varies in a predictable manner. Systematic measurement error, and its causes, can be known or unknown. A correction can be applied to compensate for a known systematic measurement error.
  - *Random measurement error*: The component of measurement error that in replicate measurements varies in an unpredictable manner.

### 3.4.2 Selection of measurement instruments, methods, and standards

A number of factors can influence the accuracy and validity of a measurement result and these must be considered when deciding on the suitability of the selected measurement instrument for the intended purpose, the reference or standard to be used for the calibration of the chosen instrument, the calibration and measurement procedures to be adopted, and the confidence that can be placed in subsequent measurements using the calibrated instrument (i.e., the factors that must be considered when developing a measurement uncertainty budget; see Section 3.5.4). Some of the most important of these factors can be summarized as follows. (Note this is not an exhaustive list and the relative importance of these, and other factors, will depend on the actual measurement being performed.)

1. Each step in the traceability chain affects the accuracy and validity of the final measurement result. Generally the more steps in the calibration chain, the higher the measurement uncertainty becomes, and it is therefore often desirable to minimize the number of steps between the national measurement standards and the reference used for the calibration. However, the uncertainty associated with each step in the chain must also be considered:

a small number of steps each with relatively large uncertainty will often result in a higher overall uncertainty than a longer traceability chain with low uncertainty at each step in this chain.

2. The most accurate results for any calibration are obtained when comparing like with like. Conversely, every difference between the reference and test instruments, or between the reference and test artifacts, introduces additional uncertainty into the results. For example, fewer potential sources of measurement uncertainty will be introduced when measuring the luminance of a visual display screen if the measuring instrument has been calibrated by reference to a similar type of display rather than, say, a tungsten filament lamp. If possible, therefore, it is generally preferable to calibrate a measuring instrument using a reference instrument that has similar properties to the test instrument. But in any case, it must always be known what reference was used for the calibration, because without this information it is not possible to carry out a proper assessment of the measurement uncertainty.
3. The relationship between the values displayed by the test instrument and the "correct" values may vary between different ranges on the instrument ("range-change errors"), or within a range ("linearity errors"). It is therefore important to calibrate the instrument on each range over which it will be used, and for several points spanning each of these ranges.
4. Strictly speaking, a calibration only applies at the time it is carried out. Instrument performance may drift with time or with use, so the calibration must be repeated at regular intervals in order to assess and allow for such drifts. This regular recalibration allows a "calibration history" to be established, which gives confidence in the reliability (or otherwise) of the results of measurements made using the instrument. A suitable recalibration interval should therefore be specified in the calibration procedure for the instrument.
5. The results of a calibration depend on the environmental and operational conditions at the time of measurement (ambient temperature, humidity, supplied current or voltage, etc.). Changes in these conditions may have a significant impact on the results of measurements made using the instrument; the most accurate results will be obtained only if the calibration conditions are carefully reproduced during use.
6. Even if the environmental and operational conditions are well controlled, repeated measurements may not agree with each other, due to random effects associated with the measuring instrument or with the artifact being measured. For example, one source of uncertainty in electrical measurements is thermal noise, arising from the equilibrium fluctuations of the electric current inside an electrical conductor due to the random thermal motion of the charge carriers. It is not possible to eliminate such random effects by the application of correction factors, but they can be allowed for by making several repeat measurements from which a mean value and standard deviation can be calculated; increasing the number of indications will reduce the uncertainty in the mean value due to their effect.

7. Instrument resolution can have a significant impact on the results of a calibration and must be considered when choosing the points at which to perform the calibration. For example, if the instrument is only able to read with a resolution of 1 unit, performing the calibration at a point that generates a reading of 10 units will mean that the best uncertainty that can be achieved is approximately 10%, even if all other sources of uncertainty are zero. Similarly resolution influences the uncertainty in the measurements made using the instrument; it is generally preferable to change to a range with higher sensitivity when measuring values toward the lower end of a given range.

## 3.5 Evaluating measurement uncertainty

This section describes the conventional approach to evaluation of measurement uncertainty, which is applicable to a broad spectrum of measurements and will be suitable for most measurements in the field of measuring the impossible. Other approaches may be more applicable in specific cases, for example, numerical approaches such as a Monte Carlo method and those based on a Bayesian analysis. It is only possible here to give a brief introduction to the principles of uncertainty evaluation; further information can be found in Joint Committee on Guides in Metrology, 2008; United Kingdom Accreditation Service, 2007; Cox and Harris, 2006; and Bell, 2001.

### *3.5.1 Defining the measurement function*

Before carrying out any measurement it is necessary to decide what quantity $Y$ is to be measured and to select an appropriate measurement procedure for this measurand. Having defined the measurement procedure, it is then possible to identify what aspects of this procedure may influence the result of the measurement: that is, to determine all significant input quantities $X_i$ that may affect the output $Y$. Based on this information it is possible to develop a model, the so-called measurement function, that describes the functional relation $f$ between the input quantities and the output:

$$Y = f(X_1, X_2, \ldots, X_N). \tag{3.1}$$

Thus the function $f$ of Equation (3.1) expresses not simply a physical law, but a measurement process, and in particular, it should contain all quantities that can contribute a significant uncertainty to the measurement result.

The value of $Y$ cannot be known exactly; instead an estimate of this value, denoted by $y$, is obtained from Equation (3.1) using input estimates $x_1, x_2, \ldots, x_N$ for the values of the $N$ input quantities $X_1, X_2, \ldots, X_N$. Thus, the output estimate $y$, which is the result of the measurement, is given by

$$y = f(x_1, x_2, \ldots, x_N). \tag{3.2}$$

### *3.5.2 Calculating the measurement uncertainty*

The uncertainty of the measurement result $y$ can be evaluated from knowledge of the uncertainties $u(x_i)$ (sometimes referred to as $u_i$ for brevity) of the input estimates

$x_i$ that are used in Equation (3.2). These uncertainties for the input quantities can be determined in two different ways:

- *Type A uncertainties* are evaluated by the statistical analysis of a series of indications.
- *Type B uncertainties* are evaluated by other methods, and are usually based on scientific judgment using all the relevant information available, which may include:
  - Previous measurement data
  - Experience with, or general knowledge of, the behavior of the materials or instruments used
  - Manufacturer's specifications
  - Data provided in calibration reports

Each component of uncertainty, however it is evaluated, is represented by a standard deviation, termed the standard uncertainty $u(x_i)$, which is equal to the positive square root of the variance $u^2(x_i)$. For a Type A uncertainty component the variance can be determined directly by statistical methods. For a Type B uncertainty component the variance (and thus the standard uncertainty) is obtained from an assumed probability distribution function (PDF), which describes the range of possible values that the measured variable can attain and the probability that the value of the variable is within any subset of that range. In the majority of cases one of two PDFs can be assigned (other PDFs may apply under special circumstances; see United Kingdom Accreditation Service, 2007; and Cox & Harris, 2006):

- A normal or Gaussian distribution (see Figure 3.1). This is used, for example, when allowing for the uncertainty associated with the calibration of a measuring instrument. The calibration certificate for such an instrument will typically give the uncertainty for a stated level of confidence, usually

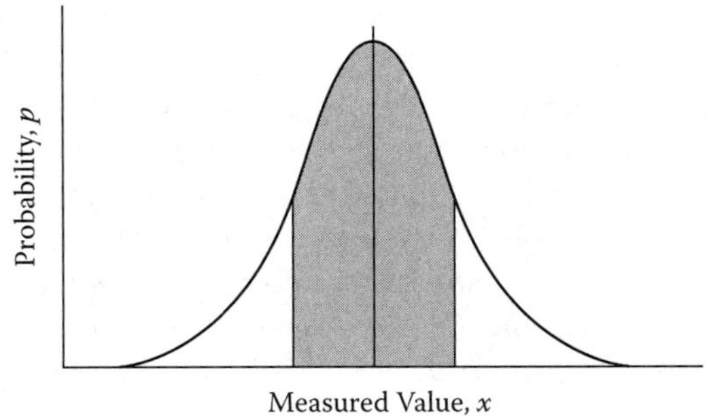


*Figure 3.1* The normal, or Gaussian, probability distribution. The size of the distribution is described in terms of a standard deviation. The shaded area represents ±1 standard deviation from the center of the distribution. This corresponds to approximately 68% of the area under the curve.

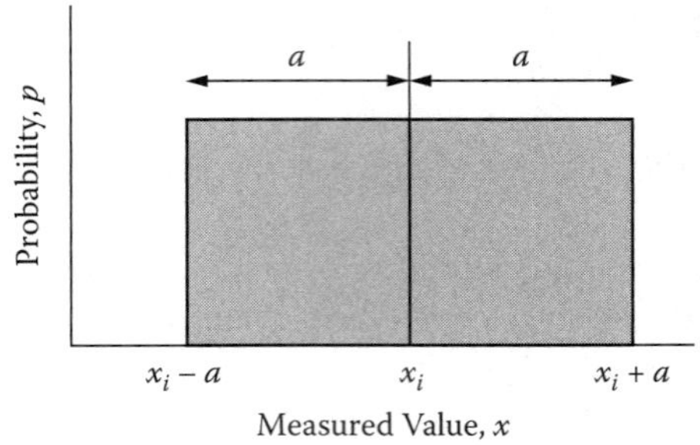


*Figure 3.2* The rectangular probability distribution. The distribution of possible values has a half-width, or semi-range, of $a$; there is equal probability of the value of $x_i$ being anywhere within the range $x_i - a$ to $x_i + a$, and zero probability of it being outside these limits. The standard deviation is given by $a/\sqrt{3}$.

95%, and the standard uncertainty can then be calculated by treating the quoted uncertainty as if a normal distribution had been used to calculate it (unless otherwise indicated) and dividing it by the appropriate factor for a normal distribution (1.96 for a 95% confidence level).

- A rectangular distribution (see Figure 3.2). This is used in situations where there is no specific knowledge about the possible values of $X_i$ between an estimated upper and lower limit and one can only assume that it is equally probable for $X_i$ to take any value within these bounds, with zero probability of being outside them. It is generally a reasonable default distribution in the absence of any other information. In this case the standard uncertainty is given by the half-width of the rectangular limits, divided by $\sqrt{3}$. Consider, for example, a meter indicating a displayed reading of 101; here the value of the quantity has equal probability of lying anywhere between 100.5 and 101.5 and the standard uncertainty is therefore $0.5/\sqrt{3}$, or 0.29.

The estimated standard deviation of the measurement result is given by the combined standard uncertainty $u_c(y)$, which is obtained by combining the individual standard uncertainties $u(x_i)$ using the law of propagation of uncertainty. This is commonly referred to as the root-sum-of-squares or RSS method of combining uncertainty components estimated as standard deviations, and is given by Equation (3.3) below. (Note Equation (3.3) gives a simplified version of the law of propagation of uncertainty, which applies when the input quantities are uncorrelated. For more detailed information the reader is referred to: Joint Committee on Guides in Metrology, 2008; United Kingdom Accreditation Service, 2007; and Cox & Harris, 2006.)

$$u_c^2(y) = \sum_{i=1}^{N} [c_i u(x_i)]^2 . \tag{3.3}$$

The parameter $c_i$ is termed the sensitivity coefficient, and quantifies how changes in the input quantity $X_i$ affect the output quantity $Y$. In other words, it describes how the output estimate $y$ varies with a corresponding small change in an input estimate $x_i$. It is obtained by calculating the partial derivative of the function $f$ with respect to $X_i$ and determining the value of this partial derivative using the estimated values of all the input quantities. However, the calculations required in order to determine sensitivity coefficients by partial differentiation can be a lengthy process, particularly when there are many input contributions and uncertainty estimates are needed for a range of values. It is often beneficial, therefore, to obtain the sensitivity coefficients directly through the practical approach of changing one of the input variables by a known amount, while keeping all other inputs constant, and noting the change in the measured output (the sensitivity coefficient is then given by the change in the measured output divided by the change in the input quantity).

It should also be noted that if the functional relationship between the input and output quantities is a simple addition or subtraction of the input quantities, then all the input quantities are directly related to the output quantity and the partial derivatives will all be unity. If the functional relationship is a product or quotient (i.e., the output quantity is obtained from only the multiplication or division of the input quantities), this can be simplified by the use of relative values, for example, those expressed in percentage terms or in parts per million. The general form of such a relationship is:

$$Y = X_1^{p_1} X_2^{p_2} \ldots X_N^{p_N}, \tag{3.4}$$

where the exponents $p_i$ are known positive or negative numbers. The *relative* standard uncertainty is then given by

$$\frac{u_c(y)}{|y|} = \sqrt{\sum_{i=1}^{N} \left[ \frac{p_i u(x_i)}{|x_i|} \right]^2}. \tag{3.5}$$

The use of relative uncertainties can often simplify the calculations and is particularly helpful when the input quantities and the uncertainties are already given in relative terms. However, sensitivity coefficients may still be required to account for known relationships, such as the influence of a temperature coefficient. Relative uncertainties should not be used when the functional relationship is already an addition or subtraction.

### 3.5.3 *Reporting measurements and uncertainties*

As explained in Section 3.4, the result of a measurement is only complete when the measured value (i.e., the estimate of the measurand) is accompanied by a statement of the associated uncertainty. Sometimes this is done by simply stating the measured value together with the combined standard uncertainty. More commonly, however, what is required is a measure of uncertainty that defines an interval about the measured value $y$ within which the true value of the measurand $Y$ is confidently believed to lie. This is termed the expanded uncertainty $U$, and is obtained by multiplying $u_c(y)$ by a coverage factor $k$. In other words:

$$U = ku_c(y) \tag{3.6}$$

and it is confidently believed that

$$y - U \leq Y \leq y + U \text{ (usually written as } Y = y \pm U). \tag{3.7}$$

Most commonly a coverage factor of 2 is used, which corresponds to a "level of confidence" or "coverage probability" of approximately 95% under a Gaussian assumption. In other words, the interval $y \pm U$ is expected to contain 95% of the values that could be attributed to the output quantity on the assumption that the uncertainty distribution is Gaussian. Where a result is quoted with an expanded uncertainty instead of a standard uncertainty, the coverage factor used must always be stated. An example is given in Section 3.5.4 below.

### *3.5.4 Calculating uncertainty: An example*

Consider the problem of measuring the current flowing through an electrical circuit by measuring the voltage drop across a calibrated reference resistor using a calibrated digital voltmeter (DVM). The current $I$ is given by the equation $I = V/R$ where $V$ is the voltage drop measured across the standard resistor $R$. Suppose that the following conditions apply:

1. The standard resistor was calibrated at a temperature of 20 °C.
2. The calibrated resistance for the standard resistor is 1.060 Ω with an expanded uncertainty of 0.001 Ω for a coverage factor of $k = 2$.
3. The operating temperature of the resistor at the time of measurement is 30 °C and the temperature coefficient for this resistor is known to be +0.001 Ω $°C^{-1}$ with a standard uncertainty of 0.0001 Ω $°C^{-1}$.
4. The manufacturer's data sheet for the standard resistor states a maximum drift in resistance of ±0.0005 Ω per year; the resistor was calibrated within the previous year and no correction for possible drift has been applied.
5. The DVM has been calibrated and adjusted so that it needs no correction to the displayed values on the 1 V range for an ambient temperature of 20 °C, with a stated expanded uncertainty for the calibration of 0.01% for a coverage factor of $k = 2$.
6. The ambient temperature at the time of measurement is 25 °C and the manufacturer's data sheet for the DVM states that the temperature coefficient does not exceed ±0.001% $°C^{-1}$; no correction is applied for the difference in temperature between the ambient conditions and the calibration conditions because a best estimate of zero is implied by the information.
7. The readout resolution of the DVM is 0.1 mV.

8. The manufacturer's data sheet for the DVM states a maximum drift in calibration of +0.8 mV per year; the DVM was last calibrated nearly one year ago and it has therefore been decided that a correction for possible drift of +0.4 mV should be applied, with a maximum uncertainty of ±0.4 mV.
9. A total of 10 independent readings are taken from the DVM on the 1 V range, with the following results: 0.8081, 0.8090, 0.8093, 0.8096, 0.8084, 0.8098, 0.8083, 0.8086, 0.8092, 0.8099.

Based on this information, the following measurement function applies:

$$I = \frac{V_m + V_d + V_t \Delta T_V}{R_c + R_d + R_t \Delta T_R}, \tag{3.8}$$

where the input quantities are as follows:

$V_m$ = voltage measured using the DVM, which has associated uncertainties arising from:
  DVM calibration, $V_c$
  Voltage measurement repeatability, $u(V) = s(\overline{V}_m)$
  DVM resolution, $V_r$
$V_d$ = drift in the DVM since calibration.
$V_t$ = temperature coefficient of the DVM.
$\Delta T_v$ = temperature difference between the ambient temperature at the time of measurement and the temperature at the time of calibration of the DVM.
$R_c$ = calibrated resistance value of the standard resistor.
$R_d$ = drift in the standard resistor since calibration.
$R_t$ = temperature coefficient of the standard resistor.
$\Delta T_R$ = temperature difference between the operating temperature of the resistor at the time of measurement and the temperature at the time of its calibration.

The mean of the measured voltage $\overline{V}_m$, and the experimental standard deviation of the mean (also known as the standard error of the mean) $s(\overline{V}_n)$, are obtained by statistical means using the following equations, where $n$ is the number of indications:

$$\overline{V}_m = \frac{1}{n}\sum_{j=1}^{n} V_{m,j} \tag{3.9}$$

$$s(\overline{V}_m) = \sqrt{\frac{1}{n(n-1)}\sum_{j=1}^{n}(V_{m,j} - \overline{V}_m)^2} \tag{3.10}$$

This gives $\overline{V}_m = 0.80902$ V and $s(\overline{V}_m) = 0.20$ mV.

This means that the best estimate of the current through the resistor is:

$$I = \frac{V_m + V_d + V_t \Delta T_V}{R_c + R_d + R_t \Delta T_R} = \frac{0.80902 + 0.0004 + 0}{1.060 + 0 + (0.001 \times 10)} = 0.7565 \text{ A}$$

This value on its own is not sufficient; the associated uncertainty must be calculated by establishing the uncertainty budget (see Table 3.5). This uncertainty budget includes an allowance for the uncertainty associated with each of the input quantities, and also states the form of the probability distribution, the divisor used to convert from the stated uncertainty value to the standard uncertainty, the sensitivity coefficient, and the degrees of freedom. In most cases the degrees of freedom is infinite, but for Type A uncertainties the degrees of freedom is one less than the number of indications on which the uncertainty evaluation is based (i.e., it is given by the value of $n - 1$ in Equation (3.10)). The effective degrees of freedom for the combined standard uncertainty $\nu_{eff}$ is calculated from the degrees of freedom for the individual uncertainty contributions $\nu_i$, using the Welch–Satterthwaite formula:

$$\nu_{eff} = \frac{u_c^4(y)}{\sum_{i=1}^{N} \frac{u_i^4(y)}{\nu_i}}, \tag{3.11}$$

where

$$u_i(y) \equiv |c_i| \, u(x_i). \tag{3.12}$$

Knowledge of the effective degrees of freedom allows the relationship between the coverage factor and the confidence level to be calculated, using the Student's *t* distribution (tabulated in UKAS M3003, 2007). For $\nu_{eff}$ greater than about 50, a coverage factor of 2 corresponds to a confidence level of approximately 95%.

For the example given above and in Table 3.5, the expanded uncertainty of the calibration is calculated to be 0.23%, or 0.0017 A, for a coverage factor $k = 2$ and with effective degrees of freedom greater than 4000. The final result of the measurement would be quoted in one of the following forms:

> The current flowing through the circuit is 0.7565 A ± 0.0017 A.
> The reported expanded uncertainty is based on a standard uncertainty multiplied by a coverage factor $k = 2$, providing a level of confidence of approximately 95%.

or

> The current flowing through the circuit is 0.7565 A ± 0.23%.
> The reported expanded uncertainty is based on a standard uncertainty multiplied by a coverage factor $k = 2$, providing a level of confidence of approximately 95%.

## 3.6 Notation

Table 3.6 summarizes the meaning of the notation used in this chapter.

*Table 3.5* Uncertainty budget for the example given in Section 5.4

| *Symbol* | *Source of uncertainty* | *Value* ± | *Value (%)* | *Probability distribution* | *Divisor* | $c_i$ | $u_i(y)$ | *Degrees of freedom* |
|---|---|---|---|---|---|---|---|---|
| $V_c$ | DVM calibration | | 0.01% | Normal | 2 | 1 | 0.005% | ∞ |
| $u(V)$ | Voltage measurement repeatability | 0.20 mV | 0.025% | Normal | 1 | 1 | 0.025% | 9 |
| $V_r$ | DVM resolution | 0.05 mV | 0.006% | Rectangular | √3 | 1 | 0.003% | ∞ |
| $V_d$ | DVM drift | 0.40 mV | 0.049% | Rectangular | √3 | 1 | 0.028% | ∞ |
| $V_t$ | Temperature coefficient of DVM | 5°C and temperature coefficient not exceeding 0.001% per °C | 0.005% | Rectangular | √3 | 1 | 0.003% | ∞ |
| $R_c$ | Resistor calibration | 0.001 Ω | 0.094% | Normal | 2 | 1 | 0.047% | ∞ |
| $R_d$ | Resistor drift | 0.0005 Ω | 0.047% | Rectangular | √3 | 1 | 0.027% | ∞ |
| $R_t$ | Temperature coefficient of resistor | 10°C and temperature coefficient uncertainty 0.0001 Ω per °C ($k = 1$) | 0.094% | Normal | 1 | 1 | 0.094% | ∞ |
| $u_c(I)$ | Combined standard uncertainty | | | Normal | | | 0.115% | >4000 |
| U | Expanded uncertainty | | | Normal ($k = 2$) | | | 0.23% | >4000 |

*Note:* The uncertainties in column 4 are relative uncertainties for the relevant input quantities (in this case voltage or resistance) and those in column 8 are relative uncertainties for the output quantity (in this case current).

*Table 3.6* Summary of notation used

| *Symbol* | *Meaning* |
|---|---|
| $c_i$ | Sensitivity coefficient used to multiply the value of an input quantity $X_i$ to express it in terms of the measurand $Y$; quantifies how changes in the input quantity $X_i$ impact on the output quantity $Y$. Given by: $$c_i \equiv \frac{\partial f}{\partial x_i}$$ |
| $f$ | Functional relationship between measurand $Y$ and input quantities $X_i$ on which $Y$ depends, and between output estimate $y$ and input estimates $x_i$ on which $y$ depends |
| $\frac{\partial f}{\partial x_i}$ | Partial derivative with respect to input quantity $X_i$ of functional relationship $f$ between measurand $Y$ and input quantities $X_i$ on which $Y$ depends, evaluated at $X_i = x_i$ where $i = 1, \ldots N$: $$\frac{\partial f}{\partial x_i} = \left.\frac{\partial f}{\partial X_i}\right\|_{x_1, x_2, \ldots, x_N}$$ |
| $k$ | Coverage factor used to calculate expanded uncertainty $U = ku_c(y)$ of output estimate y from its combined standard uncertainty $u_c(y)$ |
| $N$ | Number of input estimates $x_i$ on which the value of the measurand depends |
| $n$ | Number of repeated observations |
| $\overline{q}$ | Arithmetic mean or average of $n$ independent repeated observations $q_k$ of randomly varying quantity $q$ |
| $q_j$ | $j$th independent repeated observation of randomly varying quantity $q$ |
| $s(\overline{q})$ | Experimental standard deviation of the mean $\overline{q}$; standard uncertainty obtained from a Type A evaluation: $$s(\overline{q}) = \frac{s(q_j)}{\sqrt{n}}$$ |
| $s(q_j)$ | Experimental standard deviation determined from $n$ independent repeated observations $q_j$ of $q$: $$s(q_j) = \sqrt{\frac{1}{n-1}\sum_{j=1}^{n}(q_j - \overline{q})^2}$$ |
| $u^2(x_i)$ | Estimated variance associated with input estimate $x_i$ that estimates the input quantity $X_i$; when $x_i$ is determined from the arithmetic mean or average of $n$ independent repeated observations, $u^2(x_i)$ is obtained by a Type A evaluation: $$u^2(x_i) = s^2(\overline{q}) = \frac{1}{n(n-1)}\sum_{j=1}^{n}(q_j - \overline{q})^2$$ |
| $u(x_i)$ | Standard uncertainty of input estimate $x_i$ that estimates the input quantity $X_i$; when $x_i$ is determined from the arithmetic mean or average of $n$ independent repeated observations, $u(x_i)$ is obtained by a Type A evaluation: $$u(x_i) = s(\overline{q})$$ |

*Table 3.6 (continued)* Summary of notation used

| *Symbol* | *Meaning* |
|---|---|
| $u_c^2(y)$ | Combined variance associated with output estimate $y$ |
| $u_c(y)$ | Combined standard uncertainty of output estimate $y$ |
| $u_i(y)$ | Component of combined standard uncertainty $u_c(y)$ of output estimate $y$ generated by the standard uncertainty of input estimate $x_i$: $$u_i(y) = \lvert c_i \rvert \, u(x_i)$$ |
| $\dfrac{u(x_i)}{\lvert x_i \rvert}$ | Relative standard uncertainty of input estimate $x_i$ |
| $U$ | Expanded uncertainty of output estimate $y$ that describes the measurand as an interval $Y = y \pm U$ having a high level of confidence, equal to coverage factor $k$ times the combined standard uncertainty $u_c(y)$ of $y$: $$U = ku_c(y)$$ |
| $x_i$ | Estimate of input quantity $X_i$ |
| $X_i$ | *i*th input quantity on which measurand $Y$ depends |
| $y$ | Estimate of measurand $Y$; result of a measurement |
| $Y$ | A measurand |
| $\nu_i$ | Degrees of freedom, or effective degrees of freedom, of standard uncertainty $u(x_i)$ of input estimate $x_i$ |
| $\nu_{eff}$ | Effective degrees of freedom of $u_c(y)$ |

## Acknowledgment and copyright

The preparation of this chapter was jointly funded by the UK Department for Innovation, Universities and Skills (through the National Measurement Office's Innovation Research and Development Programme) and the European Commission (through NEST-Pathfinder Project number 043297-MINET).



## References

American Association for the Advancement of Science. (1892). *Science, 19*(474), 127.

Bell, S. (2001). *NPL measurement good practice guide no. 11 (Issue 2). A beginner's guide to uncertainty of measurement.* London: NPL. Available from www.npl.co.uk

Cox, M. G., and Harris, P. M. (2006). *Software support for metrology best practice guide no. 6. Uncertainty evaluation.* (NPL Report DEM-ES-011). London: NPL. Available from www.npl.co.uk

International Organization for Standardization. (2005). *General requirements for the competence of testing and calibration laboratories* (ISO/IEC 17025:2005). Geneva: International Organization for Standardization.

Joint Committee on Guides in Metrology. (2008). *Evaluation of measurement data—Guide to the expression of uncertainty in measurement* (JCGM 100:2008). Available from www.bipm.org/en/publications/guides/gum.html

Organisation Intergouvernementale de la Convention du Mètre. (2006). *The International System of Units (SI) (8th edition)*. Paris: Bureau International des Poids et Mesures. Available from www.bipm.org

United Kingdom Accreditation Service. (2007). *The expression of uncertainty and confidence in measurement* (UKAS Publication M3003 Edition 2). London: UKAS. Available from www.ukas.com

# 4 Meaningful and meaningless statements in epidemiology and public health

*Fred S. Roberts*

Center for Discrete Mathematics and Theoretical Computer Science
Rutgers University
Piscataway, New Jersey, USA

## 4.1 Introduction

The theory of measurement is an interdisciplinary subject that grew out of the attempt to put the foundations of measurement on a firm mathematical foundation. Building on classic examples of measurement in the physical sciences, the theory was motivated by the attempt to make measurement in economics, psychology, and other disciplines more precise. The theory traces its roots to the work of Helmholtz (1887/1930), and was widely formalized in the twentieth century in such books as Krantz, Luce, Suppes, and Tverksy (1971), Luce, Krantz, Suppes, and Tversky (1990), Pfanzagl (1968), Roberts (1979/2009), and Suppes, Krantz, Luce, and Tversky (1989). Measurement theory is now beginning to be applied in a wide variety of new areas. Little known in the fields of epidemiology and public health, the theory has the potential to make important contributions to epidemiological measurement. In turn, problems of epidemiology are posing new challenges for measurement theory.

We seek to answer questions such as the following:

- Is it meaningful to say that the malaria parasite load has doubled?
- Is the average cough score for one set of TB patients higher than that for another?
- For controlling the spread of HIV, which of abstinence education, universal screening, and condom distribution are more effective?

All of these questions have something to do with measurement. We provide a brief introduction to the theory of measurement, with an emphasis on the types of scales that can arise.

In almost every practical application in epidemiology, something is measured. Yet in many cases, little attention is paid to the limitations that the scales of measurement being used might place on the conclusions that can be drawn from them. Scales may to some degree be arbitrary, involving choices about zero points or units or the like. It would be unwise to make decisions that could turn out differently if the arbitrary choice of zero point or unit is changed in some "admissible" way. We are interested in exploring the extent to which this can happen, and in laying down guidelines for what conclusions based on scales of measurement are allowable. We make these ideas precise by introducing a key measurement theory concept of meaningfulness. Using examples from the study of diseases such as HIV, malaria, and tuberculosis, we give a variety of examples of meaningless and meaningful statements. More subtle applications include averaging judgments of cough severity or judgments of fatigue, finding measures of air pollution combining different pollutants, and evaluating alternative HIV treatments using "merging" procedures for normalized scores. We also discuss the meaningfulness of statistical tests and of answers to optimization questions in epidemiology arising from problems such as the effect of climate change on health. We then discuss general results about how to average scores to attain measures allowing meaningful comparisons and close with a discussion about measurement issues arising in the study of behavioral responses to health events.

## 4.2 Scales of measurement

It seems clear that measurement has something to do with numbers. In this chapter, it suffices to think of assigning real numbers to objects. Our approach to scales of measurement is based on the notion, going back to the psychologist S. S. Stevens (1946, 1951, 1959), that the properties of a scale are captured by studying *admissible transformations*, transformations that lead from one acceptable scale to another. For example, we transform temperature measurements from centigrade into Fahrenheit and mass measurements from kilograms into pounds. Assuming a scale assigns a real number $f(a)$ to each object $a$ being measured, an admissible transformation of scale can be thought of as a function $\phi$ that takes $f(a)$ into $(\phi \circ f)(a)$.

Our approach to scales of measurement is based on ideas introduced by Stevens. Assuming that a scale assigns a real number to each object being measured, we call a scale a *ratio scale* if the admissible transformations are of the form $\phi(x) = \alpha x$, $\alpha > 0$, an *interval scale* if the admissible transformations are of the form $\phi(x) = \alpha x + \beta$, $\alpha > 0$, an *ordinal scale* if the admissible transformations are the (strictly) monotone increasing transformations, and an *absolute scale* if the only admissible transformation is the identity. For definitions of other scale types, see Roberts (1979/2009). Thus, in the case of ratio scales, the scale value is determined up to choice of a unit; in the case of interval scales, it is determined up to choices of unit and of zero point; and in the case of ordinal scales, it is determined only up to order. Mass is an example of a ratio scale. The transformation from kilograms into pounds, for example, involves the admissible transformation $\phi(x) = 2.2x$. Length (inches, centimeters) and time intervals (years, seconds) are two other examples of ratio scales. It is sometimes argued that scales developed for loudness ("sones") define a ratio scale, but this is not universally accepted. Temperature (except where there is an absolute zero) defines an interval scale. Thus, transformation from centigrade into Fahrenheit involves the admissible transformation $\phi(x) = (9/5)x + 32$.

Time on the calendar is another example of an interval scale (to say that this is the year 2011 involves not only a choice of unit but a choice of the zero year). An example of an ordinal scale is any scale in which we give grades of materials, such as leather, lumber, wool, and so on. Expressed preferences sometimes lead only to ordinal scales, if we know our preferences only up to order. Subjective judgments in epidemiology, such as of cough or fatigue, often define ordinal scales. Counting gives an example of an absolute scale.

For many scales, the scale type can be determined by showing that the scale arises from a (numerical) representation. In the rest of this paragraph, we say a word or two about how this is done in the theory in such books as Krantz et al. (1971), Pfanzagl (1968), and Roberts (1979/2009), though the details are not needed for what follows. Specifically, one studies certain *observed relations* on a set of objects of interest, relations such as "*a* is longer than *b*," "*a* is louder than *b*," "I think the value of *b* is between the value of *a* and the value of *c*," and so on. One identifies corresponding *numerical relations*, relations on a set of real numbers, for instance, the "greater than" relation or the "betweenness" relation. Then one studies mappings that take each object of interest into a number so that objects related in a certain way in an observed relation correspond to numbers related in the same way in the corresponding numerical relation. For example, one seeks to assign numbers to objects so that *a* is judged louder than *b* if and only if the number assigned to *a* is greater than the number assigned to *b*. Such a mapping from objects to numbers is called a *homomorphism* from the observed relation to the numerical relation. In measurement theory, scales are identified with homomorphisms. Formally, an *admissible transformation* of a scale is then a transformation of the numbers assigned so that one gets another homomorphism. In some cases, one can derive a characterization of the class of admissible transformations by working from a (numerical) representation. For details on how to formalize these ideas, see Roberts (1979/2009).

It should be remarked that many scales based on subjective judgments cannot be derived from a (numerical) representation. Then, we must use the principle that the admissible transformations are those that preserve the information carried by the scale. Knapp (1990) and Thomas (1985) emphasize the difficulties involved in identifying scale type. As Stevens (1968) argues, it is often a matter of empirical judgment to determine the admissible transformations and hence the scale type.

## 4.3 Meaningful statements

In measurement theory, we speak of a statement as being meaningful if its truth or falsity is not an artifact of the particular scale values used. The following definition is due to Suppes (1959) and Suppes and Zinnes (1963).

**Definition:** *A statement involving numerical scales is* ***meaningful*** *if its truth or falsity is unchanged after any (or all) of the scales is transformed (independently?) by an admissible transformation.*

A slightly more informal definition is the following:

**Alternate Definition:** *A statement involving numerical scales is* ***meaningful*** *if its truth or falsity is unchanged after any (or all) of the scales is (independently?) replaced by another acceptable scale.*

In some practical examples, for example, those involving preference judgments or judgments of "louder than" under the "semiorder" model (Roberts, 1979/2009, 1994), it is possible to have scales where one cannot go from one to the other by an admissible transformation, so one has to use this alternate definition.

Here we avoid the long literature of more sophisticated approaches to meaningfulness. Situations where this relatively simple-minded definition may run into trouble are disregarded. Emphasis is on applications of the invariance motivation behind the theory of meaningfulness.

Consider the following statement:

**Statement S:** "The duration of symptoms in an influenza victim not treated with Tamiflu is three times as long as the duration of symptoms in an influenza victim who is so treated."

Is this meaningful? We have a ratio scale (time intervals) and we consider the statement:

$$f(a) = 3f(b). \tag{4.1}$$

This is meaningful if $f$ is a ratio scale. For, an admissible transformation is $\phi(x) = \alpha x$, $\alpha > 0$. We want Equation (4.1) to hold iff

$$(\phi \circ f)(a) = 3(\phi \circ f)(b). \tag{4.2}$$

But Equation (4.2) becomes

$$\alpha f(a) = 3\alpha f(b) \tag{4.3}$$

and (4.1) iff (4.3) because $\alpha > 0$. Thus, the statement $S$ is meaningful.

Next consider the statement:

**Statement T:** "The patient's temperature at 9AM today is 2% higher than it was at 9 AM yesterday."

Is this meaningful? This is the statement

$$f(a) = 1.02f(b).$$

This is meaningless. It could be true with Fahrenheit and false with centigrade, or vice versa.

In general, for ratio scales, it is meaningful to compare ratios:

$$f(a)/f(b) > f(c)/f(d).$$

For interval scales, it is meaningful to compare intervals:

$$f(a) - f(b) > f(c) - f(d).$$

For ordinal scales, it is meaningful to compare size:

$$f(a) > f(b).$$

Let us consider another example. Malaria parasite density is mainly obtained by reading slides under microscopes. Consider the statement:

**Statement M:** "The parasite density in this slide is double the parasite density in that slide."

Is this meaningful? Density is measured in number per microliter. So, if one slide has 100,000 per μL and another 50,000 per μL, is it meaningful to conclude that the first slide has twice the density of the second? This is meaningful. Volume involves ratio scales and counts are absolute scales. However, this disregards errors in measurement. A statement can be meaningful in the measurement theory sense but meaningless in a practical sense.

Here is still another example:

**Statement W:** "The second tumor weighs 20 million times as much as the first one."

This is meaningful. It involves ratio scales. It is surely false no matter what the unit. Note that meaningfulness is different from truth. It has to do with what kinds of assertions it makes sense to make, which assertions are not accidents of the particular choice of scale (units, zero points) in use.

## 4.4 Averaging judgments of cough severity

Suppose we study two groups of patients with tuberculosis. Let $f(a)$ be the cough severity of $a$ as judged on one of the subjective cough severity scales in use (e.g., rate severity as 1 to 5). Suppose that data suggest that the average cough severity for patients in the first group is higher than the average cough severity of patients in the second group. Is this meaningful?

Let $a_1, a_2, \ldots, a_n$ be patients in the first group and $b_1, b_2, \ldots, b_m$ be patients in the second group. Note that $m$ could be different from $n$. Then we are (probably) asserting that

$$\frac{1}{n}\sum_{i=1}^{n} f(a_i) > \frac{1}{m}\sum_{i=1}^{m} f(b_i). \tag{4.4}$$

We are comparing arithmetic means. The statement (4.4) is meaningful if and only if under admissible transformation $\phi$, (4.4) holds if and only if

$$\frac{1}{n}\sum_{i=1}^{n} (\phi \circ f)(a_i) > \frac{1}{m}\sum_{i=1}^{m} (\phi \circ f)(b_i) \tag{4.5}$$

holds. If cough severity defines a ratio scale, then (4.5) is the same as

$$\frac{1}{n}\sum_{i=1}^{n} \alpha f(a_i) > \frac{1}{m}\sum_{i=1}^{m} \alpha f(b_i), \tag{4.6}$$

for some positive $\alpha$. Certainly (4.4) holds if and only if (4.6) does, so (4.4) is meaningful.

Note that (4.4) is still meaningful if $f$ is an interval scale. For instance, we could be comparing temperatures. It is meaningful to assert that the average temperature of the first group is higher than the average temperature of the second group. To see why, note that (4.4) is equivalent to

$$\frac{1}{n}\sum_{i=1}^{n} [\alpha f(a_i) + \beta] > \frac{1}{m}\sum_{i=1}^{m} [\alpha f(b_i) + \beta],$$

where $\alpha > 0$.

However, (4.4) is easily seen to be meaningless if $f$ is just an ordinal scale. To show that comparison of arithmetic means can be meaningless for ordinal scales, note that we are asking experts for a subjective judgment of cough severity. It seems that $f(a)$ is measured on an ordinal scale, for example, 5-point scale: 5 = extremely severe, 4 = very severe, 3 = severe, 2 = slightly severe, and 1 = no cough. In such a scale, the numbers may not mean anything; only their order matters. Suppose that group 1 has three members with scores of 5, 3, and 1, for an average of 3, and group 2 has three members with scores of 4, 4, and 2 for an average of 3.33. Then the average score in group 2 is higher than the average score in group 1. On the other hand, suppose we consider the admissible transformation $\phi$ defined by $\phi(5) = 100$, $\phi(4) = 75$, $\phi(3) = 65$, $\phi(2) = 40$, $\phi(1) = 30$. Then after transformation, members of group 1 have scores of 100, 65, 30, with an average of 65, and those in group 2 have scores of 75, 75, 40, with an average of 63.33. Now, group 1 has a higher average score. Which group had a higher average score? The answer clearly depends on which version of the scale is used. Of course, one can argue against this kind of example. As Suppes (1979) remarks in the case of a similar example having to do with grading apples in four ordered categories, "Surely there is something quite unnatural about this transformation" $\phi$. He suggests that "there is a strong natural tendency to treat the ordered categories as being equally spaced." However, if we require this, then the scale is not an ordinal scale according to our definition. Not every strictly monotone increasing transformation is admissible. Moreover, there is no reason, given the nature of the categories, to feel that equal spacing is demanded in our example. In any case, the argument is not with the precept that we have stated, but with the question of whether the five-point scale we have given is indeed an ordinal scale as we have defined it. To complete this example, let us simply remark that comparison of medians rather than arithmetic means is meaningful with ordinal scales: the statement that one group has a higher median than another group is preserved under admissible transformation.

Similar considerations apply to measuring average fatigue. Fatigue is an important variable in measuring the progress of patients with serious diseases. One scale widely used in measuring fatigue is the Piper Fatigue Scale. It asks questions such as: on a scale of 1 to 10, to what degree is the fatigue you are feeling now interfering with your ability to complete your work or school activities (1 = none, 10 = a great deal)? On a scale of 1 to 10, how would you describe the degree of intensity or severity of the fatigue which you are experiencing now (1 = mild, 10 = severe)? A similar analysis applies: it is meaningless to compare arithmetic means, and meaningful to compare medians.

Let us return to cough severity, but now suppose that each of $n$ observers is asked to rate each of a collection of patients as to their relative cough severity. Alternatively, suppose we rate patients on different criteria or against different benchmarks. (A similar analysis applies with performance ratings, importance ratings, etc.) Let $f_i(a)$ be the rating of patient $a$ by judge $i$ (or under criterion $i$). Is it meaningful to assert that the average rating of patient $a$ is higher than the average rating of patient $b$? A similar question arises in fatigue ratings, ratings of brightness of rash, and so on. We are now considering the statement

$$\frac{1}{n}\sum_{i=1}^{n} f_i(a) > \frac{1}{n}\sum_{i=1}^{n} f_i(b). \tag{4.7}$$

Note in contrast to statement (4.4) that we have the same number of terms in each sum and that the subscript is now on the scale value $f$ rather than on the alternative $a$ or $b$. If each $f_i$ is a ratio scale, we then ask whether (4.7) is equivalent to

$$\frac{1}{n}\sum_{i=1}^{n} \alpha f_i(a) > \frac{1}{n}\sum_{i=1}^{n} \alpha f_i(b),$$

$\alpha > 0$. This is clearly the case.

However, we have perhaps gone too quickly. What if $f_1, f_2, \ldots, f_n$ have independent units? In this case, we want to allow independent admissible transformations of the $f_i$. Thus, we must consider

$$\frac{1}{n}\sum_{i=1}^{n}\alpha_i f_i(a) > \frac{1}{n}\sum_{i=1}^{n}\alpha_i f_i(b), \tag{4.8}$$

all $\alpha_i > 0$. It is easy to find $\alpha_i' s$ for which (4.7) holds but (4.8) fails. Thus, (4.7) is meaningless. Does it make sense to consider different $\alpha_i$s? It certainly does in some contexts. Consider the case where the alternatives are animals and one expert measures their improved health in terms of their weight gain and a second measures it in terms of their height gain.

The conclusion is that we need to be careful when comparing arithmetic mean ratings, even when we are using ratio scales. Norman Dalkey (personal communication) was the first person to point out to the author that, in many cases, it is safer to use geometric means, a conclusion which by now is "folklore."

For, consider the comparison

$$\sqrt[n]{\prod_{i=1}^{n} f_i(a)} > \sqrt[n]{\prod_{i=1}^{n} f_i(b)}. \tag{4.9}$$

If all $\alpha_i > 0$, then (4.9) holds if and only if

$$\sqrt[n]{\prod_{i=1}^{n} \alpha_i f_i(a)} > \sqrt[n]{\prod_{i=1}^{n} \alpha_i f_i(b)}.$$

Thus, if each $f_i$ is a ratio scale, then even if experts change the units of their rating scales independently, the comparison of geometric means is meaningful even though the comparison of arithmetic means is not. An example of an application of this observation is the use of the geometric mean by Roberts (1972, 1973). The problem arose in a study of air pollution and energy use in commuter transportation. (Health effects of air pollution are discussed in the next section.) A preliminary step in the model building involved the choice of the most important variables to consider in the model. Each member of a panel of experts estimated the relative importance of variables using a procedure called magnitude estimation. (Here, the most important variable is given a score of 100, a variable judged half as important is given a score of 50, and so on.) There is a strong body of opinion that magnitude estimation leads to a ratio scale, much of it going back to Stevens. (See the discussion in Roberts (1979/2009, pp. 179–180).) How then should we choose the most important variables? By the discussion above, it is "safer" to combine the experts' importance ratings by using geometric means and then to choose the most important variables as those having the highest geometric mean relative importance ratings, than it is to do this by using arithmetic means. That is why Roberts (1972, 1973) used geometric means.

## 4.5 Measurement of air pollution

There is a close relationship between pollution and health. Various pollutants are present in the air. Some are carbon monoxide (CO), hydrocarbons (HC), nitrogen oxides (NOX), sulfur oxides (SOX), and particulate matter (PM). Also damaging are products of chemical reactions among pollutants. For example, oxidants such as ozone are produced by HC and NOX reacting in the presence of sunlight. Some pollutants are more serious in the presence of others: for example, SOX are more harmful in the presence of PM. In the early days of air pollution science, there was an attempt to find a way to measure pollution with one overall measure. To compare pollution control policies, we need to compare effects of different pollutants. We might allow an increase of some pollutants to achieve decrease of others. One single measure could give an indication of how bad the pollution level is and might help us determine if we have made progress. A simple approach is to combine the weight of pollutants. Let us measure the total weight of emissions of pollutant $i$ over a fixed period of time and sum over $i$. Let $e(i, t, k)$ be the total weight of emissions of pollutant $i$ (per cubic meter) over the $t$th time period and due to the $k$th source or measured in the $k$th location. Then our pollution index is simply

$$A(t,k) = \sum_{i=1}^{n} e(i,t,k),$$

if there are $n$ pollutants under consideration.

Using this measure, Walther (1972) reached such conclusions as: (i) the largest source of air pollution is transportation and the second largest is stationary fuel combustion (especially by electric power plants); (ii) transportation accounts for over 50% of all air pollution; (iii) CO accounts for over 50% of all emitted air pollution. Statement (i) is just

$$A(t,k) > A(t,k').$$

Statement (ii) is just the statement that

$$A(t,k_r) > \sum_{k \neq k_r} A(t,k).$$

Statement (iii) is just the statement that

$$\sum_{t,k} e(i,t,k) > \sum_{t,k} \sum_{j \neq i} e(j,t,k).$$

All these conclusions are meaningful if we measure all $e(i, t, k)$ in the same units of mass (e.g., milligrams per cubic meter) and so admissible transformation means multiply $e(i, t, k)$ by the same constant.

However, although these statements are meaningful in the technical sense, we have to ask if they are meaningful comparisons of pollution level in a practical sense. A unit of mass of CO is far less harmful than a unit of mass of NOX. U.S. Environmental Protection Agency standards based on health effects for a 24-hour period allow many more units of CO than units of NOX because a unit of mass of CO is far less harmful than a unit of mass of NOX. Thus, we might wish to use a weighting factor $\lambda_i$ that measures the effect of the *i*th pollutant and then use a weighted sum

$$\sum_{i=1}^{n} \lambda_i e(i,t,k). \tag{4.10}$$

Such a weighted sum, sometimes known as *pindex*, has been used as a combined pollution index. In early uses of this measure in the San Francisco Bay Area (Bay Area Pollution Control District, 1968; Sauter and Chilton, 1970; and elsewhere), $\lambda_i$ is the reciprocal of the amount $\tau(i)$ of emissions of pollutant *i* in a given period of time needed to reach a certain danger level, otherwise called the *tolerance factor.* The reciprocal is called the *severity factor.* Using this version of pindex, Walther (1972) argues that transportation is still the largest source of pollution, but now accounting for less than 50%. Stationary sources fall to fourth place. CO drops to the bottom of the list of pollutants, accounting for just over 2% of the total. Again, these conclusions are meaningful if we use the same units of mass in each case. With these weighting factors $\lambda_i = 1/\tau(i)$, although comparisons using pindex are meaningful in our technical sense, the index does not seem to give meaningful numbers in any real sense, because reaching 100% of the danger level in one pollutant would give the same pindex value as reaching 20% of the danger level on each of five pollutants. In conclusion, we should stress again that there is a distinction between meaningfulness in the technical sense and meaningfulness in other senses.

The *severity tonnage* of pollutant *i* due to a given source is actual tonnage times the severity factor $1/\tau(i)$. In early air pollution measurement literature, severity tonnage was considered a measure of how severe pollution due to a source was. Data from Walther (1972) suggest the following. It is an interesting exercise to decide which of these conclusions are meaningful in either the technical sense or the practical sense: (i) HC emissions are more severe (have greater severity tonnage) than NOX emissions; (ii) effects of HC emissions from transportation are more severe than those of HC emissions from industry (and the same for NOX); (iii) effects of HC emissions from transportation are more severe than those of CO emissions from industry; (iv) effects of HC emissions from transportation are more than 20 times as severe as effects of CO emissions from transportation; (v) the total effect of HC emissions due to all sources is more than 8 times as severe as the total effect of NOX emissions due to all sources.

## 4.6 Evaluation of alternative HIV treatments

How do we evaluate alternative possible treatment plans or interventions for a given disease? One common procedure is the following. A number of treatments are compared on different criteria or benchmarks. Their scores on each criterion are normalized relative to the score of one of the treatments. The normalized scores of a treatment are combined by some averaging procedure and average scores are compared. If the averaging is the arithmetic mean, then the statement, "One treatment has a higher arithmetic mean normalized score than another treatment," is meaningless: The treatment to which scores are normalized can determine which has the higher arithmetic mean. Similar methods are used in comparing performances of alternative computer systems or other types of machinery.

To illustrate, consider a number of treatments/interventions in the case of HIV: universal screening, free condom distribution, abstinence education, male circumcision, and the like. Consider a number of criteria/outcomes: CD4 count (a measure of how well the body is fighting off HIV), days without poor appetite, days without profound fatigue, number of days hospitalized, and so on.

Table 4.1 shows three treatments I, II, III, and five criteria A, B, C, D, E, with the $i, j$ entry giving the score of the $i$th treatment on the $j$th criterion. Table 4.2 shows the score of each treatment normalized relative to treatment I, that is, by dividing by treatment I's score. Thus, for example, the 1,2 entry is 83/83 = 1, and the 2,2 entry is 70/83 = .84. The arithmetic means of the normalized scores in each row are also shown in Table 4.2. We conclude that treatment III is best.

However, let us now normalize relative to treatment II, obtaining the normalized scores of Table 4.3. Based on the arithmetic mean normalized scores of each row shown in Table 4.3, we now conclude that treatment I is best. So, the conclusion

*Table 4.1* Score of treatment $i$ on criterion $j$

| *Treatment/criterion* | *A* | *B* | *C* | *D* | *E* |
|---|---|---|---|---|---|
| I | 417 | 83 | 66 | 39,449 | 772 |
| II | 244 | 70 | 153 | 33,527 | 368 |
| III | 134 | 70 | 135 | 66,000 | 369 |

*Table 4.2* Normalizing relative to treatment I

| *Treatment/criterion* | *A* | *B* | *C* | *D* | *E* | *Arithmetic mean* | *Geometric mean* |
|---|---|---|---|---|---|---|---|
| I | 1.00 | 1.00 | 1.00 | 1.00 | 1.00 | 1.00 | 1.00 |
| II | 0.59 | 0.84 | 2.32 | 0.85 | 0.48 | 1.01 | 0.86 |
| III | 0.32 | 0.85 | 2.05 | 1.67 | 0.45 | 1.07 | 0.84 |

*Table 4.3* Normalizing relative to treatment II

| *Treatment/criterion* | *A* | *B* | *C* | *D* | *E* | *Arithmetic mean* | *Geometric mean* |
|---|---|---|---|---|---|---|---|
| I | 1.71 | 1.19 | 0.43 | 1.18 | 2.10 | 1.32 | 1.17 |
| II | 1.00 | 1.00 | 1.00 | 1.00 | 1.00 | 1.00 | 1.00 |
| III | 0.55 | 1.00 | 1.88 | 1.97 | 1.08 | 1.07 | 0.99 |

that a given treatment is best by taking the arithmetic mean of normalized scores is meaningless in this case.

The numbers in this example are taken from Fleming and Wallace (1986), with data from Heath (1984), and represent actual scores of alternative "treatments" in a computing machine application.

Sometimes, geometric mean is helpful. The geometric mean normalized scores of each row are shown in Tables 4.2 and 4.3. Note that in each case, we conclude that treatment I is best. In this situation, it is easy to show that the conclusion that a given treatment has the highest geometric mean normalized score is a meaningful conclusion. It is even meaningful to assert something such as: a given treatment has a geometric mean normalized score 20% higher than another treatment.

Fleming and Wallace give general conditions under which comparing geometric means of normalized scores is meaningful. It is a research area in measurement theory, with a long history and large literature, to determine what averaging procedures make sense in what situations. We return to this topic, and in particular the Fleming–Wallace conditions, in Section 4.9.

## 4.7 Meaningfulness of conclusions from statistical tests

Biostatistics is a key component of epidemiological research. However, biostatisticians know very little about measurement theory. Most have never heard about the theory of meaningfulness or limitations that meaningfulness places on conclusions from statistical tests. For over 50 years, there has been considerable disagreement on the limitations that scales of measurement impose on statistical procedures we may apply. The controversy stems from foundational work of Stevens (1946, 1951, 1959, and elsewhere), who developed the classification of scales of measurement we have described here. Stevens provided rules for the use of statistical procedures, concluding that certain statistics are inappropriate at certain levels of measurement. The application of Stevens' ideas to descriptive statistics has been widely accepted. However, their application to inferential statistics has been labeled by some a misconception.

To explore these ideas, suppose $P$ is a population whose distribution we would like to describe. We capture properties of $P$ by finding a descriptive statistic for $P$ or taking a sample $S$ from $P$ and finding a descriptive statistic for $S$. Our examples suggest that certain descriptive statistics are appropriate only for certain measurement situations. This idea, originally due to Stevens, was popularized by Siegel (1956) in his well-known book *Nonparametric Statistics for the Behavioral Sciences.* Our examples suggest the principle that arithmetic means are "appropriate" statistics for interval scales, and medians for ordinal scales. On the other side of the coin, it is argued that it is always appropriate to calculate means, medians, and other descriptive statistics, no matter what the scale of measurement. The well-known statistician Frederic Lord made this argument with a famous example of a group of first-year college football players who were upset that the average (arithmetic mean) number on their uniforms was less than that of the more advanced players. He argued that it is meaningful for the first-year players to average uniform numbers because "the numbers don't remember where they came from." Marcus-Roberts and Roberts (1987) agree. It is always appropriate to calculate means, medians, ... But, they ask: is it appropriate to make certain statements using these descriptive statistics?

The rest of this section summarizes the conclusions of Marcus-Roberts and Roberts. They argue that it is usually appropriate to make a statement using descriptive statistics if and only if the statement is meaningful. A statement that is true but meaningless gives information that is an accident of the scale of measurement used, not information that describes the population in some fundamental way. So, it is appropriate to calculate the arithmetic mean of ordinal data. It is just not appropriate to say that the mean of one group is higher than the mean of another group.

Stevens' ideas have come to be applied to inferential statistics, inferences about an unknown population *P*. They have led to such principles as the following:

- Classical parametric tests (e.g., *t*-test, Pearson correlation, analysis of variance) are inappropriate for ordinal data. They should be applied only to data that define an interval or ratio scale.
- For ordinal scales, nonparametric tests (e.g., Mann–Whitney U, Kruskal–Wallis, Kendall's tau) can be used.

Not everyone agrees. Thus, there has been controversy.

Marcus-Roberts and Roberts argue that the validity of a statistical test depends on a statistical model. This includes information about the distribution of the population and about the sampling procedure. The validity of the test does not depend on a measurement model. That is concerned with the admissible transformations and scale type. The scale type enters in deciding whether the hypothesis is worth testing at all, whether it is a meaningful hypothesis. The issue is: if we perform admissible transformations of scale, is the truth or falsity of the hypothesis unchanged?

As an example, suppose we have data on an ordinal scale and we consider the hypothesis that the mean is 0. This is a meaningless hypothesis. Can we test meaningless hypotheses? Marcus-Roberts and Roberts say, "Yes." But they question what information we get outside of information about the population as measured. To be more precise about this, consider how we test hypothesis $H_0$ about *P*. We do this through the following steps:

- Draw a random sample *S* from *P*.
- Calculate a test statistic based on *S*.
- Calculate the probability that the test statistic is what was observed given $H_0$ is true.
- Accept or reject $H_0$ on the basis of the test.

Calculation of probability depends on a statistical model, which includes information about the distribution of *P* and about the sampling procedure. But, validity of the test depends only on the statistical model, not on the measurement model. Thus, you can apply parametric tests to ordinal data, provided the statistical model is satisfied. The model is satisfied if the data are normally distributed. Where does the scale type enter? It enters in determining if the hypothesis is worth testing at all, that is, if it is meaningful.

For instance, consider data on an ordinal scale and let $H_0$ be the hypothesis that the mean is 0. The hypothesis is meaningless. But, if the data meet certain distributional requirements such as normality, we can apply a parametric test, such as the *t*-test, to check if the mean is 0.

Similar analyses can be developed for other kinds of statistical tests for data on other types of scales.

## 4.8 Optimization problems in epidemiology

The impact of climate change includes potential effects on the health of humans, animals, plants, and ecosystems. Some early warning signs of climate change include major heat events such as the 1995 extreme heat event in Chicago that led to 514 heat-related deaths and 3,300 excess emergency room admissions and the 2003 heat wave in Europe that led to 35,000 deaths. With anticipated change in climate could come an increase in the number and severity of extreme events, including more heat waves, floods, hurricanes, and the like. One response to extreme heat events is the evacuation of the most vulnerable individuals to climate-controlled environments. Here, there are modeling challenges, such as: where to locate the evacuation centers, whom to send where, finding ways to minimize travel times from home to evacuation center, and so on. Among the problems arising here is the shortest route problem: find the shortest route from home to evacuation center. This is an example of an optimization problem, more specifically a combinatorial optimization problem. We now consider the meaningfulness of conclusions about optimality in such problems.

Consider a network with vertices and edges and numbers on the edges representing some sort of strength or level or weight or length of the connection. The problem is to find the shortest path in the network from vertex $x$ to vertex $z$, where the strength of a path is the sum of the weights of edges in it. This problem occurs widely in practice. In the United States, just one agency of the U.S. Department of Transportation in the federal government applies algorithms to solve this problem literally billions of times a year (Goldman, 1981). Consider a simple network with vertices $x$, $y$, and $z$ and edges from $x$ to $y$ with strength 2, $y$ to $z$ with strength 4, and $x$ to $z$ with strength 15. What is the shortest path from $x$ to $z$ in this network? The shortest path is the path that goes from $x$ to $y$ to $z$, with a total "length" of 6. The alternative path that goes directly from $x$ to $z$ has total "length" 15. Is the conclusion that $x$ to $y$ to $z$ is the shortest path a meaningful conclusion?

The conclusion is meaningful if the strengths define a ratio scale, as they do if they are distances or times as in the evacuation problem. However, what if they define an interval scale? Consider the admissible transformation $\phi(x) = 3x + 100$. Now the weights change to 106 on the edge from $x$ to $y$, 112 on the edge from $y$ to $z$, and 145 on the edge from $x$ to $z$. We conclude that going directly from $x$ to $z$ is the shortest path. The original conclusion was meaningless.

The shortest path problem can be formulated as a linear programming problem. Thus, the conclusion that $A$ is the solution to a linear programming problem can be meaningless if cost parameters are measured on an interval scale. Note that linear programming is widely used in public health as well as in other areas of application. For example, it is used to determine optimal inventories of medicines, assignments of patients or doctors to clinics, optimization of a treatment facility, and amount to invest in preventive treatments, among other applications.

Another very important practical combinatorial optimization problem is the minimum spanning tree problem. Given a connected weighted graph or network, we ask for the spanning tree with total sum of strengths or weights as small as possible. (A *spanning tree* is a tree that includes all the vertices of the network.) This problem has applications in the planning of large-scale transportation, communication, and distribution networks. For example, given a network, we seek to find usable roads that allow one to go from any vertex to any other vertex, minimizing the lengths of the roads used. This problem arises in the case of extreme events that leave some roads flooded and when we require routes that emergency vehicles can take. Again, it is natural to ask if the conclusion that a given set of edges defines a minimum spanning tree is meaningful. It is surprising to observe that even if the weights on the edges define only an ordinal scale, then the conclusion is meaningful. This is not a priori obvious. However, it follows from the fact that the well-known algorithm known as Kruskal's algorithm or the greedy algorithm gives a solution. In Kruskal's algorithm (Kruskal, 1956; Papadimitriou and Steiglitz, 1982), we order edges in increasing order of weight and then examine edges in this order, including an edge if it does not form a cycle with edges previously included. We stop when all vertices are included. Any admissible transformation will not change the order in which edges are examined in this algorithm; therefore, the same solution will be produced.

Many practical decision-making problems in public health and other fields involve the search for an optimal solution as in the shortest path and minimum spanning tree problems. Little attention is paid to the possibility that the conclusion that a particular solution is optimal may be an accident of the way that things are measured. For the beginnings of the theory of meaningfulness of conclusions in combinatorial optimization, see Mahadev, Pekeč, and Roberts (1998), Pekeč (1996a, 1996b), and Roberts (1990, 1994, 1999).

## 4.9 How should we average scores?

We have seen that in some situations comparing arithmetic means is not a good idea and comparing geometric means is. There are situations where the reverse is true. Can we lay down some guidelines as to when to use what averaging procedure? A brief discussion follows.

Let $a_1, a_2, \ldots, a_n$ be $n$ "scores" or ratings, for example, scores on criteria for evaluating treatments. Let $u = F(a_1, a_2, \ldots, a_n)$. $F$ is an unknown averaging function, sometimes called a *merging function*, and $u$ is the average or merged score.

Fleming and Wallace (1986) take an axiomatic approach to determining appropriate merging functions. They take the case where the domain and range of $F$ are the positive real numbers and consider the following axioms:

- *Reflexivity:* $F(a, a, \ldots, a) = a$.
- *Symmetry:* $F(a_1, a_2, \ldots, a_n) = F(a_{\pi(1)}, a_{\pi(2)}, \ldots, a_{\pi(n)})$ for all permutations $\pi$ of $\{1, 2, \ldots, n\}$.
- *Multiplicativity:* $F(a_1b_1, a_2b_2, \ldots, a_nb_n) = F(a_1, a_2, \ldots, a_n)F(b_1, b_2, \ldots, b_n)$.

They show that if $F$ satisfies these three axioms, then $F$ is the geometric mean, and conversely. It is fairly simple to understand the first two axioms. Reflexivity says that if all ratings are the same, then their average is the same. Symmetry says that the average is independent of the names or order given to the criteria (which might not be true in some applications). The multiplicative property says that the average of the products of the ratings is the same as the product of the averages of the ratings. Fleming and Wallace motivate this axiom by saying that if $a_i$ measures the relative strength of treatment I to treatment II on criterion $i$, and $b_i$ the relative strength of treatment II to treatment III on criterion $i$, then $a_ib_i$ measures the relative strength of treatment I to treatment III on criterion $i$. If "strength" is speed, as in the Fleming–Wallace applications, then there is some justification for this conclusion and, moreover, to the conclusion that the average over criteria of the relative strength of treatment I to treatment III is the product of the average of the relative strength over all criteria of treatment I to treatment II times the average of the relative strength over all criteria of treatment II to treatment III. However, more generally, it is harder to be sure that Multiplicativity is a desired property of an averaging procedure.

An alternative approach uses functional equations and is based on either assumptions about scale type of some of the scales or about meaningfulness of some statements using the scales. Consider an unknown function $u = F(a_1, a_2, \ldots, a_n)$. We use an idea due to Luce (1959) that he once called the *principle of theory construction*: If you know the scale types of the $a_i$ and the scale type of $u$ and you assume that an admissible transformation of each of the $a_i$ leads to an admissible transformation of $u$, you can derive the form of $F$. (We disregard some of the restrictions on applicability of this principle, including those given by Luce [1962, 1964, 1990].)

To illustrate the ideas, let us take a simple case where $n = 1$, $a = a_1$ is a ratio scale, and $u$ is a ratio scale. An admissible transformation of scale in both cases is multiplication by a positive constant. By the principle of theory construction, multiplying the independent variable $a$ by a positive constant $\alpha$ leads to multiplying the dependent variable by a positive constant $A$ that depends on $\alpha$. This leads to the functional equation

$$F(\alpha a) = A(\alpha)F(a),\ A(\alpha) > 0. \tag{4.11}$$

By solving this equation, Luce (1959) proves that if the averaging function $F$ is continuous, $a$ takes on all positive real values, and $F$ takes on positive real values, then

$$F(a) = ca^k.$$

Thus, if the independent and dependent variables are ratio scales, the only possible way to relate them is by a power law.

This result is very general. In early writings of Luce, it was interpreted as very strictly limiting the "possible scientific laws" in all disciplines. For example, other examples of power laws are given as follows. One is

$$V = (4/3)\pi r^3,$$

where $V$ is volume and $r$ is radius (both ratio scales). A second is Newton's law of gravitation:

$$F = G(mm^*/r^2),$$

where $F$ is the force of attraction, $G$ is a gravitational constant, $m$, $m^*$ are fixed masses of bodies being attracted, and $r$ is the distance between them (everything being a ratio scale). A third is Ohm's law: under fixed resistance, voltage is proportional to current (voltage and current being ratio scales).

To illustrate the ideas when the number of independent variables (ratings being averaged) is larger than 1, suppose that $a_1, a_2, \ldots, a_n$ are independent ratio scales and $u$ is a ratio scale. Let $F$ be a merging function defined on all $n$-tuples of positive real numbers and outputting a positive real. By the principle of theory construction,

$$F(a_1,a_2,\ldots,a_n) = u \leftrightarrow F(\alpha_1 a_1,\alpha_2 a_2,\ldots,\alpha_n a_n) = \alpha u,$$

where $\alpha_1 > 0$, $\alpha_2 > 0$, …, $\alpha_n > 0$, $\alpha > 0$, and $\alpha$ depends on $\alpha_1, \alpha_2, \ldots, \alpha_n$. Thus we get the functional equation:

$$F(\alpha_1 a_1,\alpha_2 a_2,\ldots,\alpha_n a_n) = A(\alpha_1,\alpha_2,\ldots,\alpha_n)F(a_1,a_2,\ldots,a_n), A(\alpha_1,\alpha_2,\ldots,\alpha_n) > 0. \quad (4.12)$$

Luce (1964) shows that if $F$ is continuous and satisfies Equation (4.12), then

$$F(a_1,a_2,\ldots,a_n) = \lambda a_1^{c_1} a_2^{c_2} \ldots a_n^{c_n} \quad (4.13)$$

for constants $\lambda > 0$, $c_1, c_2, \ldots, c_n$. Aczél and Roberts (1989) show that if, in addition, $F$ satisfies reflexivity and symmetry, then $\lambda = 1$ and $c_1 = c_2 = \cdots = c_n = 1/n$, so $F$ is the geometric mean.

There are also situations where one can show that the merging function $F$ is the arithmetic mean. Consider, for example, the case where $a_1, a_2, \ldots, a_n$ are interval scales with the same unit and independent zero points and $u$ is an interval scale. Then the principle of theory construction gives the functional equation:

$$F(\alpha a_1+\beta_1,\alpha a_2+\beta_2,\ldots,\alpha a_n+\beta_n) =$$
$$A(\alpha,\beta_1,\beta_2,\ldots,\beta_n)F(a_1,a_2,\ldots,a_n)+B(\alpha,\beta_1,\beta_2,\ldots,\beta_n),$$

where

$$A(\alpha,\beta_1,\beta_2,\ldots,\beta_n)>0.$$

Even without a continuity assumption, Aczél, Roberts, and Rosenbaum (1986) show that in this case,

$$F(a_1,a_2,\ldots,a_n)=\sum_{i=1}^{n}\lambda_i a_i+b,$$

where $\lambda_1$, $\lambda_2$, …, $\lambda_n$, $b$ are arbitrary constants. Aczél and Roberts (1989) show that if, in addition, $F$ satisfies reflexivity, then

$$\sum_{i=1}^{n}\lambda_i=1, b=0.$$

If in addition $F$ satisfies reflexivity and symmetry, then they show that $\lambda_i = 1/n$ for all $i$, and $b = 0$; that is, $F$ is the arithmetic mean.

Still another approach to determining the form of an appropriate merging function is to replace scale type assumptions with assumptions that certain statements using scales are meaningful. Although it is often reasonable to assume that you know the scale type of the independent variables $a_1$, $a_2$, …, $a_n$, it is often not so reasonable to assume that you know the scale type of the dependent variable $u$. However, it turns out that one can replace the assumption about the scale type of $u$ with an assumption that a certain statement involving $u$ is meaningful. To return to the case where the $a_i$ are independent ratio scales, instead of assuming that $u$ is a ratio scale, let us assume that the statement

$$F(a_1,a_2,\ldots,a_n)=kF(b_1,b_2\ldots,b_n)$$

is meaningful for all $a_1$, $a_2$, …, $a_n$, $b_1$, $b_2$, …, $b_n$ and $k>0$. Then we get the same result as before: Roberts and Rosenbaum (1986) prove that under these hypotheses and continuity, $F$ satisfies Equation (4.13). Moreover, if in addition $F$ satisfies reflexivity and symmetry, then $F$ is the geometric mean. For a variety of related results, see Roberts and Rosenbaum (1986).

## 4.10 Behavioral responses to health events

Governments are making detailed plans for how to respond to future health threats such as pandemic influenza, H1N1 virus, a bioterrorist attack with the smallpox virus, and so on. A major unknown in planning for future disease outbreaks is how people will respond. Will they follow instructions to stay home? Will critical personnel report to work or take care of their families? Will instructions for immunization be followed? Mathematical models are increasingly used to help plan for health events or to develop responses to them. They have been especially important in planning responses to such recent events as foot and mouth disease in Britain and SARS. Models in epidemiology typically omit behavioral responses. These are hard to quantify and hard to measure. This leads to challenges for behavioral scientists and for epidemiological modelers who want to work with them.

In building behavioral responses into epidemiological models, we can learn some things from the study of responses to various disasters such as earthquakes, hurricanes, and fires. Many behavioral responses need to be addressed. "Compliance" with things such as quarantine instructions is one example. How do we measure "compliance?" In particular, this includes such factors as "resistance" to instructions, willingness to seek or receive treatment, credibility of government, and trust of decision makers. Other things that need to be made precise and measured include movement, rumor, perception of risk, person-to-person interaction, motivation, social stigmata (such as discrimination against certain social groups), panic, and peer pressure. There is a challenge to measurement theory here: how do we measure some of these factors? How do we bring them into mathematical models? What statements using the new scales of measurement are meaningful? Some of the issues are discussed in McKenzie and Roberts (2003), which summarizes a workshop aimed at modeling social responses to bioterrorism involving infectious agents.

There is much more analysis of a similar nature in the field of epidemiology that can be done with the principles of measurement theory. The issues involved present challenges both for theory and for application.

## Acknowledgments

The author gratefully acknowledges the support of the National Science Foundation under grant number EIA-02-05116 to Rutgers University. A number of ideas and some of the examples and language in this paper are borrowed from Roberts (1994), which explores meaningful and meaningless statements in operations research.

## References

Aczél, J., & Roberts, F. S. (1989). On the possible merging functions. *Mathematical Social Sciences, 17*, 205–243.

Aczél, J., Roberts, F. S., & Rosenbaum, Z. (1986). On scientific laws without dimensional constants. *Journal of Mathematical Analysis & Applications, 119*, 389–416.

Bay Area Pollution Control District (1968). Combined pollutant indexes for the San Francisco Bay Area. Information Bulletin 10-68, San Francisco.

Fleming, P. J., & Wallace, J. J. (1986). How not to lie with statistics: The correct way to summarize benchmark results. *Communications of the ACM, 29*, 218–221.

Goldman, A. J. (1981). Discrete mathematics in government. Lecture presented at *SIAM Symposium on Applications of Discrete Mathematics*, Troy, NY, June.

Heath, J. L. (1984). Re-evaluation of RISC I. *Computer Architecture News, 12*, 3–10.

Helmholtz, H. V. (1887). Zählen und messen. *Philosophische Aufsätze* (pp. 17–52). Leipzig: Fues's Verlag (C. L. Bryan, transl, *Counting and measuring*. Princeton, NJ: Van Nostrand, 1930.)

Knapp, T. R. (1990). Treating ordinal scales as interval scales: An attempt to resolve the controversy. *Nursing Research, 39*, 121–123.

Krantz, D. H., Luce, R. D., Suppes, P., & Tversky, A. (1971). *Foundations of measurement* (Vol. I). New York: Academic Press.

Kruskal, J. B. (1956). On the shortest spanning tree of a graph and the traveling salesman problem. *Proceedings of the American Mathematical Society, 7*, 48–50.

Luce, R. D. (1959). On the possible psychophysical laws. *Psychological Review, 66*, 81–95.

Luce, R. D. (1962). Comments on Rozeboom's criticisms of "On the possible psychophysical laws." *Psychological Review, 69*, 548–555.

Luce, R. D. (1964). A generalization of a theorem of dimensional analysis, *Journal of Mathematical Psychology, 1*, 278–284.

Luce, R. D. (1990). "On the psychophysical law" revisited: Remarks on cross-modal matching. *Psychological Review, 97*, 66–77.

Luce, R. D., Krantz, D. H., Suppes, P., & Tversky, A. (1990). *Foundations of measurement* (Vol. III). New York: Academic Press.

Mahadev, N. V. R., Pekeč, A., & Roberts, F. S. (1998). On the meaningfulness of optimal solutions to scheduling problems: Can an optimal solution be non-optimal? *Operations Research, 46 suppl*, S120–S134.

Marcus-Roberts, H. M., & Roberts, F. S. (1987). Meaningless statistics. *Journal of Educational and Behavioral Statistics, 12*, 383–394.

McKenzie, E., & Roberts, F. S. (2003). Modeling social responses to bioterrorism involving infectious agents. Technical Report, DIMACS Center, Rutgers University, Piscataway, NJ, July 24. (Available at http://dimacs.rutgers.edu/Workshops/Modeling/.)

Papadimitriou, C. H., & Steiglitz, K. (1982). *Combinatorial optimization: Algorithms and complexity*, Englewood Cliffs, NJ: Prentice-Hall.

Pekeč, A. (1996a). *Limitations on conclusions from combinatorial optimization*, Ph.D. Thesis, Department of Mathematics, Rutgers University.

Pekeč, A. (1996b). Scalings in linear programming: Necessary and sufficient conditions for invariance. Center for Basic Research in Computer Science (BRICS), technical report RS-96-50.

Pfanzagl, J. (1968). *Theory of measurement*. New York: Wiley.

Roberts, F. S. (1972). Building an energy demand signed digraph I: Choosing the nodes. Rept. 927/1—*NSF*. April. Santa Monica, CA: The RAND Corporation.

Roberts, F. S. (1973). Building and analyzing an energy demand signed digraph. *Environment & Planning, 5*, 199–221.

Roberts, F. S. (1979). *Measurement theory, with applications to decisionmaking, utility, and the social sciences*. Reading, MA: Addison-Wesley. Digital Reprinting (2009). Cambridge, UK: Cambridge University Press.

Roberts, F. S. (1990). Meaningfulness of conclusions from combinatorial optimization. *Discrete Applied Mathematics, 29*, 221–241.

Roberts, F. S. (1994). Limitations on conclusions using scales of measurement. In S. M. Pollock, M. H. Rothkopf, & A. Barnett (Eds.), *Operations research and the public sector, Vol. 6 of Handbooks in operations research and management science* (pp. 621–671). Amsterdam: North-Holland.

Roberts, F. S. (1999). Meaningless statements. In *Contemporary trends in discrete mathematics*, DIMACS Series (Vol. 49, pp. 257–274). Providence, RI: American Mathematical Society.

Roberts, F. S., & Rosenbaum, Z. (1986). Scale type, meaningfulness, and the possible psychophysical laws. *Mathematical Social Sciences, 12*, 77–95.

Sauter, G. D., & Chilton, E. G. (Eds.). (1970). *Air improvement recommendations for the San Francisco Bay Area. The Stanford-Ames NASA/ASEE Summer Faculty Systems Design Workshop, Final Report*. October. Stanford CA: Stanford University School of Engineering. Published under NASA Contract NGR-05-020-409.

Siegel, S. (1956) *Nonparametric statistics for the behavioral sciences*, New York: McGraw-Hill.

Stevens, S. S. (1946). On the theory of scales of measurement. *Science, 103*, 677–680.

Stevens, S. S. (1951). Mathematics, measurement, and psychophysics. In S. S. Stevens (Ed.), *Handbook of experimental psychology* (pp. 1–49). New York: Wiley.

Stevens, S. S. (1959). Measurement, psychophysics, and utility. In C. W. Churchman & P. Ratoosh (Eds.), *Measurement: Definitions and theories* (pp. 18–63). New York: Wiley.

Stevens, S. S. (1968). Ratio scales of opinion. In D. K. Whitla (Ed.), *Handbook of measurement and assessment in behavioral sciences*. Reading, MA: Addison-Wesley.

Suppes, P. (1959). Measurement, empirical meaningfulness and three-valued logic. In C. W. Churchman & P. Ratoosh (Eds.), *Measurement: Definitions and theories* (pp. 129–143). New York: Wiley.

Suppes, P. (1979). Replies. In R. J. Bogdan (Ed.), *Patrick Suppes* (pp. 207–232). Dordrecht, Holland: Reidel.

Suppes, P., Krantz, D. H., Luce, R. D., & Tversky, A. (1989). *Foundations of measurement (Vol. II)*. New York: Academic Press.

Suppes, P., & Zinnes, J. (1963). Basic measurement theory. In R. D. Luce, R. R. Bush, & E. Galanter (Eds.), *Handbook of mathematical psychology* (Vol. 1, pp. 1–76). New York: Wiley.

Thomas, H. (1985). Measurement structures and statistics. In S. Kotz & N. L. Johnson (Eds.), *Encyclopedia of statistical sciences* (Vol. 5, pp. 381–386). New York: Wiley.

Walther, E. G. (1972). A rating of the major air pollutants and their sources by effect. *Journal of the Air Pollution Control Association, 22*, 352–355.

# 5 Toward a probabilistic theory of measurement

*Giovanni Battista Rossi*
DIMEC
Università degli Studi di Genova
Genova, Italy

## 5.1 Basic questions

Measurement plays a fundamental role in both physical and behavioral sciences, as a link between abstract models and empirical reality. So a challenge arises, concerning the possibility of developing a unique theory of measurement for the different domains of science in which it is involved. What would we expect from one such theory?

Perhaps three main questions should be addressed, namely,

- What is the meaning of measurement?
- How do we measure?
- What can be measured?

We present here a basic kernel for such a theory, organized in two main parts, the measurement scale and the measurement process, dealing, respectively, with the first two questions. An answer to the third question, concerning measurability, comes from a combination of the two main parts of the theory, rather than as a separate issue. We present each part in deterministic terms first, then, inasmuch as uncertainty is an inherent feature of measurement, we reformulate the theory in probabilistic terms.

Before starting, let us fix some language. We first need a term for denoting *what we (want to) measure*. We may call that a property, characteristic, attribute, or feature of something: we choose *characteristic*. Then we have to name *what carries* (expresses, manifests) *the characteristic under investigation*: depending upon the discipline involved, it may be an object, an event, or even a person. Here the differences are substantial, yet we still use a unique term, *object*, but make clear that this is just a conventional term for denoting what carries the property. Then we have to distinguish between *measurable* and *nonmeasurable* properties: for the former we use, again conventionally, the term *quantity*. Furthermore, objects manifest the characteristic of interest in different ways (levels, degrees) and we call *state* the way in which an object manifests a property.

We are now ready to introduce the concept of *measurement* in itself. We refer to Finkelstein's definition (1982): "Measurement is the process of empirical objective assignment of numbers to properties (characteristics) of objects or events of the real world in such a way as to describe them." Other key terms, such as measurement scale, measuring system, and measurement process, are discussed here, and at the end of the chapter a short glossary is included for ease of reference (BIPM, 2008b; Rossi, 2009b).

## 5.2 The measurement scale

### *5.2.1 The meaning of measurement and the notion of measurement scale*

In order to put measurement on a firm foundation, we need to start from a more elementary concept, the notion of *empirical relation*. Let us demonstrate this through a simple example: the measurement of hardness of minerals according to the method proposed by Mohs in 1812 (Finkelstein, 1982). The key idea of his method was that the hardness of a mineral may be characterized by its ability to scratch other minerals. This is the empirical relation in this case and (we may assume that) it is a *weak order*.[1] He then identified a series of 10 reference materials, collectively suited to express the different degrees of hardness we may encounter in nature. They were, in increasing hardness order, talc, gypsum, calcite, fluorite, apatite, orthoclase, quartz, topaz, corundum, and diamond. Then he assigned the numbers from 1 to 10 to them, thereby fully defining a *reference scale*. We call a *standard* each element in the scale and *measure* the corresponding number. Using this as a basis, it is possible to determine the hardness of any piece of mineral $a$ by comparing it to the scale in order to identify the standard $s$ to which it is *equivalent*, in the sense that it neither scratches nor is scratched by it.

This simple example is good for showing the *meaning* of measurement: the number (measure) so assigned will really represent hardness, in that we expect $a$ to have the same hardness of any other object that obtains the same measure, to be harder than any object obtaining a lesser measure, and vice versa. In other words, if two objects, $a$ and $b$, have hardness $m(a)$ and $m(b)$, respectively, the order that holds between the measures corresponds to the order that holds between the objects; that is,

$$a \succsim b \Leftrightarrow m(a) \geq m(b). \tag{5.1}$$

An expression like (5.1), linking empirical relations to numerical relations, is called a *representation theorem*. We may note that the measure of an object reveals how it compares with all the other objects that carry the same characteristic: in our example, how a mineral compares with all other minerals, in respect of hardness. The alternative for obtaining the same information would be to actually compare the object to be measured with all the others in the class. This shows how valuable the information conveyed by measurement is. How is it possible to obtain such a remarkable saving in effort? This is thanks to the construction of the reference scale (the

10 standards object, in the Mohs case), which "materialises our knowledge of the quantity under examination" (Mari, 2000). Actually in constructing the scale we have made good use of our knowledge, consisting in knowing that hardness may be characterized by the ability to scratch another material and that the main ways in which it appears in nature are well represented by the ten-standards series.

So we may now answer the question about the meaning of measurement, by saying that measurements reproduce empirical relations in a numerical domain, thanks to the existence of a measurement scale. Note that a scale may be intended in two ways, as the set of conditions that enable measurement (general meaning) or a series of standard objects with assigned values (specific meaning). To avoid confusion, we use the term reference scale in the latter case.

In general, we may have different types of empirical relations, as we have already discussed in Chapters 1 and 4, corresponding to different empirical structures and related measurement scales. A summary of the most common and useful types of scales has been reported in Chapter 1, Table 1.2. As we have discussed in Chapter 1, scales may be characterized from two different standpoints, either according to empirical properties that they are able to reproduce, expressed by representation theorems, or on the basis of the admissible transformations that they may safely undergo. This second point of view is related to *meaningfulness*, which has been amply discussed in Chapter 4.

These ideas are basic in the representational theory of measurement. For probing this subject further, we recommend Roberts (1979/2009) as an introduction, then Krantz, Luce, Suppes, and Tversky (1971), Luce, Krantz, Suppes, and Tversky (1990), and Suppes, Krantz, Luce, and Tversky (1989) for a remarkable presentation of key results. A concise overview is provided in Finkelstein and Leaning (1984), and a recent survey is offered by Luce and Suppes (2002). We also recommend reading the original essay by Helmholtz (1971/1887), for understanding how these ideas originated.

Thus far we have presented measurement scales in a "deterministic" way, that is, by assuming that all the relations involved are either "true" or "false." This is good for clarifying the meaning of measurement, but may no longer be adequate if we look for a faithful description of what happens in reality. We now discuss when this approach is no longer satisfactory.

### 5.2.2 *On the need for a probabilistic approach*

Consider again an empirical weak-order relation, as the relation "heavier than," which occurs in mass measurement. We call a *comparator* any device that performs a comparison of objects, in respect of some characteristic of theirs. Consider now a class of objects, for example, books, and a mass comparator, for example, an equal-arm balance. There are cases in which the result of the comparison may be expressed by a deterministic statement, such as $a \succ b$, where "$\succ$" means "(empirically) greater than," which implies that whenever we compare $a$ with $b$, we observe that $a$ is heavier than $b$. For example, if $a$ and $b$ are two different books in the same series, they will have undergone the same publishing standards, that is, the same kind of paper, same cover, and so on, but they may have a different number of pages, for example, 500 versus 400. Then $a$ (the book with 500 pages) will be definitely heavier than $b$ and we may correctly represent the real situation by the deterministic relation $a \succ b$.

But suppose now that $a$ and $b$ are two distinct copies of the same book in the same series; that is, they have the same kind of paper, same cover, same number of pages. Then they should be nominally equivalent and we should observe $a \sim b$, where "~" means "empirically equivalent to." Yet we cannot be sure of this, inasmuch as there may be small differences, due to the production process (inhomogeneity of the paper, small differences occurring in the binding process, etc.) or to the usage (aging, wearing, dust, etc.). If we use a comparator sensitive enough for detecting such differences and if they are of the same order of magnitude of the "noise" of the comparator (due, e.g., to internal friction, vibration, etc.), if we repeat the comparison more times we may sometimes observe $a \succ b$, some others $a \sim b$ and some others even $a \prec b$. So we can no longer describe this situation by a single, well-determined relation, rather we have to consider the *probability* of each of the possible relations; that is, $\mathbb{P}(a \succ b)$, $\mathbb{P}(a \sim b)$, and $\mathbb{P}(a \prec b)$, where the symbol "$\mathbb{P}$" denotes the probability of a relation. The following constraint holds true:

$$\mathbb{P}(a \succ b) + \mathbb{P}(a \sim b) + \mathbb{P}(a \prec b) = 1. \tag{5.2}$$

This is why the necessity of a probabilistic representation emerges: when we compare similar objects, the result of the comparison may become uncertain. If this holds true for the measurement of physical quantities, it is even more apparent in the case of perception. If we ask a single person or a jury to compare, say, the loudness of sounds or the brightness of objects, we may observe some intra- and inter-individual variability. On the other hand, the case of a well-determined order, such as the one occurring between the two different books, may be included, by assigning $\mathbb{P}(a \succ b) = 1$. The probabilistic approach may thus be considered as a generalization of the deterministic one. In this chapter we use only simple probability rules. Good introductions to this discipline have been provided in Italian by Monti and Pierobon (2000) and in English by Papoulis (1984).

### 5.2.3 More on the interpretation of the probabilistic approach

Before proceeding, let us consider some additional points concerning the use of probability. In general, if we have two objects $a$ and $b$, and a comparator $C$, and we observe some variability in the results of the comparison, how can we interpret this variability? Should we ascribe this variability to the objects, holding that the characteristic they manifest actually varies at random from one comparison to another, or should we instead ascribe it to the comparator, assuming that it is affected by random noise?

We suggest that, in general, there is no definite answer to this question: if the only evidence we have is the result of the comparison, we cannot separate the contribution of the objects from that of the comparator, or more generally, the contribution of the observer from the contribution of the observed system. This is a kind of uncertainty principle that, it is noteworthy, already emerges from this very simple model.

Second point: someone could argue that the use of a less-sensitive comparator would lead to a determined result of the comparison. Unfortunately this is only an apparent solution. In fact, suppose that the comparator has a limited resolution: it is unable to detect differences in the objects that are less than a threshold, say $\delta$. Now suppose that objects $a$ and $b$ differ by less than the threshold; then the result will be $a \sim_\delta b$, where the symbol "$\sim_\delta$" denotes the indifference condition expressed by the comparator. Suppose now that $b$ and $c$ also differ by less than the threshold; then we obtain $b \sim_\delta c$. Yet there is no guarantee that $a$ and $c$ are also within the threshold, so the relation "$\sim_\delta$" is not transitive; that is, it is no longer an equivalence relation. So the apparent benefit of having a better *repeatability* (i.e., a propensity to obtain the same result or the same set of results when repeating the same experiment in the same conditions) is balanced by a severe drawback, the loss of the equivalence relation. Remedy would be worse than malady!

Another possible question is whether the limited repeatability of comparisons is the only reason for looking for a probabilistic representation. We suggest that, although this could be a good reason in itself, it is not the only one.

Suppose we have two (and only two) comparators, $C$ and $D$, and that we have the same confidence in both of them. Suppose that we compare $a$ and b with comparator $C$ and that we always obtain, for example, $a \succ_C b$; instead let $a \sim_D b$ be the result, also confirmed through repetitions, of the comparison through $D$. So we have a *systematic* disagreement between the two comparators, and no way for deciding between them. What can we do? Again we can treat this case in probabilistic terms, considering the results of the comparisons as *conditioned* by C and $D$, respectively, and by applying the rules of probability accordingly.

In probabilistic terms, the above result may be expressed as follows:

$$\mathbb{P}(a \succ b \mid C) = 1,\ \mathbb{P}(a \sim b \mid C) = 0,\ \mathbb{P}(a \prec b \mid C) = 0,$$

$$\mathbb{P}(a \succ b \mid D) = 0,\ \mathbb{P}(a \sim b \mid D) = 1,\ \mathbb{P}(a \prec b \mid D) = 0,$$

$$\mathbb{P}(C) = 0.5,\ \mathbb{P}(D) = 0.5,$$

and we obtain

$$\begin{aligned}
\mathbb{P}(a \succ b) &= \mathbb{P}(a \succ b \mid C)\mathbb{P}(C) + \mathbb{P}(a \succ b \mid D)\mathbb{P}(D) = 0.5,\\
\mathbb{P}(a \sim b) &= \mathbb{P}(a \sim b \mid C)\mathbb{P}(C) + \mathbb{P}(a \sim b \mid D)\mathbb{P}(D) = 0.5,\\
\mathbb{P}(a \prec b) &= \mathbb{P}(a \prec b \mid C)\mathbb{P}(C) + \mathbb{P}(a \prec b \mid D)\mathbb{P}(D) = 0.0.
\end{aligned} \tag{5.3}$$

Last, let us discuss the interpretation of the above.

We may think that either $a \succ b$ or $a \sim b$ is true and one of the two comparators is wrong, but we do not know which one, and so the only logically consistent way of expressing what we know is what we have done. Yet we can also consider, as an alternative explanation, the possibility that the objects interact with the comparators in such a way that their state changes in the two comparisons, but we are unable to define their state outside these comparisons, if these comparisons are the only evidence that we have. This is another kind of the uncertainty, or rather of the *indeterminacy*, condition. In general we may see that we are using probability as a logic, for expressing different uncertainty situations.

### 5.2.4 Probabilistic relations

We should now be motivated enough to search for a probabilistic representation. This approach is based on the notion of a *probabilistic relation*, which is not common in the theory of probability, and, as far as we know, only recently has been investigated, so we discuss it in some detail.

Consider a deterministic relation first, for example, a weak order, $\succcurlyeq$. Such a relation may be understood in two ways:

- In a specific meaning: when we write $a \succcurlyeq b$, we intend that the relation $\succcurlyeq$ holds for the pair $(a,b) \in A$.
- In a general meaning: when we consider the relation $\succcurlyeq$ on A, we refer to the set of all the pairs of elements of $A$ for which it holds.

Consider, for example, the set $A = \{a,b,c\}$ and the numerical example displayed in Table 5.1. The possible weak-order relations that may hold on $A$, that is, the possible weak orderings of its elements, are listed in column 2 of the table. In the deterministic case, one and only one of such orderings holds true. In the probabilistic case, instead, more orderings are possible and a probability is assigned to each of them, with the obvious constraint that the sum of all such probabilities must be equal to one. This is what we call a *probabilistic weak order* because weak-order relations only have nonnull probabilities. Example probability values are provided in the last column of the table. In order to understand how these probabilities may be assigned, suppose that $a$, $b$, and $c$ are sounds and we ask a group of, say, 100 persons to compare them with respect to their loudness (or sharpness, pleasantness, etc.). Then, each line in the table represents one possible response from one person. If response $\succcurlyeq_1$, for example, $a \succ b \succ c$, is provided by 20 persons out of 100, we assign probability 0.2 to it, and so on.

With the numbers provided in this example, qualitatively, $a$ is in the average greater than both $b$ and $c$, and $b$ and $c$ are equivalent. From this overall probabilistic relation on $A$, it is possible to derive the probabilities of the specific relations that hold for each pair of elements. For example,

$$\mathbb{P}(a \succ b) = \mathbb{P}(\succcurlyeq_1) + \mathbb{P}(\succcurlyeq_2) + \mathbb{P}(\succcurlyeq_8) + \mathbb{P}(\succcurlyeq_{10});$$

*Table 5.1* An illustrative example of a probabilistic order structure on $A = \{a, b, c\}$

| *Weak orders* $\succcurlyeq_i$ | *Orderings corresponding to weak orders* $\succcurlyeq_i$ | $x_a$ | $x_b$ | $x_c$ | $\mathbb{P}(\succcurlyeq_i)$ |
|---|---|---|---|---|---|
| $\succcurlyeq_1$ | $a \succ b \succ c$ | 3 | 2 | 1 | 0.2 |
| $\succcurlyeq_2$ | $a \succ c \succ b$ | 3 | 1 | 2 | 0.2 |
| $\succcurlyeq_3$ | $b \succ a \succ c$ | 2 | 3 | 1 | 0.0 |
| $\succcurlyeq_4$ | $b \succ c \succ a$ | 1 | 3 | 2 | 0.0 |
| $\succcurlyeq_5$ | $c \succ a \succ b$ | 2 | 1 | 3 | 0.0 |
| $\succcurlyeq_6$ | $c \succ b \succ a$ | 1 | 2 | 3 | 0.0 |
| $\succcurlyeq_7$ | $a \sim b \succ c$ | 2 | 2 | 1 | 0.1 |
| $\succcurlyeq_8$ | $a \sim c \succ b$ | 2 | 1 | 2 | 0.1 |
| $\succcurlyeq_9$ | $b \sim c \succ a$ | 1 | 2 | 2 | 0.0 |
| $\succcurlyeq_{10}$ | $a \succ b \sim c$ | 2 | 1 | 1 | 0.3 |
| $\succcurlyeq_{11}$ | $b \succ a \sim c$ | 1 | 2 | 1 | 0.0 |
| $\succcurlyeq_{12}$ | $c \succ a \sim b$ | 1 | 1 | 2 | 0.0 |
| $\succcurlyeq_{13}$ | $a \sim b \sim c$ | 1 | 1 | 1 | 0.1 |

that is, the probability of the (specific) relation $a \succ b$ is the sum of the probabilities of the orderings in which it holds true. With these premises, we are now in a position to formulate and prove a probabilistic representation theorem.

### 5.2.5 Probabilistic representations

Consider again the deterministic representation for weak order.

$$a \succcurlyeq b \Leftrightarrow m(a) \geq m(b).$$

As we have just seen, $a \succcurlyeq b$ is now no longer a statement that must be either true or false; rather it expresses a possibility that has a degree of probability $\mathbb{P}(a \succcurlyeq b)$. As a consequence of this, the assignment of numbers to objects will no longer be unique. Rather we associate with each element, say $a$, a random variable $x_a$. What we can require now is that this probability of observing a relation between two objects is the same as the probability of obtaining the same kind of relation between the associated random variables. So, in the case of order, the representation theorem becomes, for each $a$, $b$ in $A$,

$$\mathbb{P}(a \succcurlyeq b) = P(x_a \geq x_b), \tag{5.4}$$

or, equivalently,

$$\mathbb{P}(a \succ b) = P(x_a > x_b)$$

and

$$\mathbb{P}(a \sim b) = P(x_a = x_b).$$

We now show, in an informal way, how this can work. Look again at Table 5.1; suppose that we have first assigned the probabilities to each of the possible orderings via the sound evaluation experiment, as we have explained in the previous subsection.

Now, for each of the possible orders, it is possible to find a number assignment to the random variables $x_a$, $x_b$, and $x_c$, compatible with that order. For example, for order $\succsim_1$, which implies $a \succ b \succ c$, a very natural assignment is $x_a = 3$, $x_b = 2$, and $x_c = 1$. Actually there are many other possible assignments that satisfy empirical relations, but suppose that we adopt some conventional rules and make this assignment always unique. For example, we could agree to always use the first natural numbers, 1, 2, … and in this way we get the number assignments shown in columns 3–5 of Table 5.1. Each number assignment corresponds to an order and then it obtains the same probability of the associated order. In this way it is possible to associate a probability distribution with the random variables $x_a$, $x_b$, and $x_c$. Consider, for example, $P(x_a = 1)$. The assignment $x_a = 1$ occurs in association with orders $\succsim_4$, $\succsim_6$, $\succsim_9$, $\succsim_{11}$, $\succsim_{12}$, and $\succsim_{13}$. Consequently, because such orderings are mutually exclusive, the probability of that assignment will be equal to the sum of the probabilities of the orders in which it is true:

$$\begin{aligned} P(x_a = 1) &= \mathbb{P}(\succsim_4) + \mathbb{P}(\succsim_6) + \mathbb{P}(\succsim_9) + \mathbb{P}(\succsim_{11}) + \mathbb{P}(\succsim_{12}) + \mathbb{P}(\succsim_{13}) \\ &= 0.0 + 0.0 + 0.0 + 0.0 + 0.0 + 0.1 = 0.1 \end{aligned}$$

Similarly, we may calculate the probabilities of $x_a = 2$ and $x_a = 3$, and the probability distributions of the random variables $x_b$ and $x_c$. The results are shown in Figure 5.1.

In a similar way we may also check, in the same example, that the representation theorem (5.4) holds true, without providing a formal proof, which may be found in Rossi (2006).

Consider, for example, the relation $a \succ b$: in our example it is satisfied in orders $\succsim_1$, $\succsim_2$, $\succsim_5$, $\succsim_8$, and $\succsim_{10}$ and, consequently,

$$\begin{aligned} \mathbb{P}(a \succ b) &= \mathbb{P}(\succsim_1) + \mathbb{P}(\succsim_2) + \mathbb{P}(\succsim_5) + \mathbb{P}(\succsim_8) + \mathbb{P}(\succsim_{10}) \\ &= 0.2 + 0.2 + 0.0 + 0.1 + 0.3 = 0.8. \end{aligned}$$

On the other hand, the numerical relation $x_a > x_b$ is verified in correspondence with the same orders (this is quite obvious for the very way in which we have assigned the values to the variables $x_a$, $x_b$, and $x_c$!) and so we also obtain $P(x_a > x_b) = 0.8$, as predicted by (5.4).

It is important to note that the measure value, which in the deterministic case was a function of the object, is now a random variable. This is a big change in perspective and merits some discussion. In the deterministic case each object manifests

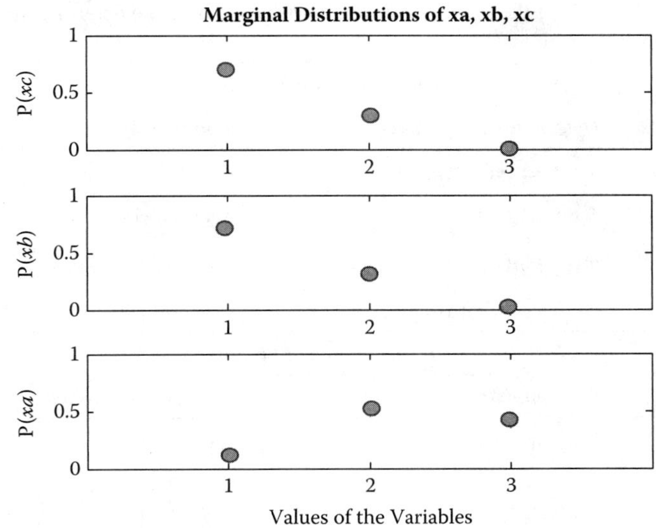


*Figure 5.1* Probability distributions for the random variables $x_a$, $x_b$, and $x_c$, associated with objects *a*, *b*, and *c*, respectively, in the example reported in Table 5.1. All these variables may take the values 1, 2, or 3. Note that for the variable $x_a$ higher values [2,3] have higher probabilities, whereas for variables $x_b$ and $x_c$ the converse holds true and they also have the same distribution.

the characteristic under investigation in one (and only one) way. We call the *state* (of the object) the way in which an object manifests a characteristic. In the deterministic case there is a one-to-one correspondence between objects and states and between states and (measure) values. In the probabilistic representation, due to the uncertainty of empirical relations, there is a one-to-many correspondence between objects and states, whereas there still is a one-to-one correspondence between states and values.

What we have so far discussed for order structures may be extended, in a similar way, to other important structures occurring in measurement, such as difference and extensive structures. A summary of results is presented in Table 5.2. The table presents an overview of the overall theory that is progressively presented, with the related notation, in the rest of the chapter.

The probabilistic approach to representations in measurement is much less developed then the deterministic algebraic one. Introductory presentations may be found in Roberts (1979/2009, Chapter 6) and in Suppes et al. (1989, Chapter 17). An early work by Leaning and Finkelstein (1980) merits mention, as well as a conspicuous contribution by Falmagne (1980). The subject has received a decisive contribution in Regenwetter (1996), where the notion of a probabilistic (there called random) relation is investigated in depth. Additional treatment is presented in Regenwetter and Marley (2001). The theory sketched here is presented in detail in Rossi (2006), where proof is provided for all the results in Table 5.2.

*Table 5.2* Synopsis of the theory considered, including both the deterministic and the probabilistic approach

| | *The measurement scale* | |
|---|---|---|
| *Scale type* | *Deterministic approach* | *Probabilistic approach* |
| Order | $a \succcurlyeq b \Leftrightarrow m(a) \geq m(b)$ | $\mathbb{P}(a \succcurlyeq b) = P(x_a \geq x_b)$ |
| Interval | $\Delta_{ab} \succcurlyeq \Delta_{cd} \Leftrightarrow$ | $\mathbb{P}(\Delta_{ab} \succcurlyeq \Delta_{cd}) =$ |
| | $m(a) - m(b) \geq m(c) - m(d)$ | $= P(x_a - x_b \geq x_c - x_d)$ |
| Ratio | $a \sim b \circ c \Leftrightarrow m(a) = m(b) + m(c)$ | $\mathbb{P}(a \sim b \circ c) = P(x_a = x_b + x_c)$ |
| | *The measurement process* | |
| *Process* | *Deterministic approach* | *Probabilistic approach* |
| Observation | $y = f(x)$ | $P(y \mid x)$ |
| Restitution | $\hat{x} = f^{-1}(y)$ | $P(x \mid y) = P(y \mid x)\left[\sum_{x \in X} P(y \mid x)\right]^{-1}$; |
| | | $\hat{x} = \mu(x \mid y)$ |
| Measurement | $\hat{x} = h(x) = x$ | $P(\hat{x} \mid x) = \sum_{y \in Y} \delta[\hat{x} - \mu(x \mid y)]\, P(y \mid x)$ |

### *5.2.6 The construction of the reference scale*

We have considered the notion of scale mainly in its general meaning, as a set of conditions necessary for measurement to be possible. Yet we have also mentioned another, more specific, meaning of the scale, that we now have to discuss. Once we have assessed, or even simply assumed, the existence of the conditions for measurability, in order to make measurement possible we have to actually construct a reference scale. Let us see what this means, both in abstract terms and through some examples.

We have already encountered an example of a reference scale, the Mohs scale for hardness, consisting of ten reference minerals, with assigned values. What is the criterion for choosing such standards? In abstract terms, in the deterministic case, for a finite set $A$ with, say, $N$ elements under an equivalence relation, we partition $A$ into its equivalence classes,[2] and then select one element in each class to form the series of standards. This series has to represent the possible manifestations of the characteristic or, equivalently, the possible states in which each object may be. Remember that in the deterministic case, each object will be in one (and only one) state.

Let us now discuss the hypothesis of *finiteness*, which is very useful for simplifying the mathematics. The rationale for this assumption is that we cannot attain, experimentally, an infinite resolution, that is, the ability of detecting infinitely small variations. Whatever the sensitivity of the comparator, there will always be a lower limit to the variations that it is able to detect and so it is reasonable to assume a finite resolution for the scale. On the other hand, for any fixed class of measurement problems, it will also be possible to assume a maximum value for the characteristic. Now, a finite resolution plus a finite maximum value makes a *finite set of possible states.* So the hypothesis of finiteness for the class of the possible states may be maintained in full generality.

Some examples may now be useful. Prior to examining them, in this regard we also have to remember that what we have called an object (something that has a stable existence), may also be an event instead (something that may be generated when needed, but that does not persist). As a first example, we consider the case of mass measurement: here the reference scale is a set of standard masses, with assigned values. How many masses may be needed in a practical case? If we want to realize, for example, the mass values from, say, 1 g to 1 kg, with resolution of 1 g, which makes 1,000 values, we do not need to have 1,000 distinct masses, but rather the following series:

$$m_{1\text{ g}},\ m_{2\text{ g}},\ \overset{*}{m}_{2\text{ g}},\ m_{5\text{ g}},$$

$$m_{10\text{ g}},\ m_{20\text{ g}},\ \overset{*}{m}_{20\text{ g}},\ m_{50\text{ g}},$$

$$m_{100\text{ g}},\ m_{200\text{ g}},\ \overset{*}{m}_{200\text{ g}},\ m_{500\text{ g}},$$

where the subscript denotes the value of the standard and the asterisk denotes a second copy of an already available standard. It is easy to check that, thanks to the addition property, it is possible to generate all the values required, with only 12 material standards! For example, we get $m_{8\ g}$ as the sum of three standards in the series; that is, $m_{8\ g} = m_{1\ g} \circ m_{2\ g} \circ m_{5\ g}$, where "$\circ$" denotes physical addition. Note also that we need two copies of $m_{20\ g}$, even though we could get $m_{20\ g}$ from other terms, because otherwise we could not get $m_{41\ g}$. This simple example demonstrates how additivity helps and that we do not need to have all the standards to exist at the same time, but rather we have to be able to generate them, by addition in this case, when they are needed.

Another example is the primary scale for length. This is obtained by a sophisticated laser system: here the scale is an electromagnetic field that propagates in the space through parallel planes. The distance between such planes, which is one wavelength, is the basic reference item for such a scale, because it is possible to realize movements parallel to the propagation direction corresponding to a certain number of wavelengths (or of fractions of a wavelength). In a sense, the reference scale is materialized by movements of a slide on a guide, so it is a collection of "events," the positions of the slides along the reference axis, which in turn are obtained as sums of elementary events, that is, small movements of the slide, of one wavelength or one fraction of wavelength each. Examples may be considered in the perceptual domain also. In the case of sound perception the reference items are carefully generated synthetic sounds having a well-defined physical intensity, spectrum, and duration. For vision, they may be reference colors, and for smell, reference odors obtained by carefully prepared solutions.

Thus far we have discussed the reference elements. We now discuss the assignment of numerical values to them. In the deterministic case we assign a single value to each element. In the case of a probabilistic representation, each object is characterized, at least in principle, by a probability distribution over a set of possible values, rather than by a single value. In practice, reference scales are accompanied by some statement about the uncertainty of the samples: the point is that such a statement has a foundation in the probabilistic representation that we have proposed. Let us consider again the example of the mass scale. One could argue that if we had a good comparator, there would be no uncertainty in distinguishing between two masses having a different value, for example, $m_{10\,g}$ and $m_{20\,g}$, so where is the uncertainty? Actually there are many causes of uncertainty, but just to have an immediate answer consider that in the scale there may be different ways of obtaining a same value, for example, $a = m_{20\,g}$ is equivalent to $b = m_{10\,g} \circ m_{5\,g} \circ m_{2\,g} \circ m^{*}_{2\,g} \circ m_{1\,g}$.

Now, elements $a$ and $b$ will be very close to each other and then it is reasonable that the comparator may compare them only in a probabilistic sense. Finally, for those samples that may be realized only in one way, for example $m_{1\,g}$, one should consider the possibility of having another independent realization of the reference scale and then, there, an element, $m_{1\,g}'$, that may be compared only probabilistically with $m_{1\,g}$. We hope that this oversimplified example may give a feeling of the uncertainty of a reference scale and how it may be characterized in terms of empirical relations.

## 5.3 The measurement process

### *5.3.1 The measuring system*

Once we have constructed a reference scale, we have to consider how to measure objects not included in the scale. First we introduce some additional language. For any object $a$, we consider its *(measure) value*, $x = m(a)$, as the number that properly describes $a$, with respect to the characteristic under consideration, that is, as the value satisfying the representation theorem (5.1 or 5.4). A direct determination of $x$ would imply actually comparing $a$ with a representative set of elements of $A$: this is what needs doing, at least in principle, for the elements of the series of standards $S$. So for each element $s \in S$, we obtain a (measure) value $m(s)$ associated with it. For an object $a$ not belonging to S, we may still consider its measure value $x = m(a)$, as the value *virtually* obtainable by comparing $a$ with a representative set of elements of $A$, but in general we proceed, for convenience, in a different way, that is, through a *measurement process*, usually carried out by a measuring system. By doing this, we obtain, for $a$, a *measurement value*, denoted by $\hat{x}$. So, to sum up, we call the "measure value," or simply "value," of an object the number that we would obtain by comparing it with (actually or virtually) all the other elements in the set $A$, and we call the "measurement value" the number that we obtain by measuring it through a proper measurement process. Let us then discuss how to obtain the measurement value $\hat{x}$.

There are two main ways of doing that, direct and indirect, illustrated, in the case of mass measurement, in Figure 5.2. We first discuss them in a deterministic context,

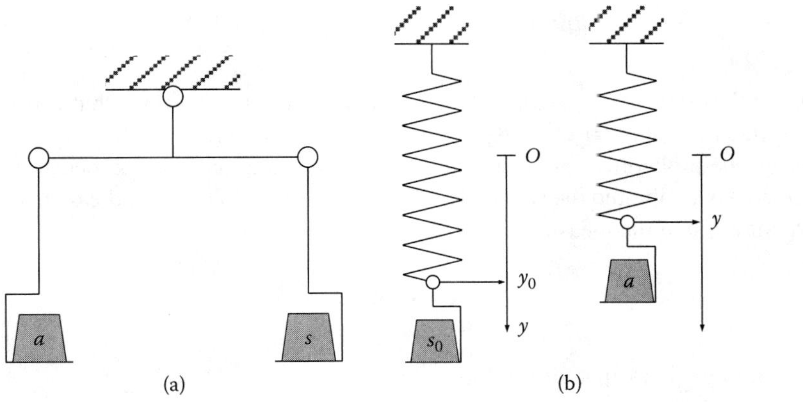


*Figure 5.2* Direct (a) versus indirect (b) measurement method.

where we assume that all the devices involved behave in a perfectly repeatable and reproducible way, then we introduce a more realistic probabilistic model, capable of accounting for the behavior of real-world devices that may present random variation or may be affected by systematic deviations.

The first simply consists in comparing the unknown object $a$ with the series of standard $S$ to find an element $s \in S$ equivalent to $a$, $s \sim a$. This is shown in Figure 5.2a, for the mass example. Let $x = m(a)$ be the unknown (measure) value of $a$. On the basis of the result of the comparison, inasmuch as we have found $a \sim s$, we assign to $a$ the measurement value $\hat{x} = m(s)$.

Note that $x$ is unknown, whereas $m(s)$ is known, because $s$ is an element of the reference scale, so we estimate $x$ by $\hat{x} = m(s)$. In the ideal case we obtain

$$\hat{x} = x,$$

that is, the measurement value equals the measure value, which in turn satisfies the deterministic representation theorem.

The second way to measure is to use a measuring system, or instrument, that has been calibrated with respect to the reference scale. In our example, Figure 5.2b, the measuring system consists of a linear spring, oriented according to the gravity field. This device may be calibrated by applying a standard $s_0$, whose value is $x_0 = m(s_0)$, and recording the corresponding displacement of the free end of the spring, $y_0$. Then, by proportionality, the object $a$ such that $m(a) = x$ will produce a displacement $y$ such that

$$y = \frac{y_0}{x_0} x = kx,$$

where $k$ is the *sensitivity* of the instrument, which must be estimated by *calibration*.[3] We call this function, that in general reads

$$y = f(x),$$

*the calibration* or *observation function* and we assume, by now, that it is a one-to-one function and consequently that it is invertible (we remove this hypothesis later on, in the probabilistic model). We know the calibration function because we have previously calibrated the spring device, therefore after observing the displacement $y$, we may assign the measurement value

$$\hat{x} = k^{-1}y = f^{-1}(y).$$

It is easy to check that also in this case

$$\hat{x} = x,$$

and the two measurements, the direct and the indirect one, are conceptually equivalent. We thus look for a common description of these two methods.

### 5.3.2 Observation and restitution

We first define a measuring system (MS) as an empirical system able to interact with the objects that carry the characteristic under investigation and to produce, as a result of such interaction, signs, that we eventually call (instrument) indications, on the basis of which it is possible to assign a measurement value to the characteristic to be measured, in agreement with a previously defined reference scale. The characteristic to be measured in a given situation is usually called the "measurand" (see the glossary at the end of the chapter) and we also use this term in the following.

In the first example of the previous subsection, the MS is made by the reference scale itself plus the comparator, and in the second by the calibrated spring. We propose to parse the measurement process in two subprocesses, *observation* and *restitution.*

In the observation phase the measurand is input to the measuring system that in turn produces an indication. In the restitution phase the indication of the MS is interpreted on the basis of the calibration function and the measurement value is obtained. Measurement is the concatenation of the observation and restitution. Note that the two phases are conceptually distinct, because observation is where information is produced, thanks to the interaction between the object and the MS that produces relevant physical or psychological transformations, whereas restitution is an information-processing phase. Restitution may be very simple, as in the case of direct measurement, where it just consists in assigning to the measurand the same known value of the standard that has been selected, in the observation phase, as equivalent to the measurand, or it may be very complicated and challenging, as in the case of image-based measurement, where it may involve sophisticated image-processing procedures. Nonetheless it is conceptually always present, inasmuch as the measurand is, by assumption, not directly observable (otherwise we would not need to measure), whereas the indication is, in the most general case, a sign, that is, something *observable*. So the measurand and the indication are two inherently different entities and in order to make a statement about the measurand, based on the observation of the indication, an interpretation process is required, which we have called restitution.

Let us now consider a deterministic model of the measurement process. As we have seen in the examples above, observation may be described by the calibration or observation function,

$$y = f(x), \tag{5.5}$$

restitution by its inversion,

$$\hat{x} = f^{-1}(y), \tag{5.6}$$

and measurement by the concatenation of the two,

$$\hat{x} = h(x) = f^{-1}[f(x)] = x, \tag{5.7}$$

where the measurement function, denoted by $h$, in this ideal case reduces to an identity. It is easy to check that this framework holds in both the cases that we have considered in the previous section. Indeed, in the case of direct comparison, if we measure the object $a$, whose (unknown) value is $x = m(a)$, and we find that it is equivalent to $s$, we obtain

$$y = f(x) = m(s) = m(a) = x,$$

$$\hat{x} = f^{-1}(y) = x.$$

In the indirect measurement example, instead, we have

$$y = f(x) = kx,$$

$$\hat{x} = f^{-1}(y) = k^{-1}y = k^{-1}kx = x.$$

Let us now illustrate graphically the general idea of observation/restitution in a simple numerical example, in which $y = f(x) = kx = 2x$, illustrated in Figure 5.3. This example is very simple, even trivial, but it is instrumental in introducing the probabilistic case, which is illustrated similarly at a later stage.

The structure of the measurement process is illustrated in Figure 5.4. It is interesting to compare this general scheme to those we have presented in Chapter 1,

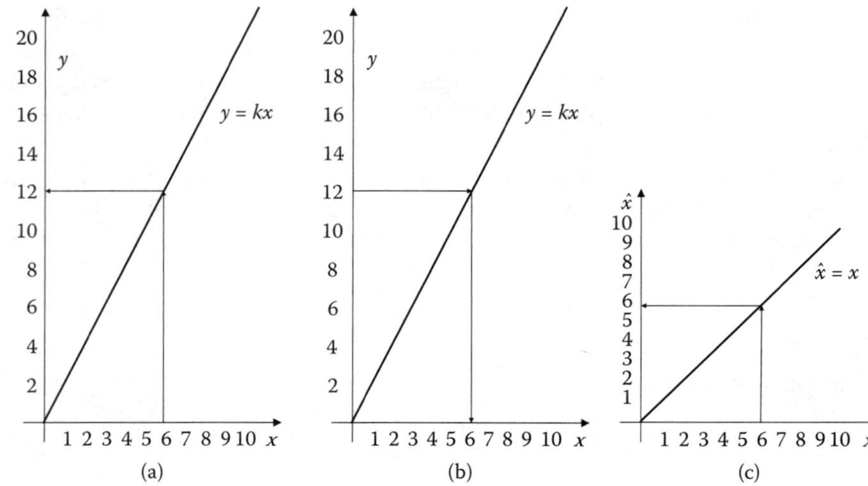


*Figure 5.3* The phases of the measurement process: (a) observation; (b) restitution: in contrast with (a) note that here the input is $y$ and the output is $x$, as indicated by the arrows; (c) measurement.

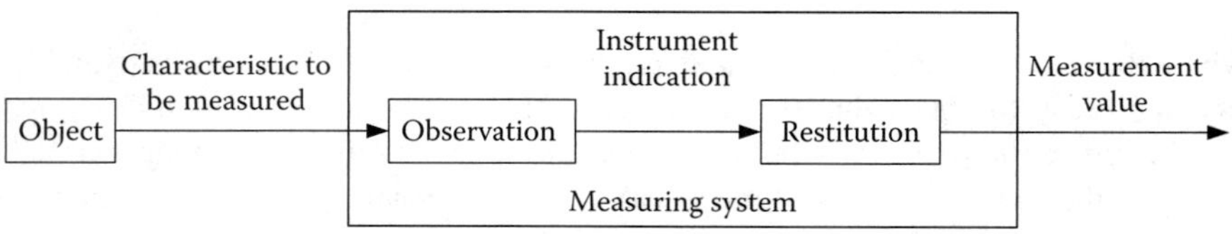


*Figure 5.4* Scheme of the measurement process.

Figures 1.1–1.5. In the case of direct measurement (Figure 1.1), the observation phase constitutes the comparison of the object with the reference scale and restitution is simply the attribution of the value of the selected standard to the measurand. Magnitude estimation (Figure 1.5) may be seen as a kind of direct measurement, with an internal reference scale. Indirect measurement occurs both in physics (Figure 1.2) and in psychophysics (Figure 1.3). Here observation includes the direct measurement of the input measured quantity(ies) or of the input stimulus and restitution is a reinterpretation of the input on the basis of the physical or psychophysical law. Lastly, in measurement in psychometrics (Figure 1.4), and probably in many applications of measurement in the behavioral sciences that use questionnaires, test items play the role of the MS, the process of administering them to subjects and collecting answers is analogous to observation, and the interpretation of the responses, in order to obtain a measurement value, is similar to restitution.

So for the above considerations we may perhaps conclude that the proposed scheme of observation/restitution is quite general and may serve as reference model. Useful references for a formal theory of the MS have been provided by Gonella (1988), Mari (2000), Morawski (1994), and Rossi (2003).

### *5.3.3 The probabilistic model*

The deterministic model describes an ideal environment. If we look for a more realistic account of what happens in reality, we may turn to a probabilistic one.

Let us reconsider observation first. In contrast with the ideal model, when we input a measurand whose value is $x$, and we repeat the experiment more times, in general we do not always obtain the same indication $y$ but rather a cluster of indications. An appropriate way to describe this behavior is to assign a probability distribution to the indications, conditioned on the value of the measurand $P(y|x)$, as shown in Figure 5.5a. In the abscissas we have the possible values $x$ of the quantity under consideration; in the ordinates the instrument indications and the corresponding conditional probability $P(y|x)$ are represented by circles: the large circles indicate a probability equal to 0.6, the small ones correspond to 0.2. For example, if the input value is $x = 6$, we may obtain three indications, whose probabilities are

$$P(y=10|x=6)=0.2,$$

$$P(y=12|x=6)=0.6,$$

$$P(y=14|x=6)=0.2.$$

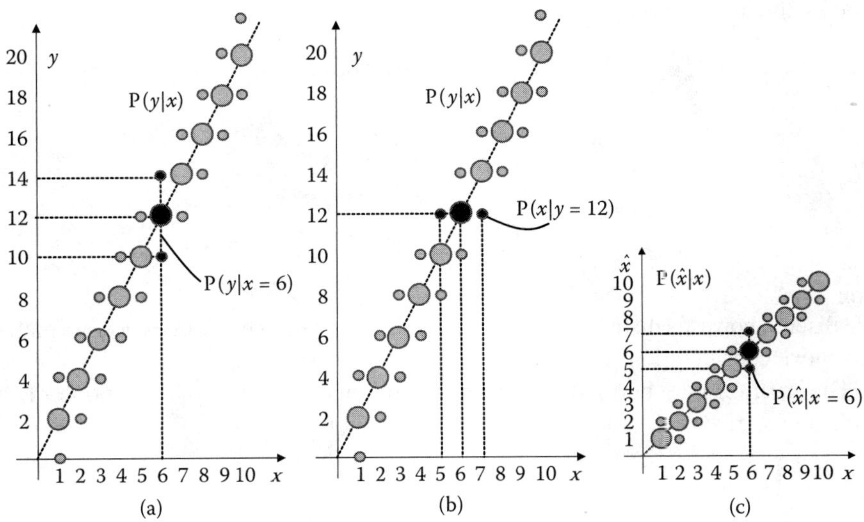


*Figure 5.5* A probabilistic model of the measurement process. The circles represent probability values: the large circle corresponds to 0.6, the small to 0.2. Phases of the process: (a) observation: note that here the input is any fixed value of $x$ and the output is a corresponding probability distribution for $y$: the example of $x = 6$ is outlined; (b) restitution: in contrast with (a), note that here the input is a fixed value of $y$ and the output is a corresponding probability distribution for $x$: the example of $y = 12$ is outlined; (c) measurement: here the input is a fixed value for $x$ and the output a probability distribution for $\hat{x}$.

This conditional distribution may still be obtained, at least in principle, by a calibration experiment and it replaces the former calibration or observation function $y = f(x)$.

How can we do restitution now? The idea, *mutatis mutandis*, is very similar to the deterministic case. Suppose that we observe $y$ = 12: from Figure 5.5b we see that such an indication may have been caused by three values of $x$, namely 5, 6, and 7, and from the same graph we may obtain the probabilities of these three causes, namely

$$P(x=5|y=12)=0.2,$$

$$P(x=6|y=12)=0.6,$$

$$P(x=7|y=12)=0.2.$$

What we have just done is a *probabilistic inversion* of the observation transformation. Analytically this may be obtained by applying the well-known Bayes–Laplace rule, as we show in a moment. Again, as in the deterministic case, we may combine observation and restitution for obtaining a description of the overall measurement process, provided by the distribution $P(\hat{x}|x)$. For example, we see in Figure 5.5c that, if $x = 6$, the measurement value $\hat{x}$ provided by the measurement process is characterized by the distribution

$$P(\hat{x}=5|x=6)=0.2,$$

$$P(\hat{x}=6|x=6)=0.6,$$

$$P(\hat{x}=7|x=6)=0.2.$$

We discuss how this distribution may be obtained in a moment. Let us now formalize the above consideration.

Observation may be modeled by the conditional probability distribution of the indications, given the value of the measurand; that is,

$$P(y|x). \tag{5.8}$$

Restitution is the probabilistic inversion of observation and it can be obtained by the Bayes–Laplace rule, as

$$P(x|y)=\frac{P(y|x)P(x)}{P(y)}=\frac{P(y|x)P(x)}{\sum_x P(y|x)P(x)}.$$

If the probability distribution for $x$ is assumed to be uniform, then the above expression simplifies as

$$P(x|y) = \frac{P(y|x)}{\sum_x P(y|x)} \propto P(y|x). \tag{5.9}$$

This expression may be explained as follows, having in mind the previous example. Our goal distribution $P(x|y)$ is the distribution assigned to the measurand $x$, once the indication $y$ has been observed. So $P(x|y)$ is a function of the variable $x$, with $y$ being a fixed value, and it may be obtained by interpreting $P(y|x)$ as a function of $x$, instead of as a function of $y$. This corresponds to what we have done in Figure 5.5b, where we have read the graph starting from the ordinates. In doing so, it may be that the values we select in this way do not sum to one; in that case we have to rescale them to ensure that the final distribution sums to one:

$$\sum_x P(x|y) = 1.$$

So for each indication $y$ we may assign a probability distribution to the measurand $x$. To describe the measurand, as usual, by a single value—the measurement value—we take a proper position parameter for the random variable $x$, conditioned by $y$, that we denote by

$$\hat{x} = \mu(x|y).$$

Usually, for an interval or ratio scale, this parameter is the *expected value*

$$\mu(x|y) = \mathrm{E}(x|y) = \sum_x xP(x|y),$$

whereas for an ordinal scale the *median* should be used instead (Stevens, 1959). Uncertainty figures can also be obtained from the final distribution $P(x|y)$ (BIPM, 2008a). Finally, we have to combine observation and restitution to obtain a description of the overall measurement process. This operation may be understood by looking at Figure 5.6.

Suppose that $x = 6$; then we may obtain $y = 10, 12, 14$, with probabilities 0.2, 0.6, 0.2, respectively. If, for example, $y = 10$, the resulting probability distribution for $x$ will be centered in $x = 5$ and thus the measurement value (the expected value of the distribution) will be $\hat{x} = 6$. This will happen with the same probability of observing $y = 10$, that is, 0.2. Analogously, if $y = 12$, we obtain $\hat{x} = 6$, which will happen with probability 0.6, and if $y = 14$, we will obtain $\hat{x} = 7$, which will happen with probability 0.2. Summarizing, we have

$$P(\hat{x} = 5|x = 6) = 0.2,$$

$$P(\hat{x} = 6|x = 6) = 0.6,$$

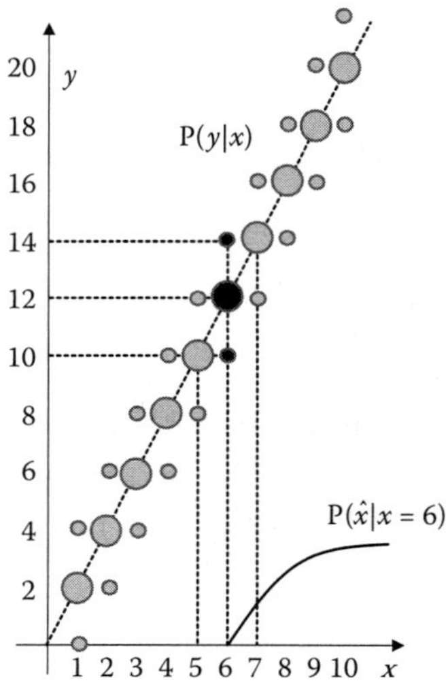


*Figure 5.6* How to obtain a description of the overall measurement process: see explanation in the text. The circles represent probability values: the large circle corresponds to 0.6, the small to 0.2.

$$P(\hat{x}=7|x=6)=0.2.$$

This is the way the graph of Figure 5.5c has been obtained. This procedure may be expressed in a formula,

$$P(\hat{x}|x)=\sum_{y\in Y}\delta[\hat{x}-\mu(x|y)]P(y|x), \tag{5.10}$$

where δ here denotes a unitary discrete impulse function; that is, for any integer $i$, $\delta(i) = 1$ for $i = 0$, and $\delta(i) = 1$, for $i \neq 0$. Let us practice applying formula (5.10) to calculate, for example, $P(\hat{x} = 6|x = 6)$. We obtain

$$\begin{aligned}P(\hat{x}=6|x=6)&=\delta[6-7]P(y=14|x=6)\\&\quad+\delta[6-6]P(y=12|x=6)\\&\quad+\delta[6-5]P(y=10|x=6)\\&=P(y=12|x=6)=0.6.\end{aligned}$$

The probabilistic description of the measurement process is summarized in the lower part of Table 5.2. For an introduction to Bayesian inference we recommend

Press (1989). Additional information on the model presented here may be found in Cox, Rossi, Harris, and Forbes (2008) and in Rossi (2003, 2006, 2009a), including possible generalizations concerning how to account for systematic effects and the extension to vector and dynamic measurements.

## 5.4 Measurability

Once the meaning of measurement has been clarified by the notion of measurement scale and the way we measure by the concepts of measuring system and measurement process, we may discuss a crucial point that has been, as we have seen in Chapter 1, a matter of strong controversy, the issue of measurability. There is no room here for a thorough discussion of this topic, and we just propose, on the basis of what we have thus far discussed, a criterion for measurability. We suggest that a characteristic *x* of a class of objects is measurable if the following four-step procedure may be successfully applied:

1. Define the *class of objects* that manifest the characteristic.
2. Identify the *empirical properties* that define the characteristic.
3. Construct a *reference measurement scale.*
4. Devise at least one *measuring system* based on that reference scale.

Simple as it may seem, this procedure involves very demanding steps to be taken; see Rossi (2007) for a discussion. Here we simply note that, at first glance, it may seem that this procedure applies to fundamental measurement only, according to Campbell's classification (Campbell, 1957/1920). As we have seen in Chapter 1, for Campbell fundamental quantities are only those for which it is possible to construct a reference scale, thanks to the "physical addition" operation, and that may be measured by direct comparison with that scale. On the other hand, derived quantities are those that may be measured indirectly, thanks to some physical law that relates them to other, independently measurable, quantities.

We may retain this classification to some extent, provided that we generalize and update it on the basis of recent irreversible results of the representational theory. So we call *fundamental* a scale that may be constructed on the basis of the *internal properties* (relations and operations) of the quantity under consideration. We call *derived* a scale obtained on the basis of interrelations linking the quantity under consideration with other quantities. For example, a scale for mass, constructed by generating the multiples and submultiples of an initial, arbitrary, unitary element, by an equal-arm balance, and by assigning values to them in accordance with the additivity property, may be considered a fundamental scale. Instead, a temperature scale based on a graduated mercury-in-glass thermometer may be considered derived from length measurement, through the property of thermal dilatation of fluids. In fact, this property is not "internal" to temperature (as would be the "warmer than" order relation) but rather relates two distinct quantities, temperature and length.

So, what can we say, in a few words, about the measurability of derived quantities?

Basically, in the case of a derived quantity $z$, the empirical properties required for constructing the scale are derived from the properties of another quantity $x$ to which $z$ is linked through a scientific law. But what is a scientific law?

We may perhaps define it, for the scope of this discussion, as a functional relation between variables, say, in our case, $z = g(x)$, that is accepted as holding true, in a given domain of knowledge and in a given historic moment.

Now, it may happen that the law $g$ has been determined, or, at least, verified, after measuring independently $x$ and $z$. In this case, we may still wish to measure $x$ indirectly through $g$, for practical convenience, but the functional relation does not have, in this case, a foundational role. For example, having previously defined temperature through thermodynamic principles (as happens now for the so-called thermodynamic temperature), we may determine the law that links temperature to the height of the mercury column in a liquid-in-glass mercury thermometer, realize that it is highly linear, and decide to make temperature measurement by that type of thermometer. Completely different is the case in which we define temperature by assuming a linear relation between it and the height of the mercury column. In this second case, temperature is intended, by definition, as that property of a body giving rise to linear variations of height in the column of a mercury thermometer, when properly coupled with it (details are inessential here). Now, in a certain stage of scientific development, one of these two solutions may be preferred, in consideration of the overall body of knowledge involved (physics, in this case), but both are, in our opinion, conceptually correct.

Thus—and this is a key point—a functional relation may be used to found the measurability of some quantity, by defining it, provided that there are good reasons for accepting that relation.

At this stage, a second problem emerges: what about the meaning of the number we associate with $z$, if empirical properties have not been directly involved in the definition of the scale of $z$? For example, in the case of temperature being defined through the mercury thermometer, what meaning would we associate with the resulting numbers?

The representational theory for derived measurement is not so advanced as the one concerning fundamental measurement, yet useful results are available. Basically, empirical relations involving both quantities come into play. Intuitively, in our example, we require first that there is an order both on temperature and on height, and then that such orders are in concordance. That is to say that if, for example, the temperature of $a$ is greater than that of $b$, then the height of the mercury column of the thermometer increases accordingly. If this happens, we may derive an order scale for temperature. If we look for an interval scale, we should also require that equivalent temperature intervals correspond to equivalent height intervals and that adjacent temperature intervals correspond to adjacent height intervals.

Therefore as a tentative conclusion, we may say that in the case of fundamental scales we construct the scale on the basis of empirical relations internal to the characteristic under consideration, whereas in the case of derived scales we take advantage of cross-relations with other characteristics. This may be more critical because the empirical structure involved is more complex, but the basic ideas remain the same. So the measurability criterion that we have proposed may still be applied, with proper adaptation.

Measurability has been recently discussed by Finkelstein (2003, 2005, 2008) and by Rossi (2007). Measurability issues are also treated by Ellis (1966), who also provides an interesting discussion of temperature measurement. An introduction to derived measurements may be found in Roberts (1979/2009); an important application of these ideas concerns magnitude estimation, on which Narens has published a thorough study (1996).

## 5.5 Final remarks

We have presented a basic kernel for a probabilistic theory of measurement, addressing three key questions, namely what is the meaning of measurement, how do we measure, and what can be measured?

We suggest that the response to the first question may be found in a theory of the measurement scale, to the second in a general model of the measurement process, and to the third in a conceptually simple measurability criterion. Further studies are required in many regards, including the problem of derived scales, a deeper characterization of the measurement process, and the extension to multidimensional measurement, to name just a few.

In developing this theory we have carefully avoided linking it to special classes of measurements or to specific measuring techniques or technologies. Thus we hope that it may constitute a good starting point for achieving a common view of measurement among different scientific disciplines.

## Glossary

Some terms in this glossary are also defined in the International Vocabulary of Metrology (VIM; BIPM, 2008b). In those cases, the definitions provided here are in essential agreement with those in the VIM, but they are differently phrased, in order to make them more suited for a foundational discussion and, it is hoped, more understandable to a multidisciplinary readership.

**Object:** the carrier of the characteristic to be measured; it may be a physical object, an event, or a person

**Characteristic or property (of an object):** what we want to measure

**Measurable characteristic (or quantity):** a characteristic that may be measured

**State (of an object, with respect to a given characteristic):** particular way in which an object manifests a characteristic

**Empirical relation:** a relation that may be observed between two or more objects, with reference to the characteristic of interest

**Comparator:** a device (or a person) that performs the comparison of objects, in respect of some characteristic of theirs

**Empirical structure (or empirical relational system):** a set of objects and a set of empirical relations on it

**Nominal, difference, interval, extensive:** different types of empirical structures
**Numerical structure (or numerical relational system):** a set of numbers and a set of numerical relations on it
**Scale:** (general meaning) the set of formal conditions for measurement (an empirical structure, a numerical structure and a measure function constituting an homomorphism between them)
**(Reference) scale:** (specific meaning) a series of standard objects with corresponding numerical values properly assigned
**Nominal, ordinal, interval, ratio:** different types of scales
**Measurand:** a characteristic of a specific object to be measured, in a specific situation
**Measuring system (or instrument):** an empirical system capable of interacting with objects carrying the characteristic under investigation and, as a result of such interaction, of producing an observable output according to which it is possible to assign a value to the object to be measured
**Calibration:** the operation by which the characteristics of the measuring system are assessed
**Measurement process:** the process by which a value is assigned to a measurand, normally based on the use of a measuring system
**(Measure) value:** a number that may be actually or virtually assigned to an object in order to express how the object compares, with respect to some characteristic, to all the other objects that carry the same characteristic
**Measurement value:** the value that is assigned to an object as the result of a measurement process
**Model:** an abstract system that, to some extent and from a certain standpoint, represents a real system (or a class of real systems); a scientific theory may be sometimes viewed as a very general model
**(Natural) law:** a functional relation (or a model) linking one or more characteristics of real objects
**Measurement model:** a model used to found the measurability of certain characteristics or to perform measurements

## Notation

| | | |
|---|---|---|
| $x$ | = | characteristic (quantity) to be measured, measurand, unknown (measure) value of the measurand |
| $A$ | = | set of objects manifesting the characteristic $x$ |
| $a, b, c, d$ | = | objects, elements of $A$ |
| $m$ | = | measure function, $m : A \rightarrow \mathbb{R}$ |
| $\Delta_{ab}$ | = | interval between elements $a$ and $b$ of $A$; it is "positive" if $a \succ b$ |
| $\succsim$ | = | empirical relation of "greater than or equivalent to;" it is a *weak-order* relation; for simplicity, we use the same symbol for denoting an order between objects, e.g., $a \succsim b$, or between intervals, e.g., $\Delta_{ab} \succsim \Delta_{cd}$ |
| $\succsim_i$ | = | $i$th weak-order relation defined on $A$ |

| | | |
|---|---|---|
| $\sim$ | = | "equivalent to," empirical equivalence relation on $A$ defined, for $a,b \in A$ by $a \sim b \Leftrightarrow a \succcurlyeq b$ and $b \succcurlyeq a$ |
| $\succ$ | = | "greater than," empirical relation of strict order |
| $\circ$ | = | binary empirical operation of addition of elements of A; it may also be considered a ternary relation on A defined, for $a,b,c \in A$ by $\circ(a,b,c) \Leftrightarrow a \circ b = c$ |
| $\delta$ | = | threshold of a comparator (see below for another meaning of the same symbol) |
| $\sim_\delta$ | = | indifference relation associated to a comparator with a threshold; it differs from an equivalence relation in that it is not transitive |
| $S = \{s_1, s_2, \ldots s_n\}$ | = | series of standards |
| $\mathbb{P}$ | = | probability of a relation |
| $P$ | = | probability function, probability distribution |
| $x_a, x_b, x_c$ | = | random variables associated to elements $a$, $b$, $c$, expressing their measure values |
| $P(x)$, $P(x = x_i)$, $P(x \leq y)$ | = | probability distribution for the random variable $x$, probability that the random variable $x$ takes the specific value $x_i$ probability that the random variable $x$ is less than or equal to random variable $y$ |
| $y$ | = | instrument indication, output of the measuring system |
| $P(y/x)$, $P(y = y_j/x = x_i)$ | = | probability distribution of $y$, conditioned by $x$; probability that $y$ takes the value $y_j$, given that $x$ has taken the value $x_i$ |
| $f$ | = | calibration or observation function of a measuring system |
| $\hat{x}$ | = | measurement value for $x$ |
| $\delta$ | = | discrete unitary impulse function: for any integer $i$, $\delta(i) = 1$ for $i = 0$, whereas $\delta(i) = 0$, for $i \neq 0$. |
| $g$ | = | function linking two quantities, $z = g(x)$, and expressing a scientific law |

## References


BIPM. (2008a). *Evaluation of measurement data—Guide to the expression of uncertainty in measurement.* (JCGM 100:2008).

BIPM. (2008b). *International vocabulary of metrology—Basic and general terms (VIM).* (JCGM 200:2008).

Campbell, N. R. (1957). *Foundations of science.* New York: Dover. (Original work, *Physics—the elements*, published 1920).

Cox, M. G., Rossi, G. B., Harris, P. M., & Forbes, A. (2008). A probabilistic approach to the analysis of measurement processes, *Metrologia, 45,* 493–502.

Ellis, B. (1966). *Basic concepts of measurement.* Cambridge, UK: Cambridge University Press.

Falmagne, J. C. (1980). A probabilistic theory of extensive measurement. *Philosophy of Science, 47,* 277–296.

Finkelstein, L. (1982). Theory and philosophy of measurement. In P. H. Sydenham (Ed.), *Handbook of measurement science* (Vol. 1, pp. 1–30). Chichester: Wiley.

Finkelstein, L. (2003). Widely, strongly and weakly defined measurement, *Measurement, 34*, 39–48.

Finkelstein, L. (2005). Problems of measurement in soft systems. *Measurement, 38,* 267–274.

Finkelstein, L. (2008, September). Problems of widely-defined measurement. Paper presented at the *12th IMEKO TC1 and TC7 Symposium on Man, Science and Measurement,* Annecy, France.

Finkelstein, L., & Leaning, M. S. (1984). A review of the fundamental concepts of measurement. *Measurement, 2,* 25–34.

Gonella, L. (1988). Measuring instruments and theory of measurement. Paper presented at the *XI IMEKO World Congress,* Houston.

Helmholtz, H. (1971). An epistemological analysis of counting and measurement. In R. Karl (Ed. and Trans.), *Selected writing of Hermann Helmholtz.* Middletown, CT: Wesleyan University Press. (Original work published 1887)

Krantz D. H., Luce, R. D., Suppes, P., & Tversky A. (1971). *Foundations of measurement* (Vol. 1). New York: Academic Press.

Leaning, M. S., & Finkelstein, L. (1980). A probabilistic treatment of measurement uncertainty in the formal theory of measurement. In G. Streker (Ed.), *ACTA IMEKO 1979* (pp. 73–81). Amsterdam: Elsevier.

Luce, R. D., & Suppes, P. (2002). Representational measurement theory. In *Stevens' handbook of experimental psychophysics* (Vol. 4). New York: Wiley.

Luce, R. D., Krantz, D. H., Suppes, P., & Tversky, A. (1990). *Foundations of measurement* (Vol. 3). New York: Academic Press.

Mari, L. (2000). Beyond the representational viewpoint: A new formalization of measurement. *Measurement, 27,* 71–84.

Monti, C. M., & Pierobon, G. (2000). *Teoria della probabilità.* Bologna: Zanichelli.

Morawski, R. Z. (1994). Unified approach to measurand reconstruction. *IEEE Transactions on Instrumentation & Measurement, 43*, 226–231.

Narens, L. (1996). A theory of ratio magnitude estimation, *Journal of Mathematical Psychology, 40,* 109–129.

Papoulis, A. (1984). *Probability, random variables and stochastic processes* (2nd ed.). Singapore: McGraw-Hill.

Press, S. J. (1989). *Bayesian statistics.* New York: Wiley.

Regenwetter, M. (1996). Random utility representations of finite m-ary relations. *Journal of Mathematical Psychology, 40,* 219–234.

Regenwetter, M., & Marley, A. J. (2001). Random relations, random utilities, and random functions. *Journal of Mathematical Psychology, 45,* 864–912.

Roberts, F. S. (1979). *Measurement theory, with applications to decision-making, utility and the social sciences.* Reading, MA: Addison-Wesley. Digital Reprinting (2009). Cambridge, UK: Cambridge University Press.

Rossi, G. B. (2003). A probabilistic model for measurement processes. *Measurement, 34,* 85–99.

Rossi, G. B. (2006). A probabilistic theory of measurement. *Measurement, 39,* 34–50.

Rossi, G. B. (2007). Measurability. *Measurement, 40,* 545–562.

Rossi, G. B. (2009a). Probability in metrology. In F. Pavese, & A. Forbes (Eds.), *Data modeling for metrology and testing in measurement science.* Boston: Birkhauser–Springer.

Rossi G. B. (2009b). Cross–disciplinary concepts and terms in measurement. *Measurement, 42*, 1288–1296.

Stevens, S. S. (1959). Measurement, psychophysics and utility. In C. W. Churchman & P. Ratoosh (Eds.), *Basic concepts of measurements* (pp. 1–49). Cambridge, UK: Cambridge University Press.

Suppes, P., Krantz, D. H., Luce, R. D., & Tversky, A. (1989). *Foundations of measurement* (Vol. 2). New York: Academic Press.

## Notes

1. A weak-order relation, $a \succcurlyeq b$, on a set A, is such that it is defined for each pair of elements of A and it is transitive; that is, if $a \succcurlyeq b$ and $b \succcurlyeq c$, then also $a \succcurlyeq c$. For the meaning of the mathematical symbols, see the Glossary and Notation sections at the end of the chapter.
2. An *equivalence class* is a set of elements all equivalent to one another. The collection of the equivalence classes of a set $A$ forms a *partition* for $A$: this means that any such class shares no element with the others and that these classes, all together, *cover* $A$; that is, they include all the elements of $A$.
3. Calibration is the process of experimentally characterizing the behavior of a measuring system. It is usually done by inputting the instrument with reference standards, whose values are known, and by recording the resulting instrument indications. The instrument behavior may thus be characterized by the calibration curve, that is, the graph of the indications versus the input values of the standards, or by some analytical curve fitted to them.

# 6 Multivariate measurements

*Gerie W. A. M. van der Heijden*[1] *and Ragne Emardson*[2]
[1]Biometris
Wageningen University and Research Centre
Wageningen, The Netherlands
[2]SP Technical Research Institute of Sweden
Borås, Sweden

## 6.1 Introduction

Measurements with persons often involve a large number of variables that have to be analyzed with statistical methods. This chapter gives a short overview of various methods that can be used. The aim is to give readers a basic understanding of the usefulness of and relations between the different methods in a condensed and accessible form. We refer interested readers to numerous multivariate statistical handbooks for a more extensive and in-depth treatment of the several methods (e.g., Mardia, Kent, & Bibby, 1979; Johnson & Wichern, 2002; Härdle & Simar, 2007; Tabachnick & Fidell, 2007).

### *6.1.1 Dataset*

In this chapter we use one example dataset of the EU-project MONAT (Measurement of Naturalness). The aim of the MONAT project is to establish a relationship between the physical attributes of an object and its perceived naturalness as assessed by humans. The dataset we use consists of a limited set of 30 samples of panels, representing wood in various degrees of naturalness. An overview of the samples is given in Figure 6.1. The samples are scored by human observers and after some processing these scores are translated to a probability score (0–1 range) for a (possibly fake) wooden panel being perceived as natural. This is done for three different perceptual modalities: (1) only by vision (VO), (2) only by touching it with a finger (TO), and (3) by both vision and touch (VT). For further details on the psychophysical aspects of the study, see, for example, Overvliet, Soto-Faraco, Whitaker, Johnstone Sorensen, McGlone, and van der Heijden (2008). Furthermore, physical attributes were measured for all the samples using different instruments (Goodman, Montgomery, Bialek, Forbes, Rides, Whitaker et al., 2008). With these instruments, vision-related attributes such as features for texture, color, and gloss

*Figure 6.1* *(See color insert.)* An overview of the 30 wood samples used in the MONAT study. The first two rows are real wood. Row one contains tiger oak panels, of which the three left panels are untreated (raw, weathered, and sanded, respectively) and the other four are waxed, oiled, varnished, and manufactured, respectively. The second row is the same for cognac oak. The bottom three rows contain artificial wood panels (3 laminates, 1 veneer, 9 vinyl, 3 paper copy, respectively).

and touch-related attributes such as features for roughness, friction, and thermal effusivity were measured. The 30 samples are shown in Figure 6.1.

### 6.1.2 Correlation and causality

In many cases an apparent correlation between two variables may be the result of a relationship between both of these two variables and a (possibly unknown) third variable. For example, in most European countries there is a correlation over time between female salaries and male average height. This does not imply that the taller the men get, the more the women are paid or vice versa. In this case both parameters have increased with time and thus a correlation is found between them. Hence, even if a statistical correlation is found between two variables, it does not always imply that there is a (direct) causal relationship between them. Furthermore even if the variables A and B are related it is not possible from a correlation analysis to determine if A causes B or if B causes A.

In controlled experiments, a limited number of factors are systematically varied and other factors are kept constant as far as possible or otherwise randomized. It is then possible to study the effect directly of a certain factor on the variable of interest and causality can often be inferred from such an experiment. However, in many studies, we cannot simply change a factor and keep all other factors constant. In the MONAT wood sample set, for example, a variety of wooden panels was chosen, but these panels did not systematically vary for a single attribute such as for color or roughness. Such a study is often referred to as an observational study. In observational studies, we need to be much more careful about conclusions we can draw, as effects could be caused by other unknown correlated factors.

In this chapter, we present some tools and methods for analyzing multivariate data sets. An assumption often made in the analysis of data is that the data come from a (multivariate) normal distribution. Therefore we first introduce the multivariate normal distribution as it is needed in several of the techniques applied later. This is followed by principal component analysis which is often used as a first tool to find systematic patterns among observations. The later sections describe several methods, including multivariate linear regression, discriminant analysis, and clustering methods.

### *6.1.3 Multivariate normal distribution*

A random variable can be described using different properties. Generally, the most important properties for a random variable are its expectation value and variance. Given measurements of a random variable it is possible to form estimators of these properties. These estimators can be of different quality.

In determining a good estimator, it is normally helpful to mathematically model the data. One common approach is to specify a probability density function (PDF) of a random variable. The PDF is a function which, for each point in the sample space, describes the density of probability that the random variable attains that specific value. The probability of a random variable falling within a given set is given by the integral of its PDF over the set.

In this chapter, we focus primarily on random variables with PDFs corresponding to a normal distribution. Because of its many convenient properties, random variables with unknown distributions are often assumed to be normal. Although potentially wrong, this is in many cases a good assumption because any variable that is the sum of a large number of independent factors is likely to be normally distributed. The probability density function for a random vector variable $x$ that has a (multivariate) normal distribution can be written as

$$f(x) = \frac{1}{(2\pi)^{p/2}|\Sigma|^{1/2}} e^{-(x-\mu)^T \Sigma^{-1}(x-\mu)/2},$$

where $p$ is the number of variables (dimensionality), $\mu$ is the expectation vector, and $\Sigma$ is the covariance matrix of $x$. For a scalar variable ($p = 1$) this reduces to the familiar expression:

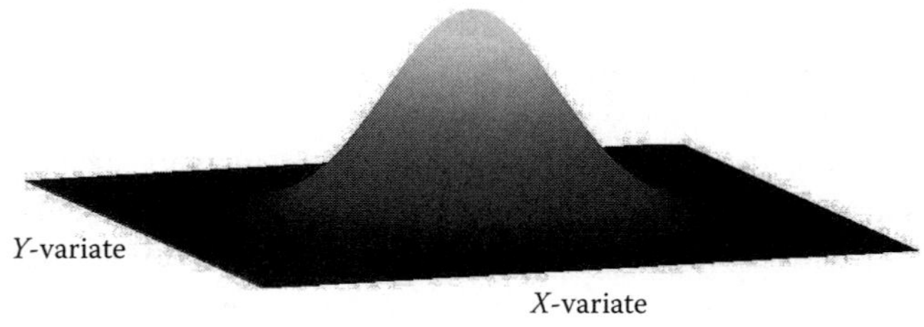


*Figure 6.2* An example of a bivariate normal distribution.

$$f(x) = \frac{1}{\sqrt{2\pi\sigma^2}} e^{-[(x-\mu)/\sigma]^2/2}.$$

An example of the two-dimensional (bivariate) normal PDF is shown in Figure 6.2.

For a random variable $x$ with a normal distribution, the probability that the distance between a vector sample $x_s$ and its expectation value $\mu$ is smaller than or equal to a specific value $\chi_p^2(\alpha)$ is $1 - \alpha$; that is,

$$P\left[(x_s - \mu)^T \Sigma^{-1} (x_s - \mu) \leq \chi_p^2(\alpha)\right] = 1 - \alpha,$$

where $\chi_p^2(\alpha)$ is the upper $(100\alpha)$th percentile of a chi-square distribution with $p$ degrees of freedom (see, e.g., Johnson & Wichern, 2002).

In a strict sense, we should distinguish between the random variable, say $x$, and its realization, say the sample vector $x_s$. However, for readability we drop the subscript $s$ and refer to $x$ both for the random vector and its realization.

Generally, we do not know the expectation $\mu$ and the covariance $\Sigma$ and we estimate these from the data. Given a specific PDF for a random vector variable, we can, for example, find a maximum likelihood estimator (MLE), which is the estimator of the property of the random variable with the highest probability given a set of measurements. This is not necessarily the best unbiased estimator for that property, but when the dataset is large enough it tends to the true value (it is an asymptotically unbiased estimator).

When we have $n$ number of observations, we can estimate $\mu$ as $\bar{x}$, the vector of mean values of the $p$ variables where

$$\bar{x}_k = \frac{1}{n} \sum_{i=1}^{n} x_{ki} \text{ for } k = 1, \ldots, p.$$

We can find an unbiased estimator of $\Sigma$ by the sample covariance matrix $S$ with each element $s_{kl}$ in $S$ as

$$s_{kl} = \frac{1}{n-1}\sum_{i=1}^{n}(x_{ki} - \bar{x}_k)(x_{li} - \bar{x}_l).$$

Given the data, we can construct the multidimensional confidence interval for μ using the following probability.

$$P\left[n(\bar{x} - \mu)^T S^{-1}(\bar{x} - \mu) \leq \frac{p(n-1)}{n-p} F_{p,n-p}(\alpha)\right] = 1 - \alpha,$$

where $F_{p,n-p}(\alpha)$ is the upper (100α)th percentile of the F-distribution with $p$ and $n - p$ degrees of freedom. The region defined by the above equation is a 100(1 – α)% confidence region for μ.

Using the MONAT dataset described above, $x$ can, for example, be the scores of human observers on the three different perceptual modalities, vision only, tactile only, and by both vision and touch for one specific wood sample. Hence, in that case $p$ equals three and μ is the expected score that any observer from a population would produce for the three modalities.

### *6.1.4 Principal component analysis*

Principal component analysis (PCA) is a useful tool for extracting and displaying systematic variations in a data matrix $X$. The main idea behind PCA is to project the data matrix $X$, containing $n$ measurements of $p$ variables, onto a new space with usually a lower dimension, $n \times k$. This is achieved by rewriting $X$ as

$$X = TA^T + E,$$

where the matrix $E$ is the model misfit. The matrices $T$ and $A$ are found by determining the eigenvalues of $X$. Hence, the matrix $A$ is chosen as the eigenvectors of $S$, the sample covariance matrix of $X$. That is, $A$ consists of the vectors $a_1, a_2, \ldots, a_k$ satisfying the equations

$$Sa_n = \lambda_n a_n,$$

and $T$ is found from

$$T = X \cdot A.$$

In order to reduce the number of variables, we can choose to form $A$ of the $k$ first eigenvectors corresponding to the $k$ largest eigenvalues. Studying the MONAT

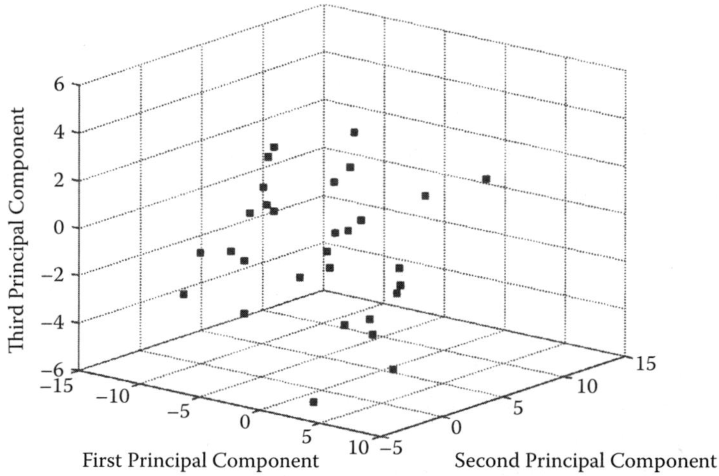


*Figure 6.3* MONAT visual features reduced from 58 to 3 dimensions.

dataset, we can use PCA to reduce the dimensions of the measured parameters. The measurements of the physical attributes corresponding to visual features contain 58 different variables. From a PCA, we find that approximately 70% of the variations can be found in the first three principal components corresponding to the three largest eigenvalues. We can thus reduce the matrix from 58 to 3 dimensions and illustrate the measurements for the 30 different objects in a 3-dimensional space instead of in 58 dimensions (see Figure 6.3).

PCA is a very useful tool in many multivariate applications, which we show later. It helps in dealing with collinearity and helps separate the regularities from the noise. These features are useful both in classification and in multivariate regression.

## 6.2 Regression

### *6.2.1 Linear regression*

In many cases we want to predict or explain a response variable $y$ from a set of predictor (or regressor) variables $x_1, x_2, \ldots, x_p$. Usually the goal is to find a relationship between a response variable that is very time consuming to obtain and predictor variables that are relatively easy to measure. Often we can assume that the relation between $y$ and $x_1, x_2, \ldots, x_p$ is linear. Then we can formulate the following linear regression model:

$$y = \beta_0 + \beta_1 x_1 + \cdots + \beta_p x_p + \varepsilon,$$

where the vector $\varepsilon$ is the random error component. Generally the errors are assumed to have mean zero and unknown variance $\sigma^2$. Furthermore the errors are assumed to be uncorrelated.

More conveniently such a model can be written in matrix notation as

$$y = X\beta + \varepsilon,$$

where the matrix $X$ is the combination of the vectors $1$, $x_1, x_2, \ldots, x_p$ and where $\beta = (\beta_0, \beta_1, \ldots, \beta_p)^T$ is the vector of coefficients and $1$ indicates a vector of ones.

If we have a set of $n$ observations $y = (y_1, y_2, \ldots, y_i, \ldots, y_n)^T$ and corresponding $X$, we can estimate the coefficients $\beta$ using the least squares method, that is, by trying to minimize the sum of squared residuals

$$RSS = \sum_{i=1}^{n} [y_i - X_i\beta]^2 .$$

The solution is

$$\hat{\beta} = (X^T X)^{-1} X^T y .$$

We can further generalize this linear regression by considering multiple response variables simultaneously and write the relation as

$$Y = XB + E,$$

where $Y$ and $E$ are matrices. In analogy with a single response variable, we can find an estimator for $B$ using general linear regression as

$$\hat{B} = \left(X^T X\right)^{-1} X^T Y .$$

If the error matrix $E$ is multivariate normal distributed with a vector of variances $\sigma_E^2$ and uncorrelated between the variables, the least squares estimator of $B$ is also normally distributed and it is also the MLE of $B$. Using $\hat{B}$, it is now possible to predict new sets of observations. Choosing new arbitrary sets of measurements $X_0$ we can predict the response variables:

$$Y_{pred} = X_0 \hat{B} .$$

The error of the prediction is then the difference between the prediction, $Y_{pred}$, and the true value $Y_0$; that is, $Y_{pred} - Y_0$. Normally, we do not know the size of the error because $Y_0$ is not known to us. We can, however, calculate the variance of this error as

$$Var\left[Y_{pred} - Y_0\right] = \sigma_E^2 \left(1 + X_0 \left(X^T X\right)^{-1} X_0^T\right),$$

which we can use to evaluate the measurement uncertainty of $Y_{pred}$.

Using the example with the MONAT dataset, we want to establish the relation between physical attributes of an object and its perceived naturalness. Hence $Y$ contains the values of the perceived naturalness and $X$ contains the measurements of the physical attributes. Finding a relation between these $X$ and $Y$ (i.e., an estimate of $B$) is then useful for predicting perceived naturalness of objects based on physical measurement only.

### 6.2.2 Prediction and validation

If we want to fit a (possibly nonlinear) regression model to a single response variable $y$ we can write the model: $y_i = f(X_i,\beta) + \varepsilon_i$, for $i = 1, \ldots, n$ observations, where $f(X,\beta)$ indicates any function of regressor matrix $X$ and coefficients $\beta$. In analogy with the linear regression case, we can estimate the coefficients $\beta$ as $\hat{\beta}$ by using the least squares method, that is, minimize the sum of squared residuals:

$$RSS = \sum_{i=1}^{n} \left[ y_i - f(X_i,\beta) \right]^2 .$$

The mean squared error ($MSE$) of the model can be calculated as

$$MSE = \sum_{i=1}^{n} \left[ y_i - f\left(X_i,\hat{\beta}\right) \right]^2 \Big/ n$$

and can be seen as an estimate of the error rate of the model.

Often we are interested in the general applicability of the model and we would like to know how well the model will perform with other data; that is, we are interested in the error rate of the model in a more general sense.

If we had access to an unlimited number of observations, we could fit the model on the entire population and, of course, the $MSE$ would then be the true error rate. In real applications we only have access to a finite set of observations. One approach to obtain an estimate of the error rate of the model is to use the entire dataset to fit the model and estimate the error rate as $MSE$. However, this error rate estimate will be overly optimistic (lower than the true error rate).

A way to solve this problem is to split the dataset in two parts: one for training the model and one for testing it. The testing of the model is often referred to as model validation. If we have an observation $y_j$ at $X_j$, we can get an impression of the lack of fit of the model for observation $j$ by looking at the residual, that is, the difference between the true observation and its predicted value: $r_j = y_j - \hat{y}_j$, where $\hat{y}_j = f(X_j,\beta)$.

In analogy with the above, we can now calculate a mean squared error of prediction ($MSEP$) for $m$ test observations as

$$MSEP = \sum_{j=1}^{m} \left[ y_j - \hat{y}_j \right]^2 / m.$$

If the dataset is large enough, we can, for example, split the dataset 50% for training and 50% for testing and hence estimate the error rate on the testing set as *MSEP*.

In many cases, we cannot afford to discard data for the model fitting: we may need more samples to fit the model properly as well as to estimate the *MSEP*. In such a case, we can use cross-validation by repeatedly dividing the data in a disjoint training set and test set. One popular approach is *K*-fold cross-validation. For this, we divide the dataset in *K* disjoint parts. We start with using $k = 2, \ldots, K$ for training the model and part $k = 1$ for testing the model. Then we repeat this procedure by using part $k = 2$ for testing and the others for training, and so on for all *K* parts. Each time the squared residuals are calculated and in this way the *MSEP* is calculated.

The most extreme case of *K*-fold cross-validation is when *K* is equal to *N*; that is, the test set has a size of 1. This is also called leave-one-out cross-validation. Several other approaches exist for performing model validation, including bootstrapping, but these fall outside the scope of this book.

The *MSEP* is a much more reliable estimate of the error rate of the model than the *MSE* of the training set and is a useful measure in order to evaluate the measurement uncertainty which is an important quantity in, for example, decision making (see also Chapter 16). Note that validation does not only apply to linear models, but to any kind of model, such as neural networks, which are described in Chapter 10.

### 6.2.3 *Curse of dimensionality: Small n, large p*

When we have a large number of regressor variables ($p$) and only a small number of observations $n$, it is often easy to obtain an apparently good fit of the model. A commonly used indicator of model fit is

$$R^2 = \frac{\sum \left[ y_i - \hat{y}_i \right]^2}{\sum \left[ y_i - \bar{y} \right]^2},$$

where $\bar{y}$ is the overall mean of the observations. Note that $R^2$ is closely related to *MSE*, but it is normalized by dividing it by the sum of squared differences from the overall mean. The value of $R^2$ is between 0 and 1, where a higher value indicates a better fit ($R^2 = 1$ indicates perfect fit).

In Figure 6.4 (left) it can be seen that $R^2$ is rather high for perceived naturalness VO ($n = 30$) using 20 arbitrary regressor variables from the MONAT dataset. However, in Figure 6.4 (right) we can see what happens if we estimate the model coefficients using 29 of the 30 observations and predict the other one with it and repeat this for all 30 points (30-fold or leave-one-out cross-validation). In this case the goodness-of-fit is called $Q^2$ and is similar to $R^2$. The main difference is that the

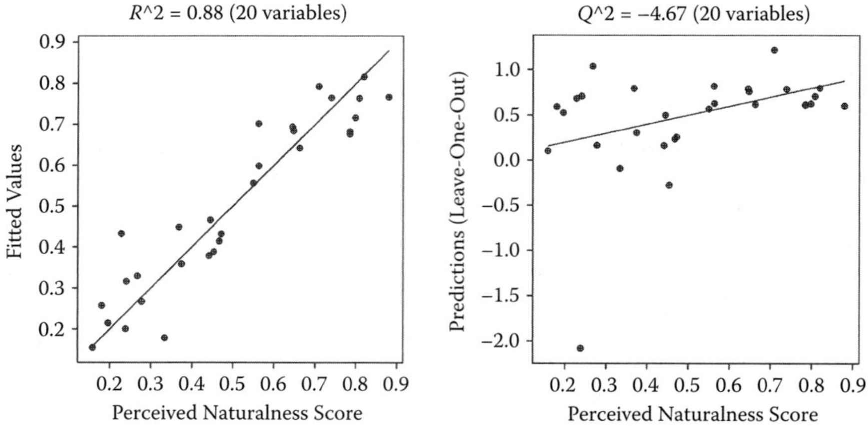


*Figure 6.4* Using 20 arbitrary variables of the vision-related X-features and the visually perceived naturalness (VO), a model can be built that describes the data well (left), but which is a very poor predictor (right) when tested on data that were not used for fitting the model.

observation $i$ was not used in the model estimation (similar to the difference between *MSE* and *MSEP*). If the model fits the data used in the training well, but is too specific for the data, the predicted value $\hat{y}_i$ can be far from the observed value $y_i$ if the $i$th observation was not in the model fit. This can clearly be seen in Figure 6.4 (right), where some predictions have several negative values and one value is really very far off (–2). Hence $Q^2$ can take negative values (this is impossible for $R^2$), which indicates that this model is even worse than the overall mean. It is clear that the model was fitted "to the noise" of the data.

If we have a large number of regressors and only a limited number of observations, it is always possible to obtain a good fit ($R^2$), because we have so many possibilities to fit the data in the high-dimensional space. However, the model thus obtained can be totally useless. So a high-dimensional space generally also requires a very high number of observations for a reliable fit, because the high-dimensional space is so empty. This is often referred to as the "curse of dimensionality."

A high number of observations is often not possible and procedures have been developed to cope with a large number of regressor variables and a limited number of observations. Particularly worth mentioning are partial least squares (PLS) and least absolute shrinkage and selection operator (LASSO; see, e.g., Hastie, Tibshirani, & Friedman, 2009). With PLS, all regressor variables are taken into account in the model, and this method is often used in highly correlated $X$-data, for example, as obtained from a spectrometer. With LASSO, the criterion is to minimize a penalized residual sum of squares:

$$\hat{\beta}^{LASSO} = \arg\min_{\beta} \sum_{i=1}^{N} \left\{ [y_i - X_i\beta]^2 + \lambda \sum_{j=1}^{P} |\beta_j| \right\},$$

where the *RSS* of the linear model gets a penalty equal to the sum of the absolute values of $\beta_1, \ldots, \beta_P$, multiplied with a shrinkage parameter $\lambda$. If $\lambda$ is zero, this is the normal linear regression; if $\lambda$ is infinite, all coefficients except the overall mean ($\beta_0$) become zero. This slight modification has a considerable impact, as it effectively functions as a variable selection procedure. In the MONAT project, the LASSO has been used to establish the relation between the response variable and the most relevant regressor variables.

### 6.2.4 Canonical correlation

Given a set (matrix) *X* and *Y* consisting of *p* and *q* variables, respectively, canonical correlation tries to find the linear relations within *X* and within *Y*, which give maximum correlation between them. The objective is to find a linear combination of the *x*-variables, say $u_1$, and a (different) linear combination of the *y*-variables, say $v_1$, so that the correlation between $u_1$ and $v_1$ is the highest attainable correlation of all possible linear combinations *u* of *X* and *v* of *Y*. In the next step, we try to find a second pair of linear combinations $(u_2,v_2)$, uncorrelated with the first pair, such that the correlation of this second pair is (conditionally) maximal, and so on, but of course no more than min(*p*,*q*) pairs can be found. An example of canonical correlation is given in Figure 6.5, where the three *y*-variables (VO, TO, and VT) were correlated with the touch-related variables of the *X*-matrix.

The figure shows the relation between the first canonical pair (left) and second canonical pair (right), with the linear combination of *X* on the *X*-axis and the linear combination of *Y* on the *Y*-axis. In Table 6.1 the correlation between the pair (*CA_Corrs*) and the % correlation (*%Corrs*), respectively, the cumulative percentage correlation (*Cum%Corrs*) is shown. Obviously, because *Y* has only three variables in this example, there can be no more than three pairs of canonical variables.

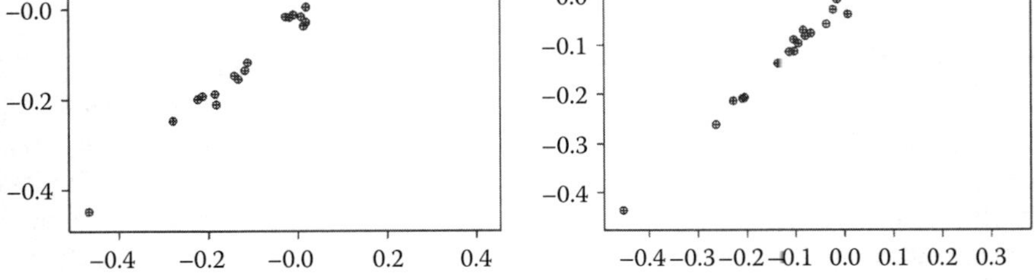


*Figure 6.5* The relation of the first (left) and second (right) canonical correlation pair is shown for the perceived naturalness Y (vision-only, touch only, and visiotactile) and the touch-related features XT are shown for 30 samples of the MONAT wood dataset.

*Table 6.1* Coronical correlation of MONAT dataset. (See also Figure 6.1.)

| *Pair* | *CA_Corrs* | *%Corrs* | *Cum%Corrs* |
|---|---|---|---|
| 1 | 0.9910 | 33.67 | 33.67 |
| 2 | 0.9893 | 33.61 | 67.28 |
| 3 | 0.9629 | 32.72 | 100.00 |

Canonical correlation produces maximally correlated linear combinations of $X$ and $Y$, but we should note these can be poor representations of the true structure of $X$ and $Y$. Furthermore, canonical correlation involves linear combinations of $y$-variables, but often you are interested in the variables themselves and in that case, you can better use linear regression.

## 6.3 Classification and clustering

### *6.3.1 Supervised classification—Linear discriminant analysis*

In many cases the response variable is not a continuous variable, but a grouping variable. For example, we can classify the MONAT wood samples in three groups: untreated wood, treated wood, and artificial products (imitation wood). For the analysis of data in groups, classification methods can be applied. The most often used classification method is linear discriminant analysis (LDA).

In LDA we assume that the different groups have different means/centroids for the $X$-variables, but the groups share a common covariance matrix $S$. The aim is to maximize the between-groups to within-groups variation. The covariance matrix $S$ is calculated by pooling the individual covariance matrices within each group $g$, that is, by forming a $p \times p$ matrix $S_g$ per group and pooling these covariance matrices $S_g$ over all groups (taking account of differences in $n_g$, the number of samples within each group $g$). The between-groups covariance matrix $G$ is calculated, using only the means for each group as data.

Next we try to maximize the ratio of the between-groups over the within-groups covariance:

$$\max_a \frac{a^T G a}{a^T S a}.$$

Put differently, try to find the largest eigenvectors for the nonsymmetric matrix $S^{-1}G$ using generalized eigenvector decomposition, taking into account the special structure of this matrix. The eigenvalues and eigenvectors can now be used to rotate and scale the original data to a space that maximizes the between-groups to within-groups variation. This can be referred to as canonical variate analysis as compared to principal component analysis. In this transformed space we can now calculate the distance of each observation to the group mean and classify the data point to the group that has the smallest distance to this point.

In Figure 6.6, a plot is shown for the wood sample data divided in three groups (untreated wood, treated wood, and artificial wood), with the scores for the first two

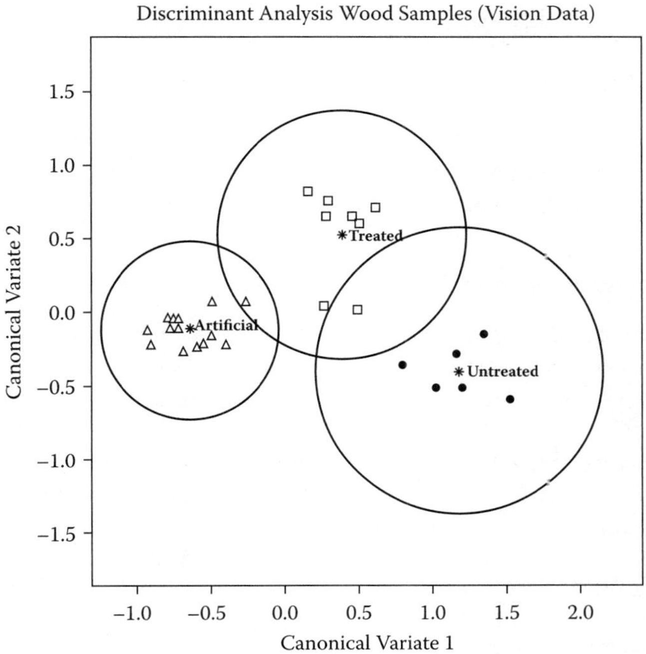


*Figure 6.6* In discriminant analysis we transform the data so that the between-groups to within-groups variation is maximized. The 30 samples of the MONAT wood dataset were divided into three classes: class 1 includes untreated wood panels (3 × 2 top left panels in Figure 6.1), class 2 includes the treated wood panels (4 × 2 top right panels), and the artificial woods on the bottom three rows are group 3. The scores for the first two canonical variates are shown for the vision-related physical features.

canonical variates of the vision-related features of the *X*-dataset. The plot also shows the corresponding group means and their 95% confidence intervals.

If we have many, often correlated, variables ($p$ is large), the matrix $S$ might not be of full rank. This means that its inverse is not defined. A solution to this is to regularize the matrix $S$ with the regularization parameter $\gamma$ as $S(\gamma) = \gamma S + (1 - \gamma)\hat{\sigma}^2 I$, where $\hat{\sigma}^2 I$ indicates the elements on the main diagonal of the matrix $S$, that is, the variances of the $p$ variables.

Many other classification methods exists, including

- *Quadratic discriminant analysis*, which allows for different covariance matrices per group instead of a common pooled covariance matrix W. Because the number of parameters is very large, $p(p - 1)/2$ for each class or group, regularization is often needed, for example, as: $S_g(\alpha) = \alpha S_g + (1 - \alpha) S$ with $S_g$ the previously mentioned covariance matrix within group $g$.
- *k-Nearest-neighbor classifier*, which classifies an object to the same class as the majority of closest points of group-size $k$. Note that the definition

of distance (closest) is not straightforward. See also the next paragraph on clustering and dissimilarity.

- *Artificial neural networks*, which allow for nonlinearity of the classifier. See also Chapter 10 in this book.

Most classification methods with a large number of variables (high $p$) are rather sensitive to noise, therefore it is strongly advised to always use (cross-)validation.

### 6.3.2 Unsupervised classification—Clustering

In supervised classification such as LDA, prior information on the class labels of the objects is needed. Sometimes, such information is not available and class labels need to be assigned to the objects without prior information; that is, we want to infer the class labels from the data themselves. A logical approach is to form clusters of data points that are considered to be close together. The clusters can then be regarded as classes formed by the data, hence the term unsupervised classification.

Different clustering approaches exist, but in this paragraph we only consider hierarchical clustering. In hierarchical cluster analysis we wish to perform the clustering in such a way that objects in the same cluster are more like each other (i.e., more similar) than they are to other objects in other clusters. The notion of similarity or dissimilarity is crucial in this context. The method forms clusters consisting of subclusters in a hierarchical way, with the individual objects as the lowest level of clusters of size 1.

### 6.3.3 Dissimilarity measure

Hierarchical clustering starts with a measure of dissimilarity $d$ between the objects or clusters. If we have measured attributes of objects, we can calculate dissimilarities between objects, taking into account the scale of the variables. Many different measures of (dis)similarity exist (Gower, 1985). For interval and ordinal scale variables, common measures are the Cityblock (L1) or Euclidean (L2) distance, divided by the range (difference between largest and smallest object) to obtain a value between 0 and 1. For binary variables, the Jaccard dissimilarity is often used: if both objects have a score 1, the dissimilarity is 0; when the scores are opposite, the dissimilarity is 1 and if both scores are 0, the entry is ignored. For nominal variables, the most common dissimilarity measure is simple matching: if both objects have the same score, the dissimilarity is 0, else it is 1.

In some cases, we do not obtain measurements of attributes of the objects, but we directly assess distances between objects. This gives rise to the direct construction of a dissimilarity or distance matrix. In Chapter 9, a special method dealing with subjective (Fechnarian) distances is described.

After having obtained a dissimilarity matrix between all pairs of objects, we can group (clusters of) objects together based on their dissimilarity. Different criteria exist for merging clusters, such as

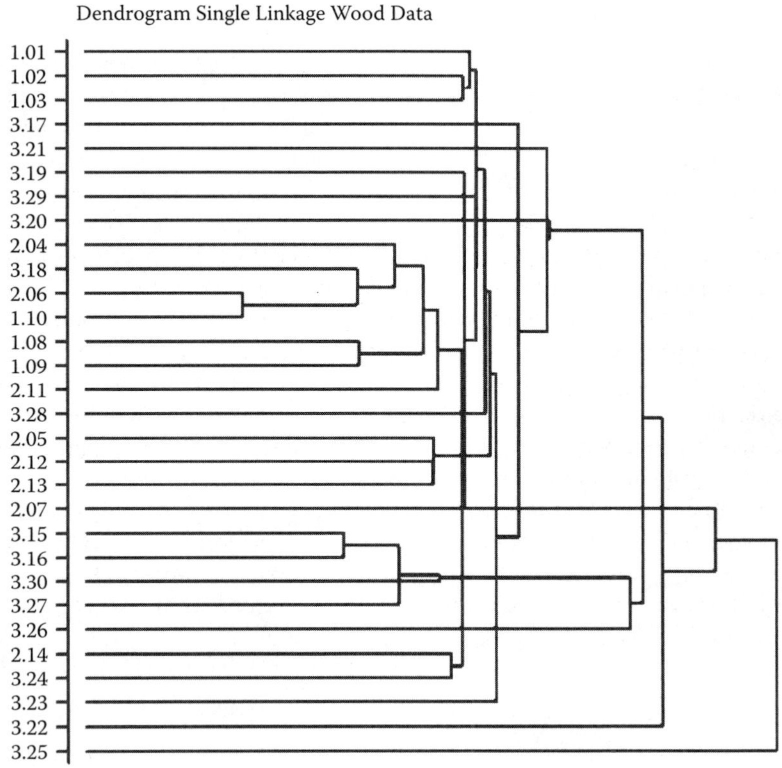


*Figure 6.7* From the MONAT wood samples, the vision-related physical variables have been selected to calculate a Euclidean distance matrix among the 30 objects. The distance matrix is used for hierarchical single-linkage clustering, which means that clusters are based on the minimum distance between any two objects in the clusters. The integral part of the numbers (e.g., 1 in 1.01) refers to (1) untreated wood, (2) treated wood, and (3) artificial wood. The decimal part refers to the panel number (1, …, 30) in Figure 6.1.

- *Single linkage:* Minimum distance between any two objects in the clusters.
- *Complete linkage:* Maximum distance between any two objects in the clusters.
- *Group average linkage:* Average distance is taken over all the objects in the two merging clusters.

In Figure 6.7 the result of hierarchical clustering is shown for the MONAT dataset. Setting a certain threshold (vertical line in the dendrogram) can give an objective criterion for grouping, but this is not always straightforward. Another disadvantage of dendrograms is that the positions of clusters and objects within clusters are not unique.

Other popular clustering approaches include K-means, fuzzy C-means and neural network approaches as self-organizing maps. If the data within a cluster can be assumed to follow a normal distribution, powerful methods exist to deal with such mixtures of normal distributions, such as the expectation-maximization algorithm.

### 6.3.4 Principal coordinates analysis

The dissimilarity matrix that was calculated in the previous paragraph can be visualized in a dendrogram. Another approach is to map the matrix into a lower-dimensional space, much like trying to reconstruct a 2-D roadmap from a city-distance table. This is the topic of multidimensional scaling, where the objective is to find a set of coordinates whose interpoint distances match, as closely as possible, those of the dissimilarity matrix. The coordinate system can be interpreted in much the same way as a map: for example, if the distance between objects in the data matrix is small, their points will appear close together in a graph using these coordinates.

In Figure 6.8 a metric scaling method is shown for the wood samples dissimilarity matrix: principal coordinates analysis. The class 1 wood samples are close together in this map, although this information is, of course, not used in the construction of the map. The calculation of principal coordinates does not require an iterative approach and is therefore fast and unique. It can be used as a starting point for many other (nonmetric) multidimensional scaling methods.

In the same graph, the minimum spanning tree is shown connecting the $n$ objects, where every object is linked to the same tree (connected network). The tree does not contain closed loops and, of all trees with one object at every node, it is the one whose links have minimum total length. The links include all those that join nearest

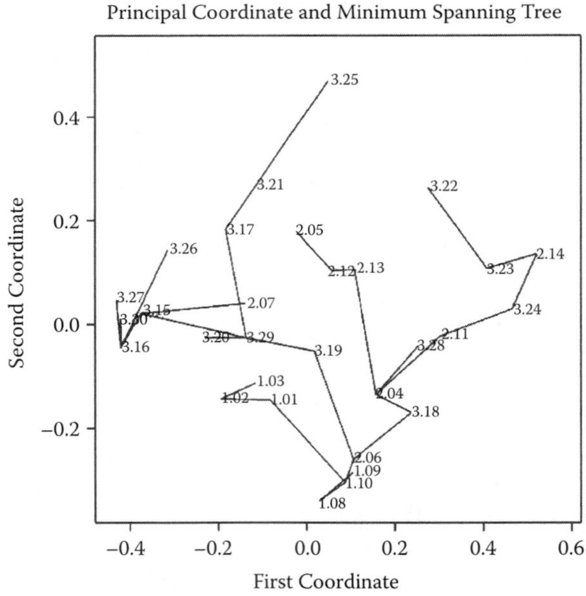


*Figure 6.8* The distance matrix used for clustering is shown here in a principal coordinate system. Also shown is the minimum spanning tree, connecting close neighbors. The tree can reveal regions in the coordinate system in which distance is badly distorted and is closely related to the single linkage dendrogram of Figure 6.7.

neighbors and the minimum spanning tree is closely related to the single linkage dendrogram. Minimum spanning trees are useful to reveal regions in the coordinate system in which distance is badly distorted.

## 6.4 Conclusions

In the previous sections we have given an overview and application of several common multivariate data analysis methods. Some methods are predominantly aimed at gaining insight to the data at hand, for example, by reducing the dimensionality of the data. PCA is very popular for this. Other methods are aimed at relating one set of features to another. One approach is to relate a single continuous $y$-variate with many $X$-measurements, which is the case in linear regression. This can be extended to model multiple $y$-variates simultaneously. If we have a large number of (possibly highly correlated) regressor variables and a small number of objects, it is better to refer to methods such as LASSO or PLS. If the objects form groups and we have that information available, we can use classification methods, such as linear discriminant analysis.

In canonical correlation the aim is to find pairs of linear relations in a multivariate $X$- and $Y$-dataset, instead of trying to predict one or more $y$-variates from the $X$-data.

If no prior information is present and the aim is to classify or cluster objects, cluster methods such as hierarchical clustering can be used. For hierarchical clustering a dissimilarity matrix is needed. Such a matrix can be constructed directly in the experiment (e.g., using pairwise comparisons) or can be formed from a set of measurement data. Dissimilarity matrices can be visualized and interpreted using multidimensional scaling methods.

When dealing with multivariate data, it is important to realize that high-dimensional spaces are generally very sparse and special care needs to be taken when interpreting the results. Methods specifically developed for use in high-dimensional data, such as PLS and LASSO, are to be preferred and (cross-)validation has to be used at all times if possible.

## References


Goodman, T., Montgomery, R., Bialek, A., Forbes, A., Rides, M., Whitaker, A., Overvliet, K., McGlone, F., & Heijden, G. W. A. M. van der. (2008). The measurement of naturalness. In *12th IMEKO TC1& TC7 Joint Symposium on Man Science & Measurement*, Annecy, France.

Gower, J. C. (1985). Measures of similarity, dissimilarity, and distance. In S. Kotz, N. L. Johnson, & C. B. Read (Eds.), *Encyclopaedia of statistical sciences* (Vol. V, pp. 397–405). New York: Wiley.

Härdle, W., & Simar, L. (2007). *Applied multivariate statistical analysis* (2nd ed.). Berlin: Springer.

Hastie, T., Tibshirani, R. & Friedman, J. (2009). *The elements of statistical learning: Data mining, inference, and prediction* (2nd ed.). Springer, Berlin.

Johnson, R. A., and Wichern, D. W. (2002). *Applied multivariate statistical analysis*. Upper Saddle River, NJ: Pearson.

Mardia, K. V., Kent, J. T., & Bibby, J. M. (1979). *Multivariate analysis*. London: Academic Press.

Overvliet, K. E., Soto-Faraco, S., Whitaker, T. A., Johnstone Sorensen, L., McGlone, F., & Heijden, G. W. A. M. van der (2008). Measuring perception of naturalness. In A. J. Spink, et al. (Eds.), *Proceedings of Measuring Behavior 2008* (Maastricht, The Netherlands, August 26–29), pp. 86–87.

Tabachnick, B. G., & Fidell, L. S. (2007). *Using multivariate statistics* (5th ed.). London: Allyn & Bacon.

# 7 The prospects for measurement in infinite-dimensional psychological spaces

## *Modern notions for geometric person measurements in finite and infinite dimensional spaces*

*James T. Townsend, Devin Burns, and Lei Pei*
Department of Psychology
Indiana University Bloomington
Bloomington, Indiana, USA

## 7.1 Introduction

This chapter is about certain spatial types of measurement of people, as carried out in the social and biological sciences. The global issue for us is perceptual classification and we specialize on spatial, for instance, geometric or topological, aspects. We offer more detail below, but for now, we simply note that classification is the assignment of an object, typically presented to one or more of our sensory modalities, to one of some number (perhaps infinite!) of classes or designated sets, often names. Because in general terms, this is neither more nor less than a function or mapping of a set of things (stimuli, memories, etc.) into another (the names or classifications), this makes this concept extremely broad. Thus, classification covers many specific activities of psychological interest. Some important ones are the following:

1. A famous form of classification is that of *categorization*, where a bunch of objects is partitioned so that each object is separately assigned to a single (typically) unique category. There are many kinds of categorization but one of special importance is usually given its own title.
2. *Identification* is where each category has exactly one member (this may be rare in the real life). We can perform an experiment where each person has exactly one name and each name is given to exactly one person, but of course, in the real world, the name of "John" is given to thousands of people. In most of the interesting psychological situations, classification is

made difficult by any number of factors. This could be because learning of the assignments is incomplete, such as in a recognition memory experiment. In this case the presented stimulus may be very easy to perceive, but the learned patterns may have become quite noisy, making the recognition task challenging. Other situations include some kind of added noise, randomness, or even very brief exposure periods.

3. *Yes–no signal detection* is the specification by an observer of whether a signal has been presented. There are only two responses: "YES" versus "NO" could be used either with faulty memory (the celebrated "Old" versus "New" memory-recognition experiment) or with simply "hard-to-detect" physical stimuli.
4. Typically with *psychological scaling*, the observer gives ratings on one or more aspects of the stimuli. For instance, one might simply be asked to report a number that seems to represent the psychological magnitude of an aspect of a stimulus, such as how happy a particular face looks (see below for more on this). Or, as is often the case in multidimensional scaling (explained a bit later), the observer might be asked about the psychological similarity of two or more objects. An old anthology, but one still held in high esteem, with several chapters that are relevant to our present enterprise is Volume I of the *Handbook of Mathematical Psychology* (Luce, Bush, & Galanter, 1963). The philosophy of science of the present authors regarding measurement and modeling of people and an expansion of some of themes, can be located in Townsend and Thomas (1993).

All the chapters in this volume on "person measurement" present and discuss valuable types of measurement of people, a number of them involving classification, usually pertaining to a finite number of aspects or dimensions. Section 7.2 starts by discussing the foundational aspects of measurement on people and considers such finite situations. Section 7.3 concerns multidimensional scaling, and also focuses on a finite number of psychological dimensions. It is meant not only to set the stage for what is to come, but also provide an elementary tutelage on the subject and to guide the prospective user of these tools to some of the classical literature.

That being said, it is our belief that almost none of the interesting aspects of perception refer at their most basic level to finite spaces. Rather, we feel that infinite-dimensional spaces are required for a suitably theoretical milieu for human perception and beyond that, to cognition and action as well! For clarity we solely emphasize perception in this chapter. The topic of finite- versus infinite-dimensional spaces is taken up in Section 7.4. As a consequence of this stance, an important topic is the mathematical issues that might arise when we inquire about the ability of people to extract finite-dimensional information, even the value on a single dimension, from objects that by their very nature reside in infinite-dimensional spaces. This question is addressed in Section 7.5.

A huge literature exists in mathematics (mostly for physics and engineering) on infinite dimensional spaces with particular relevance to functions in spaces that possess coordinates at right angles to each other. It is called *functional analysis.* Such spaces typically are inherently flat, without curvature. A revolutionary movement took place in the late nineteenth and early twentieth centuries concerned with spaces that could be curved, even with spaces whose curvature could change from point to point. We refer to Riemannian manifolds. Section 7.6 introduces the concept of manifolds as gently as possible. This kind of space proved to be exactly the appropriate setting for Einstein's theory of general relativity. We go out on a limb and suggest that manifolds may be important for human perception and cognition and action as well.

Section 7.7 takes up the potential extension of probability theory and stochastic processes to infinite-dimensional spaces: Everything we know about people, from the level of a single neuron (and lower) to the actions of the people of an entire nation are probabilistic. Hence, any theory or model whether finite or infinite must sooner or later broach this topic. There is a knowledge base for probabilities in infinite-dimensional spaces that goes back to the early part of the twentieth century, with tremendous developments occurring mid-century. This knowledge applies immediately to the types of spaces found in functional analysis, mentioned just above. There is some work going on, in addition, developing laws of probability for finite-dimensional manifolds and really cutting-edge work in probability and stochastic processes on infinite-dimensional manifolds.

Section 7.8 treats the very special and extraordinarily important case of classification models based on functional analysis, dynamic systems theory, differential equations, and stochastic processes. We then delve more deeply into the mathematics and take a look at applying these techniques to the classification field in Section 7.9. The chapter concludes with Section 7.10, which is a brief review of where we've been and why, and an attempt to set these new methods in their proper context.

The early parts of this chapter leave out the mathematics. This is not only because of somewhat limited space but also because there are scores and sometimes hundreds of articles and books on the topic. As we move along, we delve into material that is likely new to many investigators and students devoted to measurement on people. Although our greater use of mathematics as we progress may make the going a little tougher for some readers, it also affords a more rigorous and well-defined landscape for those willing to make the journey. We accompany the verbal and quantitative developments with illustrations to aid in the readers' interpretations and intuitions. In this way, we hope that everyone will gain something from our presentation.

## 7.2 Foundational measurement

A central characteristic of measurement in these regions, as opposed to vast regions of physics, is the absence of the opportunity to gather data based on strong measurement scales (e.g., Roberts, Patterson, Thomson, & Levey, 1969). This single characteristic has been the subject of hundreds of papers and books, with roots in first, from the physical science point of view, Campbell's famous book in which he develops a theory of fundamental measurement as a mapping between numerical systems and those things we wish to measure. In his theory, for something to be measurable, those things must have an ordering and the combination of those things must follow the same properties as the addition of numbers, which is often not satisfied by the things we wish to measure in psychology.

A fundamental measurement system as defined by Campbell implies a ratio scale (Suppes & Zinnes, 1963). One of the earliest proposals that the scales typically employed by physics, that is, "ratio scales" or "extensive measurement" might not be the only possibilities for rigorous application of numbers in the social or biological sciences was put forth by Stevens (1951). Later, this idea was picked up by mathematical psychologists, mathematicians, and logicians with the ensuing development of an axiomatic basis not only for extensive measurement but also the weaker (and in order of decreasing strength), absolute scale, ratio scale (extensive measurement), interval scale, ordinal scale, and so-called nominal scale. The only other scale of note is the absolute scale, which is the strongest of all (e.g., for more on these topics, see the early work and citations in Suppes & Zinnes, 1963; Krantz, Luce, Suppes, & Tversky, 1971; Pfanzagl, 1968).

A seminal concept in the theory is that numbers considered as measurements should reflect the regularities of the natural phenomena that are being measured, while retaining properties of the number system (perhaps including arithmetic conditions and the like). Hence, for some purposes, an interval scale, such as Celsius or Fahrenheit will suffice to study particular properties of a phenomenon. However, for work, say in thermodynamics, it may well be that a form of the Kelvin scale may be required. A fascinating consequent duality in the theory is that the stronger the scale, the fewer mathematical operations can be carried out on the observed measurements without distortion to the relationships between the numbers and the phenomena. An example of a permitted transformation on a ratio scale, like mass, is multiplication by a positive constant (e.g., changing pounds to kilograms). This leaves a ratio of any two measurements invariant: it is a "meaningful operation." However, calculating the ratio of yesterday's temperature with today's temperature, measured in Celsius, will not be the same as when the units are altered to Fahrenheit: meaningfulness is lost. In this interval scale we instead need to take a ratio of differences to retain meaningful results. To tersely complete the picture, absolute scales allow no transformation whatsoever and they possess no units. Counting is perhaps the prototypical example of an absolute scale: one doesn't change a "3" when one counts 3 candy bars or anything else. Of course, a change of the name of "three" from one language to another is okay! The next strongest scale is afforded the name "ordinal scale."

Ordinal measurement permits any monotonic (order-preserving) transformation to be made on the measurement numbers, but only order can be established: comparisons such as ratios or differences are meaningless. It has been debated whether the social or biological sciences may be forever confined to ordinal measurement. For now, we mainly investigate aspects of measurement that do not touch on this axiomatic theory but also a few that do. Obviously, even a modest glimpse at the entire edifice (not to mention the debates) would take several hundred pages. One of the shortcomings of the approach has been the absence of a generally accepted error theory, which would permit the erection of a statistical theory of inference within the approach. We should also mention that many statisticians, psychometricians, and others have either argued against the idea that measurement scales are needed (e.g., Lord & Novick, 1968; Townsend & Ashby, 1984) or simply ignored it. Nonetheless, from the authors' point of view, it is important to keep these considerations in mind.[1]

## 7.3 A brief introduction to multidimensional scaling

A popular method of inferring geometrical structure from data in psychology (and related disciplines) is called Multidimensional Scaling, or MDS. MDS is a set of mathematical techniques that can be used to reveal the underlying structure in data. These methods provide a spatial configuration of the data points, which allows a researcher to interpret patterns and regularities relatively easily. There are numerous (but not quite infinite!) variations of these techniques, and here we only touch on some of the most important, general, and famous methods.

To be able to represent psychological data in a geometrical form, we first need to establish a notion of "distance." There are many different ways of doing this, and careers have been spent debating which is the most appropriate. One of the most straightforward methods is to conduct a similarity experiment in which subjects rate how dissimilar different stimuli are from each other. The distance should then be a monotonic transformation of this dissimilarity, so that the more similar objects are the less distance there is between them. After establishing a matrix of all the pairwise distances between stimuli, computer programs can be used to infer where each stimulus is located in a space in relation to the others. Most modern statistical computing packages, such as SPSS, will contain a program (ALSCAL is a popular example) that displays these results for you.

But what results does it display exactly? This brings us to another topic of debate in MDS, that of dimension (The concept of which is discussed in more detail below). When the computer infers the positions of the data points in space, we have to tell it in which space to put them. Euclidean space is the most commonly used and simplest, but there is no reason why the data should necessarily be Euclidean, and various spaces and metrics have been imposed for different domain applications. Sticking with Euclidean space for now, it must be decided by the investigator how many dimensions to use. When fitting the points, MDS programs attempt to minimize the "stress" in the system, which roughly means how well the extrapolated geometric distances conform to the distances derived from the dissimilarity data. A high stress value means that the model is not fitting the data. Clearly, a model in a higher-dimensional space will always have less stress than a more constrained model. We can easily see that lower-dimensional models are included as subspaces of higher-dimensional models, so this must always be true.

So how does one know how many dimensions to use? Theoretical expectations can be brought to bear here. If your stimuli vary along only, say, $n$ dimensions, then an $n$-D model may be most appropriate (ignoring more complicated instances of interaction for now). An exception could occur if the brain is unable to separate the $n$ dimensions. In that case, a subspace consisting of $k < n$ dimensions will suffice. In no case would we expect the estimated dimension to be $k > n$, although an inappropriate metric might make it appear to be so. For example, suppose the psychological space corresponding to two physical dimensions is a 2-D hemisphere embedded in 3-D coordinate system. Then, the inappropriate Euclidean metric could make it seem that three dimensions are better than two. If one has the correct metric in hand, the stress of the two-dimensional model should be almost as small as that for three- or greater-dimensional models. This subjective comparison among the stresses of different models can be used as the deciding factor even in the lack of theoretical expectations. In this uninformed case, the experimenter should pick the model such that all subsequent models of greater dimensionality yield only a small reduction in stress relative to the previous reductions.

If all of psychological space were nicely Euclidean with separable dimensions, then all of this would be fine and we could construct high-fidelity maps for every dataset. As I'm sure you've guessed, this is sadly (but more interestingly) not the case. What if psychological dissimilarity data are not directly associated with a metric? For instance, it could be that decisional biases intrude that violate properties associated with any metric (e.g., Townsend, 1971). In such a case, it is sometimes possible to extricate the true dissimilarity apart from the decisional influences. In any event, we need to know what the properties of a valid distance measure are. The three axioms that any metric must satisfy are:

Minimality: $d(a,b) \geq d(a,a) = 0$: No pair of objects is more similar to each other than any object is to itself, and the latter distance is 0.

Symmetry: $d(a,b) = d(b,a)$: Nancy's face is as similar to Joan's as Joan's face is to Nancy's.

The triangle inequality: $d(a,c) \leq d(a,b) + d(b,c)$: The political distance between Obama's world-view and George W. Bush's is less than or equal to the distance between Obama's and Franklin D. Roosevelt's plus that between Roosevelt's and Bush's.

It could be that one or more of the axioms is violated due to perturbation by a decisional bias, or it could happen in a more fundamental, systematic sense. The mathematical psychologist Amos Tversky pointed out that all three of these axioms can be routinely violated in basic psychological experiments (Tversky, 1977). Minimality is violated whenever stimuli differ in their self-similarity. Symmetry is often violated in similarity data as well, especially if one stimulus is seen as more broad or general than the other, perhaps including the latter as a subclass. For example, the word "poodle" would be seen as more similar to the word "dog" than the reverse.

The triangle inequality is harder to refute, because it is a quantitative statement, and similarity data is inherently ordinal. It has been shown that trivial manipulations of data can produce satisfaction of the first two assumptions, so the triangle equality often plays a major role in testing for the presence of a metric. Although there have been more rigorous expositions of the subject, Tversky gives a quick intuitive argument for why we shouldn't believe that the triangle equality will necessarily hold in all cases. Assume that the perceptual distance from Cuba to Russia should be small for political reasons (remember, 1977), and the perceptual distance from Cuba to Jamaica should be small for geographic reasons. The triangle inequality would then force the distance from Jamaica to Russia to also be fairly small, which we would not expect.

One reaction to these arguments has been to impose a different metric on the space. Instead of using the standard Euclidean metric to compute distances, many other functions have been used. A common family of metrics takes the form:

$$d_{ij} = \sum_{m=1}^{n} \left| \left( x_{im} - x_{jm} \right)^{r} \right|^{\frac{1}{r}}.$$

These are commonly called power metrics. When $r = 2$ we have the standard Euclidean metric, and $r = 1$ is what is known as the city block metric. In this metric distances are computed as the sum of the projected distances in each orthogonal dimension (as in a city, when you can only travel in orthogonal dimensions, instead of as the crow flies). In this metric, the triangle inequality becomes an equality. If we consider values of $r < 1$, the triangle inequality is now reversed. This can be interpreted to saying that traveling along one dimension is "faster" than traveling along a diagonal path. These metrics can be better understood if we consider graphs of unit distance, shown in Figure 7.1. In these graphs every point corresponds to an equal distance from the origin.

Tversky offered up a different approach when he rigorously developed the *feature contrast model*. In this model, the similarity between two objects is a function of the features that the objects have in common, minus the features that differ between them. The feature contrast model captures the intuitive idea that identical shared features decrease psychological dissimilarity between two objects, a property unattainable with metric-based differences. This relatively simple model is sufficient to account for each of the previously mentioned violations of the metric axioms.

One of the primary difficulties involved in modeling psychological data is that the perceptual phenomena that we seek to describe are confounded by the decisional processes inherent in any experimental situation. The classic theory designed to tease these aspects apart is known as Signal Detection Theory (SDT). This theory was established in 1966 by John Swets and David Green, building on earlier work done by radar researchers. In this methodology, participants are asked to discern

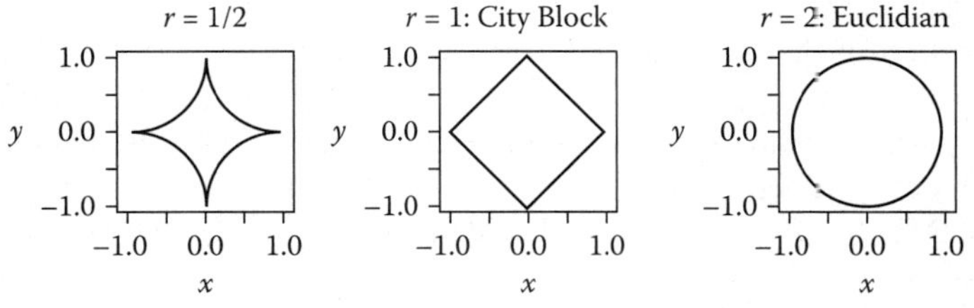


*Figure 7.1* Each graph shows all points with a unit distance from the origin.

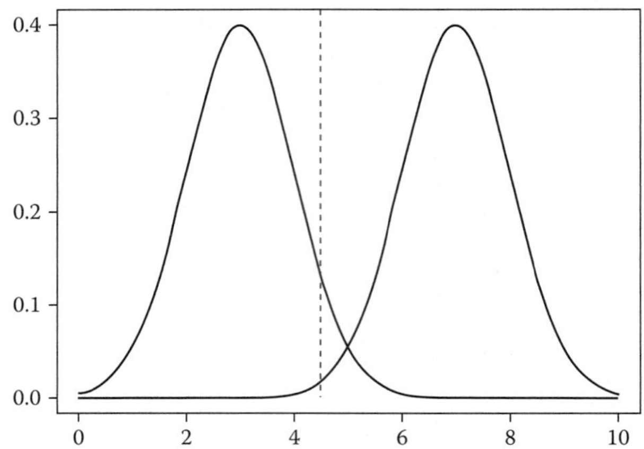


*Figure 7.2* A typical SDT graph of signal and noise densities. The dotted line is the decision criterion.

"signal" trials from "noise" trials. The experimenter can then find values for the participant's perceptual discriminability and their decision criterion. These variables can be independently manipulated to study various decisional or perceptual qualities. In SDT, stimuli are considered to be perceived probabilistically. Instead of each stimulus corresponding to a single fixed point in some space, as in MDS models, stimuli have corresponding probability density functions.

A typical example is shown in Figure 7.2. The left curve corresponds to a noise trial, and the right to a signal trial. The vertical dotted line represents a decision criterion, where a participant will change from calling everything on the left "noise" to calling everything on the right a "signal". We can see that the participant will be incorrect for the stimuli belonging to the noise distribution that fall on the right of the criterion (called false alarms) and also for the stimuli from the signal distribution that fall to the left of the criterion (called misses). Shifting the criterion left or right (which can be achieved by altering the experimental instructions) will result in a tradeoff between these two kinds of wrong answers. The only way to increase the total number of correct answers is to increase the distance between the means of the two distributions, which is referred to as $d'$. This theory offers a natural explanation for the confusions between stimuli while also elucidating the differences between perceptual and decisional effects, which are measured with $d'$ and the criterion, respectively.

A limitation of the SDT method as typically employed is that stimuli are only allowed to vary along a single dimension, making the methodology applicable to a paucity of psychological experiments. In 1986, Gregory Ashby and James Townsend developed a multidimensional extension of SDT that they call General Recognition Theory (GRT). In GRT, the probability density functions associated with stimuli are multidimensional, so stimuli can vary along as many dimensions as desired. Because of the difficulty involved in making four- or more dimensional graphs, let us consider the case where stimuli vary along just two dimensions. Figure 7.3a shows

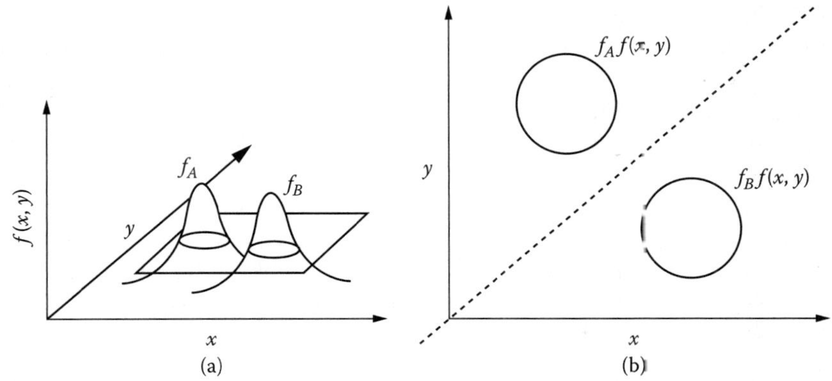


*Figure 7.3* (a) Three-dimensional densities of two distributions; (b) an equal likelihood plot of the same two densities.

the probability densities of two stimuli that vary along dimensions $x$ and $y$ (Ashby & Townsend, 1986). The plane shown passing through both functions describes the equal probability contours of the two distributions. Because the shape of the intersection of this plane with a given density (a circle in this case) does not change depending on the height of the plane (it will only expand or contract), it is useful to graph just these intersections. This is shown for our example case in Figure 7.3b.

We can see that this latter graph can easily be mapped onto our earlier understanding of signal detection theory. The dotted line once again represents the decision criterion; the only difference is that it now depends on both dimensions (the decision on the $x$ dimension depends on the level of the $y$ dimension). Even though the decision for each dimension is dependent upon the other, in this case both stimuli are *perceptually independent*. We mean by this is that the perceptual effects of one dimension do not influence those of the other dimension. If this property were violated, we would see that in the graph of equal probability contours. Instead of seeing circles, which portend perceptual independence, we would see skewed ellipses that would point up-right for positive correlation and down-right for negative. Having positively dependent variables means that the greater the perceptual effects are on one dimension, the greater they will be on the other.

It is important to note that perceptual independence is logically distinct from having a decision criterion on one dimension that is not influenced by the other dimension. This latter property is referred to in GRT as *decisional separability.* A third, also logically distinct formalization of the idea of independence is called *perceptual separability.* This property means that the perceptual effects of one dimension are not dependent on the other. This definition sounds quite similar to that of perceptual independence, but the difference is that independence is a within stimulus condition, while perceptual separability is between stimuli.

Although GRT approaches the modeling of psychological phenomena in a fundamentally different way from MDS, because of its generality and versatility it has been shown that standard Euclidean MDS is actually a special case contained within the GRT framework (Ashby, 1988). When constrained in this manner, GRT will necessarily be required to assume the metric axioms that we examined earlier. However, in the fully generalized GRT model there is no need to make these assumptions. In GRT, the overlapping regions of multiple stimulus densities correspond to where they are confused with each other, rather than relying on a distance metric. Because these confusions are a function of both the means and standard deviations of the densities, the probability of a correct recognition is not necessarily monotonic with the distance between the perceptual means. Other metric violations can also be accounted for to yield an accurate description of the data in a wide variety of circumstances (e.g., Ashby, 1992; Kadlec & Townsend, 1992; Thomas, 1999, 2003).

## 7.4 Dimensions: Finite and infinite

The concept of dimension really only began to assume a rigorous treatment in the late nineteenth century. There are now several mathematical approaches to dimensionality. First, let us just define *space* as some set of points, where a point is a *primitive*, that is, an undefined entity. The point may in fact, be given in more immediately comprehensible terms, but need not: often it can gain its meaningfulness through a list of axioms about what structure it exists within (e.g., on the space itself) or operations that can be done on it, and so on. The easiest approach to understand is probably the one that defines dimension as "the minimum number of real numbers that can be employed to define a point in the space."[4] Then an infinite-dimensional space is one that requires a *denumerable* (i.e., can be put in one-to-one correspondence with an infinite set of integers) or *nondenumerable* set of numbers (e.g., the irrational numbers, products of such sets and so on), to indicate a specific point in the original space. Of course, this definition requires some sort of function that relates the points in the space to numbers, and that is far from always the most natural tack to take with some spaces. Nonetheless, it is the most straightforward definition for our purposes. Our definition of a physical or psychological dimension is that it be representable by a possibly bounded interval on the real line.

Infinite-dimensional spaces, although frequently obeying many precepts found in finite spaces, sometimes demand special care and tactics, and occasionally simply act in seemingly bizarre ways relative to finite spaces. A natural question from readers is likely to be why we need infinite-dimensional concepts and especially in spatial terms. Thus there appear to be a finite, if unbelievably huge, number of fundamental particles in the universe. (However particles are defined by modern physics, and in spite of the particle-wave duality of quantum theory, and the definition of "fundamental" has altered over the past century with, string theory notwithstanding, no clear end in sight.) However, infinite-dimensional spaces are a necessity for theory in modern science, including physics. One of the arguments for infinite-dimensional models is that mathematical descriptions when the points number in the millions or billions, are simpler or more elegant, depending on the uses of the model. The same goes for spaces of very high dimension. Thus, Newtonian mechanics enjoys the artifice of continuous trajectories (where a trajectory contains a nondenumerable number of points) of objects in, say, 3-D space, although a modern quantum description might look quite different.

Most functions that even high school students meet are defined on an infinite space, that of the real numbers (the latter being nondenumerable as we saw above, for it is made up of a denumerable set, the integers plus the rational numbers and the irrational numbers). Furthermore, the most useful of functions, such as the set of all continuous functions on the real line, are themselves infinite, with the latter set having the same dimensionality as the real line itself! In fact, the ubiquitous appearance of continuous (and often, smooth, i.e., differentiable to a high or infinite degree) functions in science by itself forms a powerful argument for the inclusion of infinite-dimensional spaces in psychology. Whether or not the theorist looks to functions, and we welcome it (e.g., see Townsend, Solomon, Wenger, & Spencer-Smith, 2001; Townsend & Spencer-Smith, 2004; Townsend, Aisbett, & Busemeyer, 2005), even a kind of common-sense consideration of such objects as the set of all faces seems to call for infinite-dimensional spaces (see especially the first of the list immediately above). Even though the number of faces on earth is finite, it is clearly possible in principle to create an infinite number of faces. Interestingly, even the modern approaches to approximation and numerical analysis, employ as a fundamental underpinning, the structures of infinite-dimensional function spaces. And, psychologists and statisticians are beginning to work out statistical procedures and theories that are appropriate for interesting sets of functions (see, e.g., Ramsay & Silverman, 2006).

## 7.5 Inserting or extracting finite psychological dimensions into (out of) an infinite-dimensional space

Now, there are many directions we could take from here. An important one is: Is it possible to think of finite-dimensional spaces as sub-parts of infinite-dimensional spaces? This would be a boon for psychophysical scaling because it means that it would not be unnatural to think and work with finite psychological spaces, even if the "real" description demands infinitude. In fact, given that almost all real stimuli appear to be objects from infinite-dimensional spaces, it is clear that our 150 years or so of finite-dimensional psychophysics would lie on a very shaky foundation indeed if, say, a dimension such as visual area or hue were not, first of all, mathematically separable in some sense from the more complex (infinite-dimensional) signal of which it is a part, and secondly, the biological entity (e.g., the reader) was not able to pluck this information from the signal. Thus, visual area of the surface of a dinosaur is not only computable from the complicated space of all dinosaurs but the visual system of a human can approximate that size, thus extricating the size dimension from this point of that space. In the case of hue, the actual signal may be a continuum of wave lengths from the light spectrum, yet the visual system computes a composite hue obeying the laws of color perception.

Due to space concerns here (not infinite-dimensional!), we only concern ourselves with the situation where a psychological dimension corresponds to a physical dimension. Of course, a physical dimension itself may or may not be very useful in science. For instance, products of powers of measurements, with the power being a rational number of basic physical dimensions (usually mass, length, and time) constitute new dimensions but only a relatively small number of these are useful in physical laws (see, e.g., Chapter 10 in Krantz et al., 1971).

Consider a space $X$ that is infinite-dimensional according to the above discussion. Then to elicit a physical dimension that might (or might not) make up a psychological dimension, we simply need to map an interval $(a,b)$ into $X$ as in $f(x)$ where $x$ is contained in $(a, b)$ and $f(x)$ is contained in $X$. We write this more compactly as $f$: $(a,b) \rightarrowtail X$. Although perfectly logical, this definition of a dimension as contained in $X$ is not very intuitive. To unpack this situation a bit more, consider a depiction of infinite-dimensional spaces based on a generalization of a so-called Cartesian product of dimensions. Thus, $\mathbb{R}^2 = \mathbb{R} \times \mathbb{R}$, the combination of 2 selections from the set of real numbers. We can think of these combinations as a 2-place vector.

This concept can be extended first to arbitrary finite combinations of $\mathbb{R}$, where we use the pi symbol to indicate a *Cartesian product*, that is, all conceivable combinations as in

$$\prod_{1}^{n} \mathbb{R}^i$$

and in this particular case, $\mathbb{R}^i = \mathbb{R}$ for $i = 1, 2$. In general then, consider an index set that, instead of $i = 1, 2, \ldots, n$, $n$ is either countably (i.e., equal to the number of integers) or uncountably (equal to the number of all real numbers) infinite. Instead of using products of $\mathbb{R}$, we can use any kind of space; these spaces do not even have to be the same as one another. We can even take a combination of some finite and some infinite spaces. Then we have our space

$$X = \prod_{\alpha} X_\alpha,$$

which means that we take all the possible combinations of the spaces $X_\alpha$, one value for each possible value of $\alpha$. In addition to the apparent description of a generalized point in this space as an infinite-dimensional vector (with position in the vector indicated by the value of $\alpha$), we can also think of it as a function $f$: $\{\alpha\} \rightarrowtail X_\alpha$. For instance, when each $X_\alpha$ is $\mathbb{R}$ and $\{\alpha\}$ is also in $\mathbb{R}$, and $f$ is continuous, then each vector is a member of the set of all continuous functions defined on the interval $(a,b)$.

Now that we have a fairly intuitive idea of this highly useful type of space, we can simply form a new function that assigns a value in $X$ for each member of the interval $(a,b)$. In a special case, it might be that, say $X_{237}$ contains a 1–1 image of $(a,b)$, $f$: $(a,b) \rightarrowtail X_{237}$, and this either is a useful dimension for psychologists (e.g., loudness) or physicists, or both. So far, even with the foregoing explanation, the situation may seem abstract and of little use. But consider the more interesting example

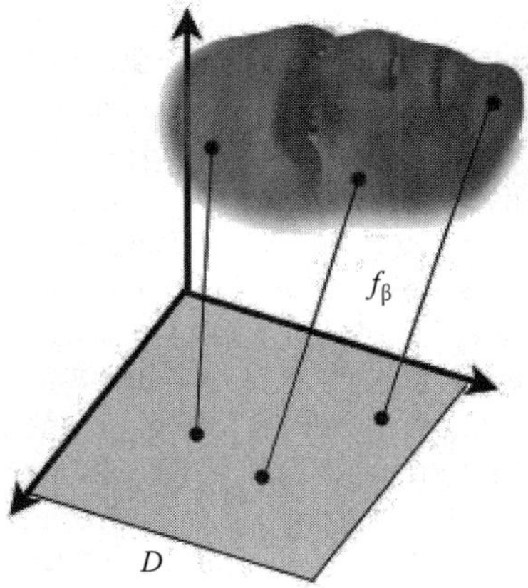


*Figure 7.4* $f_\beta$ is the mapping from the domain D onto a specific face in the face space.

of the space of all faces and call it *F*. We postulate that *F* is contained in the space of all 2-D surfaces, considered as continuous functions of a bounded subset of some cross-product of intervals. It won't hurt to simply pose our mapping as a function from some domain *D* realized as the pair of intervals $(0, 1) \times (0, 1) = D$ into this face space, *F*. We focus, for simplicity, on the front half of the face. Basically, we can do the same kind of thing on the rear of the faces.

Let the face function be $f_\beta: D \rightarrowtail F$, over a non-denumerable set $\{\beta\}$, and we can without harm think of a particular face as being associated with a particular map, say $f_\beta$. Each face will be a different $f_\beta$ mapping the domain into the face space such that every point in the domain corresponds to a point on the face. Figure 7.4 shows a face constructed in this fashion. Now, we mustn't lose track of our first goal, which was indicating how psychological dimensions can be exhibited in an infinite-dimensional space, such as our current face space *F*. Suppose we wish to experiment with the psychological dimension of mouth size (*ms*) and the set of all mouth sizes: $MS = \{ms\}$, contained naturally in $\mathbb{R}$. Of course, there is a true physical dimension of surface area of the mouth in this case, but that may well not be linearly related to the psychological dimension. We can include $ms = 0$, even though we may never actually observe that in reality. Anyhow, we embed *MS* in *F* by, for instance, taking all members of *F* but without a mouth and then forming the total $F = F_{-mouth} \times MS$.

This operation constructs all possible faces with all possible mouth sizes. In actuality, some faces may not accommodate some, perhaps particularly large mouth sizes. This type of constraint does no real harm to our deliberations here, and in fact, a more sophisticated theory based on the idea of manifolds can readily encompass this type of constraint (see, e.g., Townsend et al., 2001). In any event, any 1-D curve in *F* can, for every face-point traversed, be indexed by a value of *ms*. In fact, any such trajectory through *F* can be modified so as to measure mouth size at each of its points (i.e., at each face). Of course, a subset of trajectories will possess a constant *ms* while other facets of the faces vary, and so on. From the reverse perspective, we can think about how as attention is directed toward a mouth, perceptual operators are filtering the psychological mouth size from each face to which it is attending.

The present theory may seem intriguing (or too complex to exert any effort for), but is there any hope for disentangling psychological dimensions from an infinite-dimensional space? The answer is apparently "yes" in any cases we have seen. The Shepard–Kruskal approach and its many relatives might seem to apply most immediately to stimuli that are themselves exhibiting and varying the finite dimensions under study. A real-life, often employed case is a set of rectangles with varying length and width (Schonemann, Dorcey, & Kienapple, 1985). Although the Shepard–Kruskal approach has never been given an axiomatic underpinning, nonetheless it seems clear that humans and probably many in the animal world can attend to a small number of dimensions at a time from stimuli that are inherently from an infinite-dimensional space, especially when a finite set of 1-D dimensions are varying across the stimuli. In fact, even the set of rectangles can be interpreted as a very special subset of the set of all 2-D surfaces. The dimensions of psychological length and width would then be extracted by the Shepard–Kruskal procedures. It should be noted, though, that some individuals abstract the dimensions of size (length × width) and shape (length ÷ width). In addition, the fact that infinite-dimensional spaces are not incompatible with 1-D psychological dimensions helps weld together the various psychological tasks and processes, from unidimensional psychophysics (e.g., Fechner, Adler, & Boring, 1966; Falmagne, 2002; Baird, 1997; Link, 1992) to higher order mental functions such as symbol and language identification (e.g., Townsend & Landon, 1982, 1983; Pelli, Farell, & Moore, 2003; Rumelhart & McClelland, 1987), to categorization (e.g., Nosofsky, 1986; Ashby, 1992) and beyond.

Perhaps even more interestingly, by bringing to bear principal component analysis (closely related to singular value decomposition), it is feasible in principle to dissect a set of perceived patterns, even faces, into a set of objects from the same dimensional space, that can (at least so the wish goes) be interpreted as a set of faces that serve as a foundation from which all the faces in the stimulus set and, one hopes, many more, can be built up. In the example case of our face space, these foundational "basis" faces are called *eigenfaces*. More rigorously, this approach originally stems from the theory of vector spaces.

Many of the present readers may have taken a basic linear algebra course, where they learned about sets of independent basis vectors (possibly, but not necessarily at right angles to one another), weighted sums of which can produce any vector in the space (of course, we have to omit a lot of detail here!). It turns out that, say, the space of continuous differentiable functions, which can be multiplied by numbers and then added, subtracted, and so on, form a valid, but infinite-dimensional vector space. Nonetheless, the property of infinitude does not rule out the possibility of finding a set of eigenvectors (in this case, actually eigenfunctions), infinite in number, which can, with the proper numbered weights, exactly reproduce any of the original stimulus functions.

In fact, in continued analogy with the common vector spaces to which readers are undoubtedly accustomed, there are many ways of selecting a usually infinite, but discrete, set of basis vectors that perform the foregoing service. Furthermore, it also happens that these functions (or in the present case eigenfaces) can be ordered in their importance for producing human behavior, for instance, similarity judgments, confusion probabilities, and so forth. Hence, the investigator will take a finite set of these eigenfaces as being the most important, down to a certain but arbitrary level of precision, and use them as hypothetical representations of the basic faces of which "all" others can be reconstructed. Naturally, because we end with a finite number, these will only approximate the original faces to some degree. Anyhow, this seemingly kind of exotic and unpromising approach has actually been carried out with great success by a number of laboratories. An auspicious example is found in the research of Alice O'Toole and her colleagues (see, e.g., O'Toole, Wenger, & Townsend, 2001; Deffenbacher, Vetter, Johanson, & O'Toole, 1998), where eigenfaces have been employed to discover many intriguing aspects of face perception.

Our only word of caution here is that often the eigenfaces may not resemble real faces to a high degree. This facet is important in our overall discussion, inasmuch as even though the space of continuous functions is a legitimate vector space (e.g., a weighted sum of two continuous functions is again a continuous function), the space of all faces is not. This is because not all faces would necessarily be representable as some sort of combination of basis faces. This lack of nice vector space qualities leads us to consider a more general framework, in fact, one where locally, that is, within a small region, one has vector space characteristics (in fact, Euclidean properties), but where globally, the space will not be either Euclidean or a vector space. A natural setting to consider is that of a manifold, which is also the framework within which Einstein's theory of general relativity came to be expressed. In order to help the reader develop some intuition for these rich spaces, we actually need to take a step back to rather primitive, but extremely useful concepts, such as a topology.

Finally for this topic, we observe that the question of independence of psychological dimensions has long been of interest in perceptual science. For instance, the dimensions of loudness and intensity (commonly, and somewhat oddly, called "volume" in English) are mutually dependent, although their physical sources are not. Within a more complex setting, social psychologists have found that perceived intelligence and attractiveness are correlated although, of course, they are not in reality. Ashby & Townsend (1986) proposed a general theory of perceptual dependence among psychological dimensions embedded in a multidimensional pattern recognition setting. Many supplements to the theory and associated methodology have been made and applications in various areas of perception and action (e.g., Kadlec & Townsend, 1992; Thomas, 2003; Maddox, 2001; Wenger & Ingvalson, 2003; Amazeen, 1999).

## 7.6 Manifolds for psychological spaces

We put aside for now, the property of having an infinite number of dimensions to pursue a different course. Of the virtually infinite number of possible generalizations of Euclidean geometry, there is another one that stands out which has been hardly explored at all in psychological domains. We are referring to "manifold theory". The concept of a space plus a topology is so important that we have to deal with it, at least informally, before beginning in earnest. First, a *space* is any set (collection) of entities we call *points*. These can, as in the kinds of spaces with which the reader is likely most familiar, be approximated by dots. In more complicated situations, however, such as the space of all continuous functions, a point would be an entire continuous function. The space is then the collection of all of these points. Anyhow, a mathematician usually quickly imposes more structure on the space. This catapults us to the idea of topological spaces.

A topological space $X$ is a set of points with a special collection of subsets of points called *basis sets*. One then takes all possible finite numbers of intersections of these sets along with all possible finite or infinite unions of these sets to produce the so-called "set of open sets" (we also must include $X$, the set of all points that make up the space, plus the empty set, Ø). That is, every set in this possibly very big set of sets is by definition *open*. The so-called *closed* sets can then be elicited by taking the complement $X - O_\alpha = C_\alpha$ where $O_\alpha$ is open and $C_\alpha$ is then closed. With this structure and little else, one can immediately define continuous functions from one topological space $X$ to another $Y$ along with many other valuable concepts. If $X$ and $Y$ are topologically equivalent, one can find a bicontinuous function that carries every point in $X$ to one in $Y$ and vice versa, and one already has the justification for the oft-repeated topology joke that "A topologist is a person who can't tell the difference between a tea cup and a doughnut," because, of course, the stretching and shrinking allowed in such a function preserves the topological properties (e.g., how many holes a space possesses) of either space. Topology is extremely powerful for the relatively small set of assumptions on which it rests. For even more interesting properties, we now proceed to topological manifolds.

The essence of a topological manifold $M^n$ rests on three vital properties:

1. $M$ is Hausdorff. This means that for any two points, two sets can be formed containing those points which have no intersection (overlap).
2. $M$ has a countable basis.
3. $M$ is locally Euclidean. That is, any point in $M$ is contained in a small open set $O_M$ (called a *neighborhood*) that can be mapped bicontinuously (both the original function and its inverse are continuous) and in a 1–1 (each point in $O_M$ maps to exactly point in an open set $O_E$ of $E^n$) and onto (all points in $O$ have an inverse point in $O_M$) fashion.

This means that a small region of our manifold can be treated approximately (and totally in the limit as the original set gets smaller and smaller) like a Euclidean space. We can now use the Euclidean metric locally,

$$d(x_1, x_2) = \sqrt{\left(\sum_1^n (x_{1,i} - x_{2,i})^2\right)}$$

where $x_1 = (x_{1,1}, x_{1,2}, \ldots, x_{1,n})$, an $n$-place vector in Euclidean $n$-D space, and similarly for $x_2$. It can be shown that a topological manifold can always be granted a global metric. However, without more assumptions, that metric may not be the one we wish, a Riemannian metric, named after the great mathematician Bernard Riemann. Riemann furthered the drive toward non-Euclidean geometry, and worked out a type of metric that generalized the one invented by another mathematical genius, Karl Friedrich Gauss for special cases, and which included as special cases, those posed by Lobachevsky and Bolyai (negative curvature), but long before the invention of the curvature concept. Riemann's manifolds and his measure capture both positive as well as negative curvature.

Some bright mathematicians met this need and bestowed the drive for a generalized metric with great force, by inventing a kind of differentiation that works on manifolds instead of just in Euclidean space. This topic is much more recondite than we can detail here but basically we can view the operations in a simple case to get a feeling for what is going on. Basically (and very roughly), we can think of bundles of vectors that sit on a manifold and starting at any single point, direct us to the next point. With some care, we can provide differentiation operations on these vectors such that the "output" of the differentiation operator remains in the original manifold (e.g., in a manifold that appears as a surface in $\mathbb{R}^3$, the derivative vectors might stick out away from the surface we are studying). Without care taken to confine them to the manifold at hand, we can't represent speed and acceleration to provide for a Newton-like mechanics in our novel space.

Closely associated with our setup is a matrix (or quadratic operator) that maps velocity vectors into a speed number. This result can be integrated over a path to produce a path length. Even better, we can put conditions on the paths such that we can evoke the closest possible analogue to straight lines in Euclidean spaces (formally called *geodesics*). We define the Riemannian metric as an $n \times n$ matrix (where $n$ is the dimension of the manifold), which is usually written $g_{ij}(x)$, with $i, j$ running from 1 to $n$ and $x$ being a point on the manifold. It tells how fast distance is accumulating at different places in the space (signified by $x$) and how the different dimensions, $i$ and $j$, affect that accumulation at each point. For instance, suppose that our manifold is shaped like a mountain and that we wish our metric to take into account not only distance in our usual sense but also perhaps the effort (e.g., power) that is expended in moving around on this manifold. Hence, when the grade is fairly flat, we can make $g_{ij}(x)$ small but when the going gets steep we can make it much larger. Suppose too that our journey starts at a point where, when we move in the direction of both increasing dimension $i$ as well as dimension $j$ we are heading up the steepest part of the slope. If we momentarily hold one dimension constant, the effort is considerably less (due to not actually climbing upward). This situation is pictured with a large $g_{ij}(x)$ close to the starting point and $g_{ii}(x)$ and $g_{jj}(x)$ being smaller (in Euclidean space, these are the only entries in the matrix that are appropriate, and all are equal to 1 for all points $x$).

Note the strong interaction between dimensions here, which is absent in Euclidean space. Interestingly, this (relatively) simple function is all that is required to investigate the curvature in our space, a fact that was prefigured by Gauss and made general and rigorous by Riemann. (Gauss was a senior professor and sat on Riemann's habilitation exam, which is something like an advanced doctoral dissertation in Germany but currently being dissolved) Even with this brief (and quite nonrigorous) tutorial, we can perhaps see that manifolds increase the generality and scope of the kinds of spaces we could consider for psychology magnificently.

As a simple, finite-dimensional example, consider the traditional shape used in color theory to capture some important aspects of color: A. Hue; B. Brightness; C. Saturation (or its opposite, Complexity). When we don't worry too much about the precise shape, the surface looks like two ice cream cones with their tops (the biggest part of the cone) stuck together. This is a manifold that can, of course, be embedded in Euclidean 3-D space. The middle, widest portion is used to depict the optimal brightness level, where the full range from gray (in the very center of the circle) to the brightest hues is possible. As we descend toward the bottom apex, all is dark, and up at the other apex the stimulus light is so bright that no hue can be discerned. This little space is very well behaved (except at the apexes, where strange geometric things happen, so we put those aside for now). Using Riemann's techniques, we quickly learn that although "in the large," the space is not globally like a Euclidean space (e.g., it is bounded rather than unbounded), locally around a given point, its curvature is 0 just like in Euclidean space. Intuitively, this is because our double cone, with a cut from bottom to top, and one through the center, unrolls to make a portion of a Euclidean plane.

## 7.7 Probability theory in infinite-dimensional spaces

So now we are in possession of elementary topology, manifolds, metrics, differentiability (what mathematicians like to call *smoothness*), and finite- and infinite-dimensionality. Next we need a way to induce *randomness,* that is probability, on our finite- or infinite- dimensional manifolds. Fortunately, there is a well-trodden pathway that allows us to retain our desirable generality. This comes by way of utilizing the resident topology to our own ends. First, we observe that probability is a form of the rigorous concept of measure. A *measure* is constituted by a function that maps sets (often called *classes*) of sets into the real numbers in a regular fashion. The conditions to satisfy the tenets of a measure, and again we cannot reach detail here, are things such as (1) additivity of the measure of non-overlapping sets in the topology, and (2) finiteness of the measure (i.e., the measure is always bounded by some fixed real number). There are several others that we don't talk about here, but with the added stipulation that if we have a probability measure, the measure on the entire set of points (i.e., the points in the topological space) is equal to 1 (i.e., something has to happen). Hence, we simply form an appropriate topology, then take its sets and assign a probability measure to them.

A class of sets (along with certain operations) meeting these and other technical tenets is called a *sigma field.* Basically, one can assess the probability of an event by computing the measure associated with appropriate sets in the sigma field. This general argument applies to finite- or infinite-dimensional spaces. As might be expected, peculiarities can arise in the latter case, but usually they don't unduly perturb the pathways to the theorist's goals. These deliberations should convince us that infinite-dimensional spaces can possess probability distributions, particularly when a metric is present. In many cases, some of which are standard in such fields as electrical engineering (although the rigorous underpinnings might be found only at the graduate-school level), one may employ tools from other fields, such as functional analysis, or stochastic processes, to avoid the explicit production of an appropriate sigma field. We discuss more on this topic later.

Any topological manifold can do this, but we are especially interested in (infinitely differentiable) Riemann manifolds, which are all metrizeable, and in fact, we wish to only work with those that are complete metric spaces. A nice property of metrics is that any metric generates a topology but not all topologies admit a metric. The finite cases are dealt with elsewhere (e.g., Townsend et al, 2001), so we want to see what happens with infinite-dimensional manifolds or other infinite-dimensional spaces. Perhaps the most straightforward infinite-dimensional space is the space of all continuous functions on an interval I on the real line, which may itself be infinite (i.e., [0, 1]), say $f\colon I \rightarrowtail \mathbb{R}$. Of course, the graph of each of these functions yields the usual picture of a typical function as taught to us in elementary math. Interestingly, it has been shown that this class of objects (i.e., the set of functions) is of the same dimensionality (the jargon term is *cardinality*) as the points on the real line itself! There are lots of metrics we could use but an extremely useful type is the so-called $\mathcal{L}^2$ metric

$$d(f,g) = \int_0^i \left[ (f(x) - g(x))^2 \, dx \right]^{1/2},$$

where $f$ and $g$ are two such functions. It should be obvious that this is the analogue of the Euclidean metric in finite spaces. Even more intriguing is the fact that it is the only power metric in function space that satisfies the conditions required to be a Riemannian metric. Thus, the infinite-dimensional twin of the city block metric (see above),

$$d(f,g) = \int_0^1 |(f(x) - g(x))| \, dx$$

is not a type of Riemannian metric on any manifold.

We back up for a moment in order to examine the finite $n$-dimensional metric and a path length in $n$-dimensional space. The general infinitesimal displacement in $n$-dimensional Riemannian manifold is

$$ds = \left\{ \sum_{i,j=1}^{n} \left[ g_{ij}\left(x_1, x_2, \ldots, x_n\right) dx_i dx_j \right] \right\}^{1/2}.$$

Observe that $g_{ij}$ is simply an $n \times n$ matrix and that it can depend, in general, on the specific point in space, $(x_1, x_2, \ldots, x_n)$, where we are currently. However, in the special case where $g_{ij} = I$, the identity matrix at all points in the space, this expression reduces to the Euclidean metric. Likewise, the path length of a path through Euclidean $n$-space is

$$\int \cdots \int \left\{ \sum_{i,j=1}^{n} \left[ g_{ij}\left(x_1, x_2, \ldots, x_n\right) dx_i dx_j \right] \right\}^{1/2}$$

where $n$ integrals are taken tracking the appropriate path. Perhaps it is even more intuitive when the displacements $dx_i$ are converted to velocities, $dx_i/dt$, for then we can simply consider the path in terms of the velocities of each coordinate. Here we evaluate, say $dx_i$, as being a tiny motion in the $x_i$ direction, for $i = 1, 2, \ldots, n-1, n$. This obviously pushes us to a new point $(x_1', x_2', \ldots, x_n')$ where $g$ can take on a new value, and so on. All this will come in handy in the infinite dimensional case just following.

Moving back to functions in one variable, inasmuch as it is more intuitive to confine ourselves to this "space of differentiable functions in one dimension," let us indicate the general Riemannian metric on this elementary manifold:

$$ds = \int_0^{t'} \left( \int_0^1 \int_0^1 g_{\alpha\beta}(h)\left(\partial f(\alpha,t)/\partial t\right)\left(\partial f(\beta,t)/\partial t\right) dx_a dx_\beta \right)^{1/2} dt.$$

Now, we have to adjust our thinking a bit. Instead of considering $dx_a$ as an miniscule motion in the $x_a$ direction, we can think of it in the following way. Take a look at the two facial profiles in Figure 7.5, drawn as a function on $x$ from 0 to 1. Now, for every $\alpha$, $x_a$ is a number between 0 and 1. However, we now need to think of $dx_a$ as a motion from, say face $f_1$ to face $f_2$, that is, moving up or down vertically between the two designated faces. Because of the possibility of noise, we can only assume that each function along the path, that is, $h$ is "face-like", not that it is necessarily a true face. Indeed, in a pattern identification situation one or both of $f_1$ and $f_2$ could

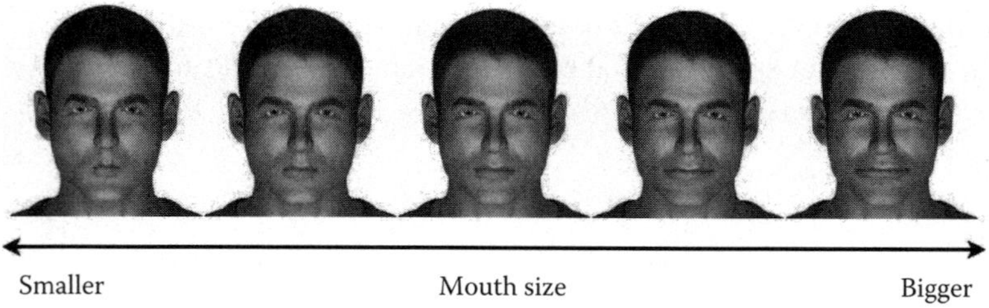


*Figure 7.5* Here is a series of faces that vary across one isolated dimension, mouth size, but there are infinitely many other dimensions in the space of all faces.

be noisy renditions of faces. The extra complexity here must be explained a bit more. We are representing a function as a gigantic (and dense!) vector, $\gamma = f(x)$, $x \in \mathbb{R}$, and because $f$ is our current point, we have to let the metric $g$ depend on it, which is why it appears in the argument of $g$. In addition, instead of $dx_i$ for a finite $i = 1, 2, \ldots, n$, we must extend this notation to $dx_a$ where a runs over the interval [0,1], and the same is true for β. So, the overall idea is that we are depicting the movement of $f$ by way of how it changes with each coordinate of $f$. And, because we are using a general quadratic metric of the coordinates, whether finite or infinite, we have to take the two-way products of all possible coordinate changes, that is, $dx_a$ and $dx_\beta$. Finally, then the path length through this function space, explicitly using our velocity representation, is just

$$d^R(f,g) = \int_0^{t^*} \left[ \int_0^1 \int_0^1 g_{\alpha\beta}(h)\left(dx_\alpha/dt\right)\left(dx_\beta/dt\right) \right]^{1/2} dt.$$

Of course, when we seek the shortest path length between two faces, we can define that as the distance and the ensuing path as the geodesic between them. Again, the reader may wish to confirm that when α, β are both identical to 1 and don't depend on $f$, we get back to the analogue to the Euclidean metric, the $\mathcal{L}^2$ metric (and see Townsend et al, 2001, for more on this and other issues pertaining to face-geodesics). In any event, all this can be (with some tedium) expanded to functions in any finite-dimensional space. It is important to observe before we go further that just because we use the term "path" here, as is common, we do not imply a temporal factor. All the above, for instance computing the distance between two faces, might take place simultaneously along the path, although some paths might nonetheless take longer to compute than others. A more abstract and general notation is possible (e.g., Boothby, 1975; Townsend et al, 2001). Such notations are very useful because they capture the principal ideas in a markedly clear fashion without sometimes mind-numbing profusions of indices. On the other hand, when the scientist wishes to actually compute something, the evil indices must be present and accounted for.

## 7.8 A special case of great importance

Of course, infinite-dimensional manifolds have not yet seen much application in most of science, especially the life sciences. Yet, it seems worthwhile to mention a special case of our quantitative apparatus that has been of enormous value in the basic and applied sciences. The theory goes by many names, but one term is the "mathematical theory of communication" (which we simplify to MTC), used for example by Norbert Wiener. As worth virtually everything, including mathematics, there are roots in the distant past for this theory, but a real explosion of new results from mathematicians, physicists, and engineers, occurred in the mid-twentieth century. To a major extent, this work accompanied the amazing scientific and technological effort expended in and around the time of World War II. We recall the names of formidable mathematicians such as Norbert Wiener, John von Neumann, and electrical engineer Claude Shannon. The sphere of mathematical communications theory intersects huge regions of mathematics and physics, including functional analysis, stochastic processes, and probability, waveform analysis (e.g., Fourier and Laplace transforms), electrical engineering, differential equations, and deterministic and stochastic dynamic systems, and so on. In the present writers' opinion, the whole of this work is as important to modern technology and science (if not usually so lethal in application) as the splitting of the atom.

In most applications of MTC, we employ various types of function spaces. These may be deterministic or probabilistic, but usually do not require manifold theory per se. When needed, differentiation can be extended to so-called Fréchet or Gauteaux derivatives, and usually ordinary Lebesgue or Riemann integration suffices for integration. For many purposes, the function space is itself a vector space, sometimes with a norm (as in Banach spaces: the norm of a function is the analogue of the magnitude of a vector in a finite-dimensional vector space) or an inner product (the analogue of the dot product in a Euclidean vector space). The inner product, the analogue of the dot (or ineptly called by non-mathematicians the "cross product") of two functions of a real variable is just

$$\int_{-\infty}^{\infty} f(x)g(x)dx$$

The accompanying metric, which by now will probably not shock the reader, is simply

$$d(f,g)=\left[\int_{-\infty}^{\infty}(f(x)-g(x))^2\,dx\right]^{1/2},$$

which naturally looks very much like our good friend, the Euclidean metric, but stretched out along the real-line continuum. We can then think of

$$d^R(f,g)=\int_0^{t^*}\left[\int_0^1\int_0^1 g_{\alpha\beta}(f)\left(dx_\alpha/dt\right)\left(dx_\beta/dt\right)\right]^{1/2}dt,$$

which we formulated above, as weighting distinct parts of figures such as faces differently, depending on their importance. For instance, it is well known that the eyes play a critical role in face perception and hence we would expect $g_{\alpha\beta}$ to be large when transversing that part of the face.

## 7.9 Applying these ideas to classification

Now, suppose that a person is confronted with a pattern from an infinite-dimensional space. As pointed out above, almost everything seen or heard is from such a space, not a finite-dimensional one. In applying the above concepts to this situation, we have to make sure that our space is big enough to contain not only patterns arising in a noiseless, perfect perception environment, but also the patterns that are perturbed by some type of noise, or that are simply randomized in some way. Thus, the theoretical system we propose is an analogue to the fact that probabilistic identification in a noisy environment (e.g., Ashby & Townsend, 1986), demands a very similar type of theoretical structure as does categorization of a set of patterns that are associated with a probability distribution (e.g., Ashby, 1992). First, let us agree that some kind of representation is constructed of each pattern to be classified, whether it is categorized by a set of exemplars (see Nosofsky, 1988) or a template. In identification, it might be a memory of each object to be uniquely identified. Let us concentrate on the case of identification inasmuch as one can readily generalize that situation to categorization or reduce it to signal detection. The reader may refer to detailed developments and discussion of this material for the finite vector case in Townsend & Landon (1983).

Let us conceive of the input as a random function in some $n$-dimensional space (e.g., a perturbed two-dimensional surface plus noise placed in a three-dimensional Euclidean space with an $\mathcal{L}^2$ metric ). It is standard to use an $\mathcal{L}^2$ metricized function space for physical signals so we continue that here (but cf. Cornish & Frankel, 1997). Let $U_i$ be the random function describing the probabilistic input for stimulus $S_i$ and $U = \{Ui\}_1^N$ the set of $N$ randomized inputs. We take $X$ as the perceptual image space. $X$ is considered as an infinite-dimensional function space, but may be embeddable in some finite-dimensional space. So, the perceptual map is $U_i \rightarrow X$, and each realization $f$ of the set $F$, where $F \sqsubseteq X$ is assumed to be continuous. The memory pattern set $Y$, with which the input is matched, is taken as a deterministic set of functions. That is, $g \in Y$ is well memorized with no noise attached. In certain cases, not having both be random can substantially simplify matters such as calculations.

Next, we need an evidence space $Z$ to represent the evidence for each resulting comparison of an input with the $N$ memory items from $Y$. The simplest, yet very natural space to employ here is just $\mathbb{R}^+$, that is, the positive real numbers. Hence, we must have a map $e$: $(F,G) \rightarrow \mathbb{R}_0^+$, that is, $e(f,g) = r \in \mathbb{R}_0^+$,with the "0" subscript indicating that 0 is included (naturally, this set can easily be generalized to include the negative real numbers if required). The evidence function could be calculating distance, Bayesian likelihood, or some other measure of acceptability of a memory alternative. In any event, $z \in Z = \mathbb{R}_0^+$ will be a real-valued random variable, and the image of a particular $(f,g)$. Now, within $X$ every point function, except for ties, will be in favor of one response alternative over the others, say the $j^{th}$. Then, for a perceptual signal $f$ in such a set, $e(f,g_j) = MAX_1^n[e(f,g_k)]$, again except for ties. This means that outside of ties, $X$ will be partitioned into sets of points (i.e., functions) that favor one of the alternatives. Then the probability of responding $R_j$ when the stimulus was $S_i$ requires determining the probability assessed across the various percepts, $f$, that can appear when $S_i$ is presented. This probability will be $P(R_j|S_i) = P[e(f,g_j) = MAX_1^n[e(f,g_k)]S_i]$.

Interesting facts about the evidence functions:

1. As noted, under very weak conditions (e.g., there exist points in $X$ where $e(f,g_k)$ favors $R_k$ for all $k$; and so on) $e$ will partition the space into mutually exclusive regions that favor each of the alternatives plus points where ties may occur.
2. Consider pairs of, say, $g_i$ and $g_j$, distinct memory patterns and the set of $f \in F$ such that $h(f,g_i,g_j) = e(f,g_i) - e(f,g_j) = 0$. Then, in most circumstances, the border separating whether $R_i$ wins versus where $R_j$ wins, will be a closed submanifold in $X$. We can call the set $\{f\}$ such that $h(f,g_i,g_j) = e(f,g_i) - e(f,g_j) = 0$, the kernel of h, and again they are equidistant from faces $g_i$ and $g_j$. On either side of this boundary one or the other wins. Now, the same things happens when any pair is considered and we can also look for ties among three, four or more of the set of $N$ faces. Under fairly weak conditions, the distinguished set $\{f\}$ (e.g., designated by the tied distance) will even be a nice sub-manifold of the original face space, inheriting its topology from that of the parent space. Sometimes the region of face space where, say, $g_i$ wins over its competitors, will be connected. However, devotees of signal detection in a single dimension will recognize that even there, the region of points where YES dominates the NO decision will not be connected: When the distributions of signal + noise.versus noise-alone are normal with unequal variances, this disconnection always occurs under a maximum likelihood decision rule. Yet another nice property ensues if the equidistant boundaries all have probability = 0 of occurring, for then we don't have to worry about jumping outside of our evidence space to adjudicate ties. This is quite a natural occurrence for finite-dimensional spaces.

What happens when the situation is stochastic? Suppose the human observer or signal processor, let's call her Sheila, is at least to a first approximation a linear filter, and that she is attempting to recognize one of $N$ patterns. Suppose that the observer is deterministic (i.e., her filtering mechanisms act the same way each time they are called into play) and that a specific signal $i$ ($i$ = 1, 2, ..., $N$) is itself a continuous function ($s_i(t)$) with Gaussian noise ($-(t)$) added in. Then, the signal pattern can be expressed as $U(t) = s_i(t) + -(t)$. The observer's filter for each signal possibility (e.g., the $j^{\text{th}}$) can be written also as a function of $t$, $h_j(t)$. It turns out (see, e.g., Luenberger, 1979; Padulo & Arbib, 1974) that her output on her $j^{\text{th}}$ perceptual template is

$$x_{ij}(t) = \int_0^t h_j(t-t')\left[s_i(t') + \tilde{N}(t')\right]dt',$$

under some reasonable conditions. That is, Sheila is using a template across time represented by $h$ to filter or compare with the input. In fact, when the noise has certain properties, $h_j(t) = s_j(t)$, which means the filter-template is a replica of the $j^{th}$ pattern itself and the filtering action is basically a correlation of the input with each one of these $N$ stored replicas. This action produces

$$x_{ij}(t) = \int_0^t s_i(t')\left[s_i(t') + \tilde{N}(t')\right]dt'.$$

There are several decision structures that could be imposed, but given our space considerations, we take the most straightforward: we suppose that Sheila samples information for a fixed interval, say, $[0,t^*]$ and then selects the maximum correlation provided by $x_{ij}(t^*)$, as calculated across $j$ for a given present signal $i$. Under some restrictions, this strategy is optimal and is called a *matched filter*. Indeed, if $-(t')$ is stationary Gaussian white noise with variance $\sigma_N^2 = 1$ and mean $\mu_N = 0$, $x_{ij}(t)$ will be itself normal with mean

$$\mu_x = \int_0^t s_i^2(t')\,dt'$$

and variance

$$\sigma_x^2 = \int_0^t s_i^2(t')\,dt'$$

the very same thing![11]

What happened to our metric? Well, with the same sampling rule but now using the simplest Riemannian metric, the $L^2$ metric, we would compute

$$d\left(s_i(t'), x_{ij}(t^*)\right) = \left[\int_0^{t^*} \left\{s_i(t') - \left[s_j(t') + \tilde{N}(t')\right]\right\}^2 dt'\right]^{1/2}.$$

Now this quantity is monotonic with its square which is easier to deal with so we examine $d^2(s_i(t'), x_{ij}(t^*))$ instead. We find that its mean of expectation (signified by the operator $E$) is

$$\mu_d = E\left[\int_0^{t^*} \left\{s_i^2(t') - 2s_i(t')s_j(t') + s_j^2(t') - 2\left(s_i(t') - s_j(t')\right)\tilde{N}(t') + \tilde{N}^2(t')\right\}dt'\right]$$

$$= E\left[\int_0^{t^*} \left\{s_i^2(t') - 2s_i(t')s_j(t') + s_j^2(t') + \tilde{N}^2(t')\right\}dt'\right]$$

due to the fact that the mean of $-(t') = 0$. Next,

$$\int_0^{t^*} s_i^2(t')$$

is a constant and the same for all comparisons (recall that $s(t')$ is the presented signal) and

$$\int_0^{t^*} \tilde{N}^2(t')dt'$$

is a random variable but is also the same on any one trial for all the comparisons and so neither of those quantities can discriminate the various decision/response alternatives. Hence, the only operative quantity is

$$\int_0^{t^*} \left\{-2s_i(t')s_j(t') + s_j^2(t')\right\}dt'$$

with mean

$$\int_0^{t^*} \left\{-2E\left[s_i(t')s_j(t')\right]dt'\right\} + \int_0^{t^*} E\left[s_j^2(t')\right]dt'.$$

Notice, in particular that the term

$$\int_0^{t^*} \left\{-2s_i(t')s_j(t')\right\}dt'$$

is directly proportional to the critical term from our matched filter approach above, namely involving the integral of $s_i(t')s_j(t')$. Therefore, minimizing the distance is tantamount to maximizing the correlation between the input and the decision alternatives. The only difference is that our distance approach includes a biasing term,

$$\int_0^{t^*} s_j^2(t')dt',$$

which provides a relative bias for alternative *j* according to its energy or magnitude. We won't detail the derivation of the variance this time but it is also closely related to that of the matched filter expressions. Interestingly, both these rules are also equivalent under certain constraints to a rule based on maximizing the likelihood that the presented signal pattern was *j*, given the observation.

## 7.10 Conclusion

Our itinerary on the geometric aspects of psychological classification has taken us from foundational, axiomatic measurement theory through (finite) multidimensional scaling, to concepts of dimensionality, including infinite dimensional spaces. From there, we reassured ourselves that finite dimensional subspaces of infinite-dimensional spaces are legitimate mathematical concepts, meaning that models which perform dimensional reduction can readily be applied as hypotheses about the human abstraction of psychological dimensions. This is something that is taken for granted, but its truth is not at all obvious, although we certainly find some way to filter interesting dimensions. Next, we moved on to ideas that are still relatively new in mathematics (i.e., only around 150 years old), that of non-Euclidean and Riemannian geometries, and even more ambitious, infinite-dimensional Riemannian spaces. In the social and biological sciences, probability and stochastics are a necessity, and we briefly surveyed the prospects for placing probability distributions on finite- and infinite-dimensional manifolds. It can be said that mathematicians are still in hot pursuit of the best ways of carrying out this program. Nonetheless, the next two sections exhibit important special cases and applications to classification illustrating theory and methodologies that have been around since at least the 1940s and 1950s in engineering and computer science, and have been expanded and deepened in the meantime.

We take it as a plausible working hypothesis that the gargantuan corpus of questions in social, biological, and even such areas as cognitive science, including machine intelligence and human–machine interactions, ultimately cannot all rest comfortably or rigorously within the simpler types of geometric spaces that have dominated those areas (with the exception of the special cases treated in the last two sections, which have seen extensive implementation in engineering and computer science). That is, in the final analysis, an empirical question, but we believe our present and future researchers should accouter themselves with the powerful tools that can aid in answering fundamental questions such as these. Over the centuries, the symbiosis between physics and mathematics has tremendously enriched both fields. Up to now, the social and biological sciences have largely been on the borrowing rather than lending side of the interactions, but there are strong signs that this is changing, for the better!

## Endnotes

1. The primary disciplines of the authors are psychology, and cognitive science. We shall use "psychology" as a proxy for any of the social or biological fields that cannot be readily specified in terms of physics (an example of a candidate for one that can be so described might be quantum properties of a neurotransmitter in re-uptake dynamics).
2. Modern psychology now includes a tremendous effort in neuro-sciences, especially neuro-imaging and of course, also affords a rich domain of mathematical research possibilities–thus, for the latter, see the websites for the US Society for Mathematical Psychology and the European Mathematical Psychology Group.

3. There has been much work mostly theoretical in the interim. Narens (1985) studies the critical notion of "meaningfulness" in foundational measurement. Luce & Weber (1986) provide a in-depth account of axiomatic decision making from an axiomatic measurement theory viewpoint.
4. Mathematical psychology is a subfield of psychology where, in place of verbal theorizing, mathematical theories or as they are often called, "models", are utilized to make one's assumptions rigorous, and to make strong predictions that are testable by observational data. Townsend & Kadlec (1990) offer a brief overview of the major branches of mathematical psychology and Townsend (2008) discusses challenges and prospects for mathematical psychology in the twenty-first century.
5. Tversky was not the first to think of identical features as affecting the psychological similarity of two objects. He traces his theory to seminal ideas of Restle (1961) who proposed set theoretic means of assessing similarity which could include the former. Other uses of this concept in models of pattern recognition can be found in work by Townsend & Ashby (1982). Nonetheless, Tversky's theory was by far the most quantitatively thorough and was developed in the context of the previously discussed foundational measurement theory.
6. The theory (or rather theories) of dimensionality has grown over the years. Relatively deep earlier treatments along some avenues can be found in Hurewics & Wallman (1941) and Nagata (1965).
7. A limitation of principal components analysis is that it assumes that the basis vectors be orthogonal to one another. It might well be that the basis vectors for a psychological vector space are linearly independent but not orthogonal. A methodology which assumes independence but not orthogonality which has gained much attention lately, especially in the analysis of fMRI signals (literally "functional magnetic resonance imaging," a neuroimaging method based on measurement of blood oxygen levels and their changes during psychological tasks) is called "independent components analysis" (ICA). However, this approach too, has its limitations.
8. It bears mentioning that relativity theory, even the special theory, requires adding time as a negative number in figuring the distance in the space (e.g., Minkowski, 1908).
9. The Ashby group has developed a general theory of categorization based on general recognition theory (e.g., see Chapters in Ashby, 1992).
10. A volume on applications of tensor analysis (a typically applied branch of differential geometry) by Schouten (1951) is a landmark in the applications of tensor theory to physics. However, it stands as one of the more challenging-to-read treatises in science, due to the maze of indices.
11. This nice event comes about due to stationarity, the properties of white noise, and the values of the noise mean and variance.

## References


Amazeen, E. L. (1999). Perceptual independence of size and weight by dynamic touch. *Journal of Experimental Psychology: Human Perception & Psychophysics*, *25*(1), 102–119.

Ashby, F. G. (1988). Estimating the parameters of multidimensional signal detection theory from simultaneous ratings on separate stimulus components. *Perception & Psychophysics*, *44*, 195–204.

Ashby, F. G. (1992). *Multidimensional models of perception and cognition*. Hillsdale, NJ: Lawrence Erlbaum Associates.

Ashby, F. G., & Townsend, J. T. (1986). Varieties of perceptual independence. *Psychological Review, 93*, 154–179.

Baird, J. C. (1997). *Sensation and judgment: Complementarity theory of psychophysics.* Hillsdale, NJ: Lawrence Erlbaum Associates.

Boothby, W. M. (1975). *An introduction to differentiable manifolds and Riemannian geometry.* New York: Academic Press.

Cornish, N. J., & Frankel, N. E. (1997, Aug). The black hole and the pea. *Physics Review D, 56*(4), 1903–1907.

Deffenbacher, K. A., Vetter, T., Johanson, J., & O'Toole, A. J. (1998). Facial aging, attractiveness, and distinctiveness. *Perception, 27*(10), 1233–1243.

Falmagne, J. (2002). *Elements of psychophysical theory* (Vol. 1). Oxford: Oxford University Press.

Fechner, G., Adler, H., & Boring, E. (1966). *Elements of psychophysics.* New York: Holt, Rinehart and Winston.

Hurewics, W., & Wallman, H. (1941). *Dimension theory.* Princeton, NJ: Princeton University Press.

Kadlec, H., & Townsend, J. T. (1992). Signal detection analysis of multidimensional interactions. In F. G. Ashby (Ed.), *Probabilistic multidimensional models of perception and cognition.* Hillsdale, NJ: Lawrence Erlbaum Associates.

Krantz, D. H., Luce, R. D., Suppes, P., & Tversky, A. (1971). *Foundations of measurement: Vol. 1. Additive and polynomial representations.* New York and London: Academic Press.

Link, S. W. (1992). *The wave theory of difference and similarity.* Hillsdale, NJ: Lawrence Erlbaum Associates.

Lord, F. M., & Novick, M. R. (1968). *Statistical theories of mental test scores.* Reading, MA: Addison-Wesley.

Luce, R., Bush, R., & Galanter, E. (Eds.). (1963). *Handbook of mathematical psychology* (Vols. I–III). New York: Wiley.

Luce, R. D., & Weber, E. U. (1986). An axiomatic theory of conjoint expected risk. *Journal of mathematical psychology, 30*(2), 188–205.

Luenberger, D. G. (1979). *Introduction to dynamic systems: Theory, models, and applications.* New York: Wiley.

Maddox, W. T. (2001). Separating perceptual processes from decisional processes in identification and categorization. *Perception & Psychophysics, 63*(7), 1183–1200.

Minkowski, H. (1908). "Space and time." In J. J. C. Smart (Ed.), *Problems of Space and Time* (pp. 297–312). London: Macmillan.

Nagata, J. (1965). *Modern dimension theory.* Amsterdam: North-Holland.

Narens, L. (1985). *Abstract measurement theory.* Cambridge, MA: MIT Press.

Nosofsky, R. M. (1986). Attention, similarity, and the identification-categorization relationship. *Journal of Experimental Psychology. General, 115*(1), 39–57.

Nosofsky, R. M. (1988). Exemplar-based accounts of relations between classification, recognition, and typicality. *Journal of Experimental Psychology: Learning, Memory and Cognition, 14*(4), 700–708.

O'Toole, A. J., Wenger, M. J., & Townsend, J. T. (2001). Quantitative models of perceiving and remembering faces: Precedent and possibilities. In M. J. Wenger & J. T. Townsend (Eds.), *Computational, geometric, and process perspectives on facial cognition* (p. 50). Hillsdale, NJ: Erlbaum Press.

Padulo, L., & Arbib, M. A. (1974). *System theory.* Philadelphia: Saunders.

Pelli, D. G., Farell, B., & Moore, D. C. (2003). The remarkable inefficiency of word. *Nature, 423*(6941), 752–756.

Pfanzagl, J. (1968). *Theory of measurement.* (p. 50). New York: Wiley.

Ramsay, J., & Silverman, B. (2006). *Functional data analysis.* Springer-Verlag, New York.

Restle, F. (1961). *Psychology of judgement and choice.* New York: Wiley.

Roberts, L. D., Patterson, D., Thomson, J. O., & Levey, R. P. (1969, Mar). Solid-state and nuclear results from a measurement of the pressure dependence of the energy of the resonance gamma ray of *au*197. *Physics Review, 179*(3), 656–662.

Rumelhart, D. E., & McClelland, J. L. (1987). *Parallel distributed processing.* Cambridge, MA: MIT Press.

Schonemann, P. H., Dorcey, T., & Kienapple, K. (1985). Subadditive concatenation in dissimilarity judgements. *Perception & Psychophysics, 38*, 1–17.

Schouten, J. (1951). *Tensor analysis for physicists.* Oxford: Clarendon Press.

Stevens, S. (1951). *Mathematics, Measurement and psychophysics.* S. Stevens (Ed.). New York: Wiley.

Suppes, P., & Zinnes, J. (1963). Basic measurement theory. In R. D. Luce, R. Bush, & E. Galanter (Eds.). *Handbook of mathematical psychology* (Vol. 1, pp. 3–76). New York: Wiley.

Thomas, R. D. (1999). Assessing sensitivity in a multidimensional space: Some problems and a definition of a general d'. *Psychonomic Bulletin & Review, 6*, 224–238.

Thomas, R. D. (2003). Further consideration of a general d' in multidimensional space. *Journal of Mathematical Psychology, 9*, 40–50.

Townsend, J. T. (1971). Theoretical analysis of an alphabetic confusion matrix. *Perception & Psychophysics, 9*, 40–50.

Townsend, J. T. (2008). Mathematical psychology: Prospects for the 21st century: A guest editorial. *Journal of mathematical psychology, 52*, 269–280.

Townsend, J. T., Aisbett, J., & Busemeyer, J. B. (2005). General recognition theory and methodology for dimensional independence on simple cognitive manifold. In H. Colonius & E. N. Dzhafarov (Eds.), *Measurement and representation of sensations: Recent progress in psychophysical theory.* Washington, D.C.: American Psycholgocial Association.

Townsend, J. T., & Ashby, F. G. (1982). An experimental test of contemporary mathematical models of visual letter recognition. *Journal of Experimental Psychology: Human Perception and Performance, 8*, 834–864.

Townsend, J. T., & Ashby, F. G. (1984). Measurement scales and statistics: the misconception misconceived. *Psychological Bulletin, 96*(2), 394–401.

Townsend, J. T., & Kadlec, H. (1990). Mathematics and psychology. In R. Mickens (Ed.), *Mathematics and science.* Singapore: World Scientific.

Townsend, J. T., & Landon, D. E. (1982). An experimental and theoretical investigation of the constant ratio rule and other models of visual letter recognition. *Journal of Mathematical Psychology, 25*, 119–163.

Townsend, J. T., & Landon, D. E. (1983). Mathematical models of recognition and confusion in psychology. *International Journal of Mathematical Social Sciences, 4*, 25–71.

Townsend, J. T., Solomon, B., Wenger, M. J., & Spencer-Smith, J. (2001). The perfect gestalt: Infinite dimensional Riemannian face spaces and other aspects of face cognition. In J. T. Townsend & M. J. Wenger (Eds.). *Computational, geometric and process issues in facial cognition: Progress and challenges.* Hillsdale, NJ: Erlbaum Press.

Townsend, J. T., & Spencer-Smith, J. (2004). Two kinds of global perceptual separability and curvature. In C. Kaernbach, E. Schröger & H. Müller (Eds.), *Psychophysics beyond sensation: Laws and invariants of human cognition.* Mahwah, NJ: Erlbaum.

Townsend, J. T., & Thomas, R. D. (1993). Foundations of perceptual theory. In S. C. Masin (Ed.), (chap. On the need for a general quantitative theory of pattern similarity). Elsevier Science Publishers.

Tversky, A. (1977). Features of similarity. *Psychological Review*, *84*(4), 327–352.

Wenger, M. J., & Ingvalson, E. (2003). Preserving informational separability and violating decisional separability in facial perception and recognition. *Journal of Experimental Psychology: Learning, Memory and Cognition*, *29*, 1106–1118.

# 8 Psychophysical linguistics

*Stephen Link*

Department of Psychology
University of California, San Diego
La Jolla, California, USA

## 8.1 Introduction

"I have measured out my life with coffee spoons," Prufrock declares in T. S. Eliot's (1917) famous *The Love Song of J. Alfred Prufrock*. The measure may be somewhat dubious but the meaning is plainly clear. How would the meaning change if this measure of life also changed? For example, if instead of coffee spoons we substitute teaspoons, tablespoons, soup spoons, or even sugar spoons. In terms of psychophysical measurement, how far is each of these new meanings from the meaning established by Eliot's poetic choice of "coffee spoons"? The development of a measure of distance between meanings is the focus of this chapter.

The type of judgment required in this case is one of matching or similarity. For example, does "I have measured out my life with tablespoons" have the same or different meaning from Prufrock's declaration? If different, how much different is it? Such judgments of matching or similarity are commonly used in linguistic experiments yet their theoretical basis is widely unknown. Although such judgments of similarity or dissimilarity occur as routinely as judgments of largeness or smallness they are based on a different principle. Judgments of similarity or dissimilarity require for their analysis a very different treatment, a different theoretical basis, than do judgments of largeness or smallness.

Many years after Fechner's development of the original model for the comparative judgment of two stimulus magnitudes, psychophysicists discovered that some of the judgments made in psychological experiments were not judgments of differences in stimulus magnitude at all but were, instead, judgments of equality or sameness. Seizing on this discovery Urban (1907) suggested that three different responses be employed in the typical discrimination experiment. A comparison stimulus might be judged to be smaller, larger, or equal with respect to a standard stimulus. Although experimental subjects did use these three response categories in a number of experiments, the theory of how such judgments might occur required many years of subsequent development (cf. Link, 1992). And, as the study of comparative judgment advanced, psychophysicists realized that the judgment of smaller or larger is one type of judgment and that the judgment of equality or inequality, of sameness or difference, is the only other type of judgment to be discovered since Fechner's introduction of comparative judgment in 1860.

## 8.2 Discrimination of visual angle

Let us return to a once-famous, but now virtually unknown, experiment using judgments of sameness or difference reported by Dorwin Cartwright (1941). The experimental result that differentiates such judgments from judgments of largeness or smallness is illustrated in Figure 8.1. Here are results from a typical method of constant stimuli experiment employing visual angles as stimuli. Experimental subjects decided if a presented angle varying to 160° from 10° was within a learned interval of 60° to 100°. Both response latency, the time from the presentation of the stimulus to the response, also called response time (RT), and response proportions show the existence of what Urban (1910) defined as an "Interval of Uncertainty."

The "Interval of Uncertainty" is the contiguous interval within which the probability of making the judgment equal is greater than 0.50. Cartwright's results show how, at the edges of this "interval," at the point of 50%, the mean response latency, or response time, reaches a peak. Indeed, mean response times appear to be a function of the distance of a comparison stimulus from the edges of the interval of uncertainty. This one of many results, confirmed over many decades, shows that the application of a judgment model based on monotonic changes in performance as a function of stimulus difference is not applicable to judgments of sameness and difference.

## 8.3 Numerical comparisons

Similar results from numerical comparison experiments performed in my laboratory by Anna Ventresca (1988) verify the repeated occurrence of these findings. Subjects

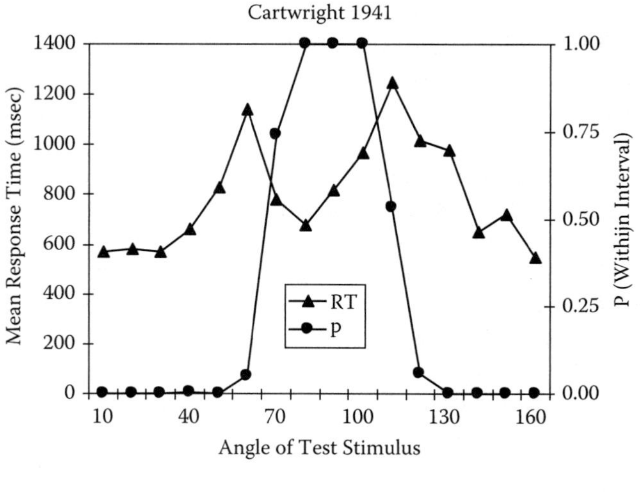


*Figure 8.1* Results from Cartwright (1941) on judging whether a test angle was within the interval of 60° to 100°. Mean response times in milliseconds.

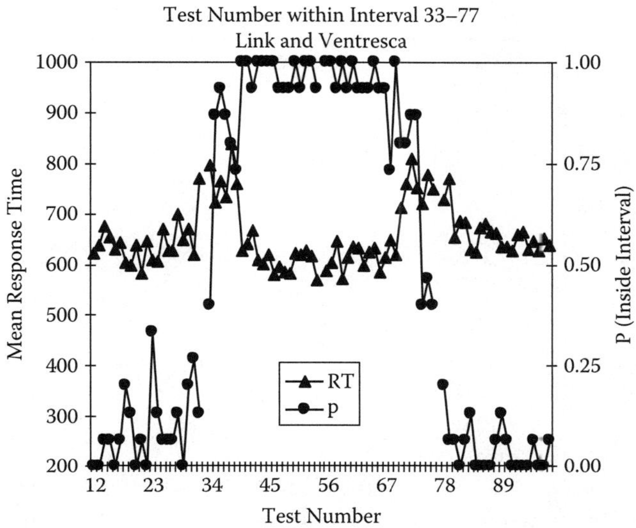


*Figure 8.2* Numerical comparisons of test numbers within or outside a specified interval. The left axis shows mean response time in milliseconds. The right-hand axis shows the proportion of judgments that the presented test number is within the interval of 33 to 77.

were given an interval defined by two numbers and were to judge whether a test number existed within or outside the interval. The size of the interval and the test numbers changed from trial to trial. Figure 8.2 shows previously unpublished results for response proportions and mean response times when the interval spanned 33 to 77 and test stimuli ranged from 12 to 99 exclusive of 33 and 77.

As is easily seen, the pattern of results is similar to that of the Cartwright experiment. Response times become largest when the response proportion is about 0.50. The results derive from an average of many trials from four very well-trained subjects who were given many different intervals and test stimuli. The relations in Figure 8.2 are typical of the results across all ranges of intervals employed, this range, 33 to 77, being the largest. A theoretical basis for numerical comparisons is described in "Measuring imageless thought: The relative judgment theory of numerical comparisons" (Link, 1990).

## 8.4 Face recognition

If any more proofs of this widely found relation were needed, Link and Lee (2009) reported similar results from experiments on face recognition. Ten subjects were to respond Same or Different to a test face presented simultaneously with an unchanging standard face. Test faces were either the same as the standard face (50% of trials) or were faces with the eyes displaced by varying numbers of pixels (1 pixel = 0.04 cm) ranging to +10 pixels from –10 pixels, each presented with probability 0.025. Faces remained present until the subject responded. Response choice and response times were measured. No feedback was given during the 1,000 trials.

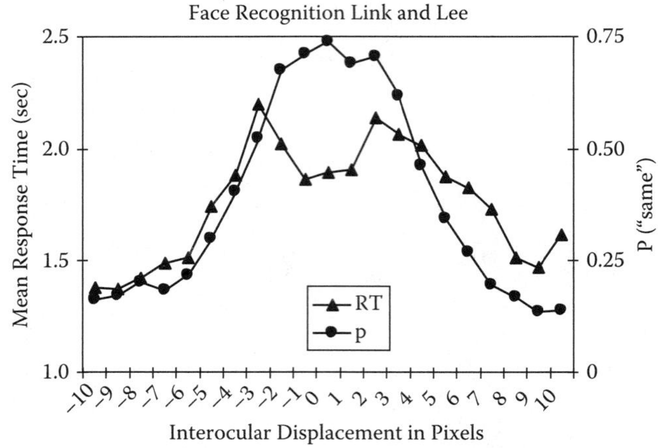


*Figure 8.3* Response times and proportions for the last 400 of 1,000 judgments of face similarity. Eyes were displaced by various numbers of pixels (0.04 cm/pixel) on the abscissa from a standard face. Results from Link and Lee (2009).

Once again the pattern of results shown in the Cartwright and Link and Ventresca experiments emerges as shown in Figure 8.3. Near the stimulus difference generating 50% responding the mean response times reach a maximum and then decrease on either edge of the "Interval of Uncertainty." These results from ten subjects use the raw data averaged across subjects. Similar results were obtained for other groups of subjects who studied the standard face at the beginning of the experiment for either 10, 20, or 30 seconds and then were tested in 1,000 trials for recognition without feedback.

## 8.5 The measurement of meaning

In these psychophysical experiments only a single dimension is altered to create different comparison stimuli. In a linguistic space defined by meaning, but of unknown topology, words may create dimensions of unknown character. Nevertheless we may assume that when a word is presented in the context of a sentence it varies in the linguistic space along some dimensions of difference. The less complex the contribution of the word to the meaning the fewer dimensions may be required for determining the distance contributed by the word to the meaning.

Cartwright (1941) provides an example of the type of experiment useful in determining the distance between meanings. In following up on the results shown in Figure 8.1 Cartwright tested the changes in meaning caused by changes in a key word in two sentences. The experiment is described by Cartwright (1941):

> At the beginning of the experiment the Ss were given a sentence with instructions to arrive at a clear formulation of the meaning of the various words in it. Then, they were shown some new words, which were to be substituted for one of the words of the sentence. Upon seeing each word, S was required to decide whether the substitution of the new word changed the basic meaning of the

sentence. Two different sentences were selected so that a word common to both would relate to different ranges of meaning, thus creating different differentiations of the test series. Ten Ss were given the two sentences and the test series on different days. Sentence I was: Yesterday I saw a huge building. Sentence II was: Yesterday I saw a huge man. The test-series contained the following 10 words: 1. immense, 2. grand, 3. great, 4. vast, 5. colossal, 6. large, 7. magnificent, 8. big, 9, mighty, 10. massive. It was supposed that a list of words which would be appropriate substitutes for huge in Sentence I would possess certain words which would not be appropriate substitutes in Sentence II. It is not proposed that Sentence II limits the total number of appropriate substitutes for huge, but rather the number of appropriate substitutes within the test series employed in this experiment. The test series was presented six times to each S. Since ten Ss were tested on both sentences, 1200 decisions were recorded.

Cartwright measured choice ("Yes" or "No") and vocal RT. He reported the percentage of "Yes" responses for each subject and sentence but only the subject's mean vocal RT for each probe word without distinguishing between "Yes" and "No" responses. At the end of the experiment Cartwright required subjects to rank order words on the basis of similarity of the resulting sentences to the standard sentence. From the individual ranks it is possible to compute the probability that a word changes the similarity between a standard and a comparison sentence by using the 60 judgments for each rank order. Although this is not a measure of distance it does provide a basis for determining a meaningful distance. Table 8.1 provides the proportions for each rank order of words in terms of similarity of the rank order word's sentence to the standard sentence.

## 8.6 A theory of similarity judgments

For each rank order these proportions are converted to logits based on the theory of comparative judgment proposed by Link (1975, 1992) but extended here to judgments of similarity. Link (1992) showed how a difference between two random variables with Poisson distributions can drive an accumulation of differences leading to one or the other of two alternative responses. In the case of similarity judgments one of these Poisson distributions, say *S*, measures similarity and the other, say *D*, measures dissimilarity between two stimuli. The magnitude of similarity is characterized by a Poisson distribution with mean value $\mu$. The dissimilarities have a Poisson distribution with parameter $\lambda$. Link proved that when these two measures are compared through an accumulation of differences between them, $S - D$, the probability of choosing a test stimulus to be similar to the standard stimulus equals

$$P = \frac{1}{1+e^{-A\theta}}, \tag{8.1}$$

where *A* is the amount of similarity required before an unbiased response can occur and $\theta = \ln(\lambda/\mu)$ is the logarithm of the ratio of the mean values characterizing the similarity and dissimilarity of the compared sentences.

*Table 8.1* Proportions *p*1 and *p*2 of choosing a test word to create a meaning similar to the standard sentence

| | *Words* | | | | | | | | | |
|---|---|---|---|---|---|---|---|---|---|---|
| *Sentence* | *1* | *2* | *3* | *4* | *5* | *6* | *7* | *8* | *9* | *10* |
| p1 | 0.995 | 0.929 | 0.896 | 0.831 | 0.615 | 0.549 | 0.385 | 0.202 | 0.087 | 0.022 |
| Aθ1 | 5.29 | 2.56 | 2.15 | 1.59 | 0.47 | 0.20 | –0.47 | –1.37 | –2.35 | –3.82 |
| RT1 | 156.8 | 180.2 | 201.3 | 294.2 | 219.5 | 231.2 | 190.1 | 216.2 | 200.4 | 159.3 |
| p2 | 0.995 | 0.979 | 0.814 | 0.583 | 0.368 | 0.120 | 0.055 | 0.022 | 0.022 | 0.005 |
| Aθ2 | 5.29 | 3.82 | 1.47 | 0.33 | –0.54 | –2.00 | –2.85 | –3.82 | –3.82 | –5.29 |
| RT2 | 145.7 | 166.6 | 199.9 | 235.7 | 192.9 | 225.1 | 197.2 | 175.3 | 149.5 | 143.0 |

*Note:* Words are in rank order of similarity within subjects.

Some algebra shows that the unknown parameters $A$ and $\theta$ can be estimated from data by using experimentally determined proportions, $p$, to estimate the theoretical probability $P$, and then computing,

$$A\theta = \ln\left(p/(1-p)\right). \tag{8.2}$$

This is a measure, called a logit in the statistical literature, of the difference between the similarity and dissimilarity of the test stimulus and the standard because

$$A\theta = A[\ln(\lambda) - \ln(\mu)] \tag{8.3}$$

is a distance measure on the scale of the natural logarithm.

Notice that by exponentiating Equation (8.3) we obtain a power law that depends on the strengths of similarity and dissimilarity; that is,

$$e^{A\theta} = \left(\frac{\lambda}{\mu}\right)^{A}. \tag{8.4}$$

But, examining Equation (8.2) we see that by exponentiating $A\theta$ the natural logarithm on the right-hand side of Equation (8.2) is removed. Therefore, there exists a power law relation between proportions of responses and the underlying strengths of similarity and dissimilarity:

$$\frac{p}{1-p} = \left(\frac{\lambda}{\mu}\right)^{A}. \tag{8.5}$$

This is called the Power Law of Similarity.

With respect to response times Link (1975, 1992) split the measured response time into two parts. The first part measured the time taken to make the eventual decision, the decision time, and the second part contained all those components that were not related to the decision process per se. Thus the observed response time can be written as

$$\text{Mean (RT)} = \text{Mean (Decision time)} + \text{Mean (Nondecision components)}. \tag{8.6}$$

Theoretical analysis of this stochastic process, often described as a bounded random walk, reveals that

$$\text{Mean (Decision time)} = \frac{A}{(\lambda-\mu)}(2P-1)$$

when there is no response bias and $\lambda \neq \mu$. As the denominator approaches zero, $\theta$ approaches 0, the value of $P$ approaches 0.50, and the mean decision time approaches a maximum of

$$\frac{A^2}{\lambda+\mu},$$

where the denominator is the variance of $S - D$.

In a carefully run experiment the nondecision components of response time should be controlled across changes in stimulus difference so that the changes in observed response time are those associated with the decision process itself. With respect to the decision times, the maximum decision time was shown to occur when $P = 0.50$. Thus, when the estimator of $P$, that is, $p$, equals 0.50 the maximum response time should be observed. This theoretical prediction is confirmed by many previous experiments.

## 8.7 Theoretical analysis of Cartwright's experiment

The proportions of similarity of meaning judgments made during the experiment appear in Table 8.1. These proportions are used to determine the values of $A\theta$ shown below each proportion. The orderly decline in these values from 5.29 to –3.82 for Sentence 1 and from 5.29 to –5.29 for Sentence 2 is sufficient evidence that values of $A\theta$ are in close agreement with the rank orderings provided after the experiment. Indeed, the rank orders may follow from the remembered magnitudes of $A\theta$, a magnitude that may be considered as the feeling of similarity.

Although the two sentences provide somewhat different measures based on their rank orders of words, the agreement between the measures is very good, producing a correlation 0.97 as shown in Figure 8.4. Notice in Figure 8.4 that the best linear fit accounts for 94% of the variance. Furthermore, the measures of meaning for these two sentences are related by the equation $0.78(S2) = S1 - 1$, where $S2$ is the measure of $A\theta$ for sentence 2 and $S1$ is the measure of $A\theta$ for sentence 1. This equation relates the similarity in meanings for the two sentences.

Cartwright also measured the individual subject vocal response times for each judgment. Although the subjects varied in terms of overall vocal response times for these judgments, the various subject times can be adjusted for individual differences by computing response time deviation values for each subject's response time for each judgment. These adjusted values are obtained by computing a $t$-value for each response time for each subject with each sentence. These values are determined by subtracting from a single response time the subject's mean response time for that sentence and dividing by the standard deviation for that subject's judgments for that sentence. These values are then free from biases due to the between-subject differences in magnitude and variability of the judgment response times. However, Cartwright's reports of the individual subject mean vocal response times for each rank-ordered word allows for computations of mean response times that parallel the computations generating Figures 8.1–8.3. Therefore the actual mean vocal times enter into the analysis of response times reported below.

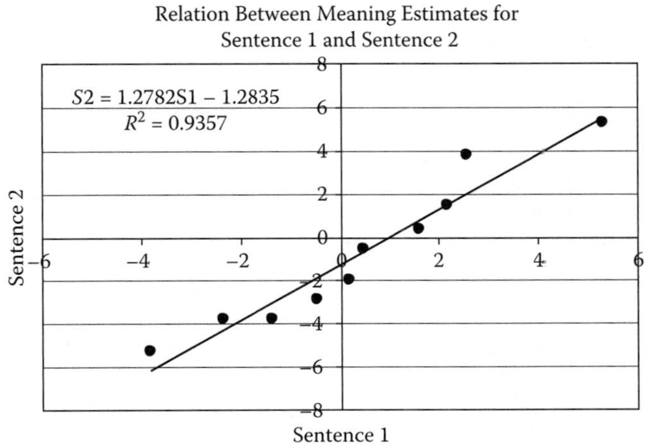


*Figure 8.4* Measures of similarity for test sentences versus two similar standard sentences compared. Correlation = 0.97.

To simplify the analysis somewhat the two sentences were combined in terms of rank order to produce a single composite of the relation between response times and response proportions. The question to be answered is whether the previous results for comparative judgments of similarity are also exhibited in Cartwright's data. In previous figures a physical measure of stimulus difference was the variable controlled by the experimenter. Both positive and negative values of stimulus difference allowed for a two-sided view of the subject's performance. Here we have only a single side because the direction of distance of the test word meanings from the standard sentence meaning is unknown. It is as if in the previous figures we folded the figures at zero stimulus difference and then viewed only a single side.

The sign of stimulus difference is in this case unknown, thus the single-sided graph somehow needs to convey the same information about the relations of response proportion and response times as in the previous analyses. Some of the words may correspond to positive stimulus differences and some to negative stimulus differences, which are currently unknown. However, if we allow some latitude in creating a useful comparison with the previous results we may expand upon the standard sentence as if two sides of the graph were actually measured in order to provide a comparison with the previous figures. This is shown in Figure 8.5 where the rank orders decrease away from the standard sentence on both sides. Of course this is symmetric but then so are the previous figures, and this proves the point of this comparison. The results with these words and sentences are similar to results obtained with physically measureable stimuli.

In conclusion these various results provide an insight into how psychophysical theory and data analysis provide a basis for the measurement of differences in meaning between two sentences. This result is a satisfactory outcome of applying psychophysical analysis to a linguistic question. The new, fundamental, ideas such as the Power Law of Similarity provide a basis for more refined experiments in the measurement of meaning.

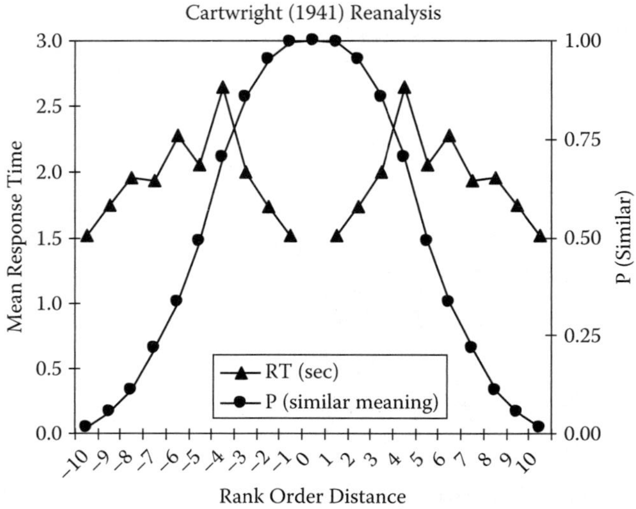


*Figure 8.5* Reanalysis of Cartwright's 1941 judgments of sentence similarity. The results are flipped across the value zero as if there were both positive and negative values of stimulus difference. No measure is available for a comparison of the standard sentence with itself, but the probability of similarity, equal to 1.0, is based on theory.

## References


Cartwright, D. (1941). Relation of decision-time to categories of response. *American Journal of Psychology, 54,* 174–106.

Eliot, T. S. (1917). *Prufrock and other observations.* London: The Egoist.

Link, S. W. (1975). The relative judgment theory of two-choice response time. *Journal of Mathematical Psychology*, *12,* 114–135.

Link, S. W. (1990). Measuring imageless thought: The relative judgment theory of numerical comparisons. *Journal of Mathematical Psychology, 34,* 2–41.

Link S. W. (1992). *The wave theory of difference and similarity.* Hillsdale, NJ: Lawrence Erlbaum.

Link, S., & Lee, K. (2009). Psychophysics of face recognition. In M. A. Elliott, S. Antonijević, S. Berthaud, P. Mulcahy, B. Bargary, C. Martyn, & H. Schmidt (Eds.), *Fechner Day 2009. Proceedings of the 25th Annual Meeting of the International Society for Psychophysics*, Galway, Ireland: The International Society for Psychophysics.

Urban, F. M. (1907). On the method of just perceptible differences. *Psychological Review*, *14*, 244–253.

Urban, F. M. (1910). The method of constant stimuli and its generalizations. *Psychological Review*, *17*, 229–259.

Ventresca, A. (1988). *Same/difference judgments of numerical comparisons: A study using an Interval of Equality*. B.A. Honours Thesis. McMaster University. Hamilton, Canada: Link Psychophysical Laboratory.

# 9 Mathematical foundations of Universal Fechnerian Scaling

*Ehtibar N. Dzhafarov*

Department of Psychological Studies
Purdue University
West Lafayette, Indiana, USA

and

Swedish Collegium for Advanced Study in the Social Sciences
Uppsala, Sweden

## 9.1 Introduction

The main idea of Fechner's original theory (Fechner, 1860, 1877, 1887) can be described as follows (see Figure 9.1). If stimuli are represented by real numbers (measuring stimulus intensities, or their spatial or temporal extents), the *subjective distance* from a stimulus $a$ to a stimulus $b > a$ is computed by *cumulating* from $a$ to $b$, through all intermediate values, a measure of *dissimilarity* of every stimulus $x$ from its "immediate" neighbors on the right. A modern rendering of Fechner's theory (Dzhafarov, 2001) defines the dissimilarity between $x$ and $x + dx$ as

$$D(x, x+dx) = c\left(\gamma(x, x+dx) - \frac{1}{2}\right),$$

where $\gamma(x, y)$ is a *psychometric function*

$$\gamma(x, y) = \Pr[y \text{ is judged to be greater than } x]$$

with no *"constant error"* (i.e., $\gamma(x, x) = 1/2$), and $c$ is a constant allowed to vary from one stimulus continuum to another. Assuming that $\gamma(x, y)$ is differentiable, and putting

$$\frac{D(x, x+dx)}{dx} = \left.\frac{\partial\gamma(x,y)}{\partial y}\right|_{y=x} = F(x),$$

the Fechnerian distance from $a$ to $b \geq a$ becomes

$$G(a,b) = \int_a^b F(x)dx.$$

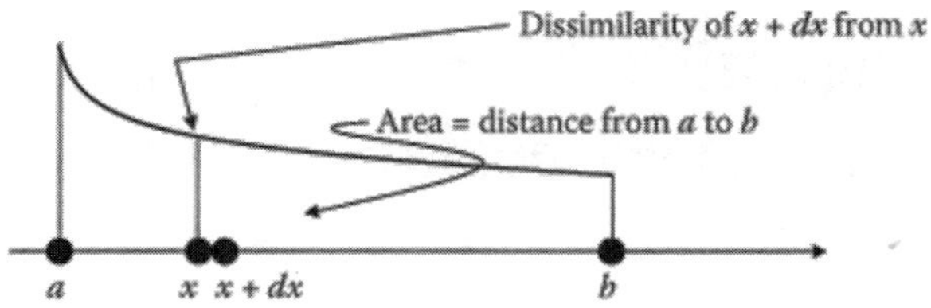


*Figure 9.1* Fechner's main idea. To compute the subjective (Fechnerian) distance from $a$ to $b$ on a stimulus continuum, one cumulates (here, integrates) the dissimilarity of $x$ from its infinitesimally close neighbors on the right as $x$ changes from $a$ to $b$.

In particular, if

$$F(x)=\frac{k}{x},$$

which is a rigorous form of *Weber's law*,

$$G(a,b)=k\log\frac{b}{a}.$$

We get the celebrated Fechner's law by setting $a$ at the "absolute threshold" $x_0$,

$$S(x)=k\log\frac{x}{x_0},$$

where $S(x)$ can be referred to as the *magnitude of the sensation* caused by stimulus $x$. If $F(x)$ happens to be different from $k/x$, the expressions $G(a, b)$ and $S(x)$ are modified accordingly. Thus, from

$$F(x)=\frac{k}{x^{1-\beta}},\ 1\geq\beta>0,$$

one gets

$$G(a,b)=\frac{k}{\beta}\left(b^{\beta}-a^{\beta}\right)$$

for the subjective distance from $a$ to $b$, and

$$S(x)=\frac{k}{\beta}\left(x^{\beta}-x_0^{\beta}\right)$$

for the sensation magnitude of $x$. In this rendering Fechner's theory is impervious to the mathematical (Luce & Edwards, 1958) and experimental (Riesz, 1933) critiques levied against it (for details see Dzhafarov, 2001, and Dzhafarov & Colonius, 1999). The main idea of this interpretation was proposed by Pfanzagl (1962), and then independently reintroduced in Creelman (1967), Falmagne (1971), and Krantz (1971) within the framework of the so-called "Fechner problem" (Luce & Galanter, 1963).

Fechner's theory launched the world-view (or "mind-view") of classical psychophysics, according to which perception is essentially characterized by a collection of unidimensional continua representable by axes of nonnegative real numbers. Each continuum corresponds to a certain "sensory quality" (loudness, spatial extent, saturation, etc.) any two values of which, *sensory magnitudes*, are comparable in terms of "*less than or equal to*." Moreover, each such continuum has a primary physical correlate, an axis of nonnegative reals representing intensity, or spatiotemporal extent of a particular physical attribute: the sensory attribute is related to its physical correlate monotonically and smoothly, starting from the value of the absolute threshold. This mind-view has been dominant throughout the entire history of psychophysics (Stevens, 1975), and it remains perfectly viable at present (see, e.g., Luce, 2002, 2004).

There is, however, another mind-view, also derived from Fechner's idea of computing distances from local dissimilarity measures, dating back to Helmholtz's (1891) and Schrödinger's (1920, 1920/1970, 1926/1970) work on color spaces. Physically, colors are functions relating radiometric energy to wavelength, but even if their representation by means of one of the traditional color diagrams (such as CIE or Munsell) is considered their physical description, and even if the subjective representation of colors is thought of in terms of a finite number of unidimensional attributes (such as, in the case of aperture colors, their hue, saturation, and brightness), the mapping of physical descriptions into subjective ones is clearly that of one multidimensional space into another. In this context the notions of sensory magnitudes ordered in terms of "greater–less" and of psychophysical functions become artificial, if applicable at all. The notion of subjective dissimilarity, by contrast, acquires the status of a natural and basic concept, whose applicability allows for but does not presuppose any specific system of color coordinates, either physical or subjective. The natural operationalization of the discrimination of similar colors in this context is their judgment in terms of "*same or different*," rather than "greater or less." (For a detailed discussion of the "greater–less" versus "same–different" comparisons, see Dzhafarov, 2003a.)

This mind-view has been generalized in the theoretical program of *Multidimensional Fechnerian Scaling* (Dzhafarov, 2002a–d; Dzhafarov & Colonius, 1999, 2001). The scope of this differential-geometric program is restricted to stimulus spaces representable by *open connected regions of Euclidean n-space* (refer to Figure 9.2 for an illustration.). This space is supposed to be endowed with a probability-of-different function

$$\psi(\mathbf{x}, \mathbf{y}) = \Pr\,[\mathbf{y} \text{ and } \mathbf{x} \text{ are judged to be different}].$$

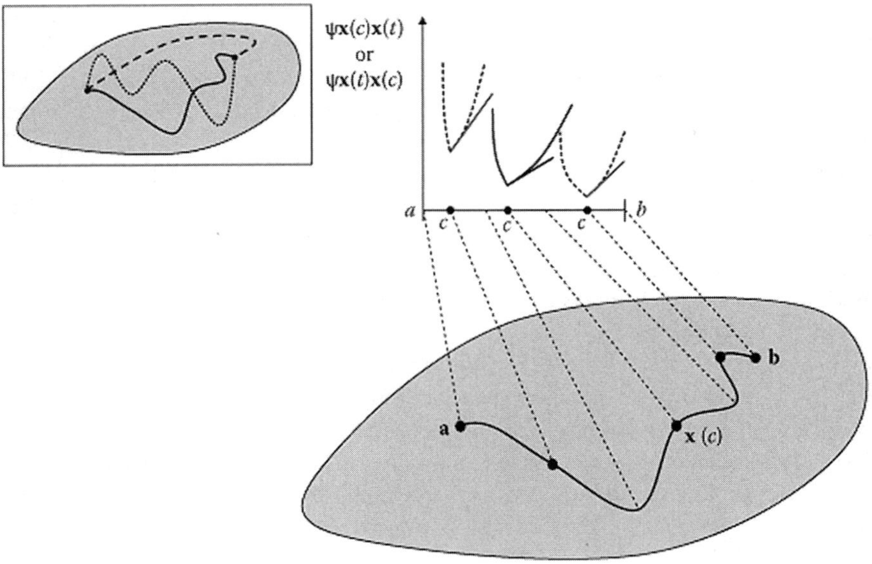


*Figure 9.2* A continuously differentiable path $\mathbf{x}(t)$ (thick curve) is shown as a mapping of an interval $[a, b]$ (horizontal line segment) into an area of Euclean space (gray area). For any point $c \in [a, b]$ there is a function $t \mapsto \psi(\mathbf{x}(c), \mathbf{x}(t))$ defined for all $t \in [a, b]$ (shown by $V$-shaped curves for three positions of $c$). The derivative of $\psi(\mathbf{x}(c), \mathbf{x}(t))$ at $t = c+$ (the slope of the tangent line at the minimum of the $V$-shaped curve) is taken for the value of $F(\mathbf{x}(c), \dot{\mathbf{x}}(c))$, and the integral of this function from $a$ to $b$ is taken for the value of length of the path. The inset at the left top corner shows that one should consider the lengths for all such paths from **a** to **b**, and take their infimum as the (generally asymmetric) distance $G\mathbf{ab}$. The overall, symmetric distance $G^*\mathbf{ab}$ is computed as $G\mathbf{ab} + G\mathbf{ba}$. [The lengths of paths can be alternatively computed by differentiating $\psi(\mathbf{x}(t), \mathbf{x}(c))$ rather than $\psi(\mathbf{x}(c), \mathbf{x}(t))$. Although this generally changes the value of $G\mathbf{ab}$, it makes no difference for the value of $G^*\mathbf{ab}$.]

Any two points **a**, **b** in such a space can be connected by a *continuously differentiable path* $\mathbf{x}(t)$ defined on a segment of reals $[a, b]$. The "length" of this path can be defined by means of the following construction. Assume that

$$\psi(\mathbf{x}, \mathbf{x}) < \min\{\psi(\mathbf{x}, \mathbf{y}), \psi(\mathbf{y}, \mathbf{x})\}$$

for all distinct $\mathbf{x}$, $\mathbf{y}$, and that for any $c \in [a, b]$ the discrimination probability $\psi(\mathbf{x}(c), \mathbf{x}(t))$ has a positive right-hand derivative at $t = c+$,

$$\left.\frac{\mathrm{d}\psi\big(\mathbf{x}(c), \mathbf{x}(t)\big)}{\mathrm{d}t}\right|_{t=c+} = F\big(\mathbf{x}(c), \dot{\mathbf{x}}(c)\big).$$

The function $F(\mathbf{x}(t), \dot{\mathbf{x}}(t))$ is referred to as a *submetric function*, and the differential $F(\mathbf{x}(t), \dot{\mathbf{x}}(t))\mathrm{d}t$ serves as the local dissimilarity between $\mathbf{x}(t)$ and $\mathbf{x}(t) + \dot{\mathbf{x}}(t)\mathrm{d}t$. Assuming further that $F$ is continuous, we define the length of the path $\mathbf{x}(t)$ as the integral

$$D(\mathbf{x}[a,b]) = \int_a^b F(\mathbf{x}(t), \dot{\mathbf{x}}(t))\,\mathrm{d}t.$$

Applying this to all continuously differentiable paths connecting **a** to **b** and finding the *infimum* of their *D*-lengths, one defines the *(asymmetric) Fechnerian distance* *G***ab** from **a** to **b** (a function which satisfies all metric axioms except for symmetry). The *overall (symmetrical) Fechnerian distance* *G****ab** between **a** and **b** is computed as *G***ab** + *G***ba**. Although this description is schematic and incomplete it should suffice for introducing one line of generalizing Fechnerian Scaling: dispensing with unidimensionality but retaining the idea of cumulation of local dissimilarities.

A further line of generalization is presented in Dzhafarov and Colonius (2005b, 2006c). It is designated as Fechnerian Scaling of Discrete Object Sets and applies to stimulus spaces comprised of "isolated entities," such as schematic faces, letters of an alphabet, and the like (see Figure 9.3). Each pair (**x**, **y**) of such stimuli is assigned a probability ψ (**x**, **y**) with which they are judged to be different from each other. Schematizing and simplifying as before, the local discriminability measure is defined as

$$D\,(\mathbf{x}, \mathbf{y}) = \psi\,(\mathbf{x}, \mathbf{y}) - \psi\,(\mathbf{x}, \mathbf{x}),$$

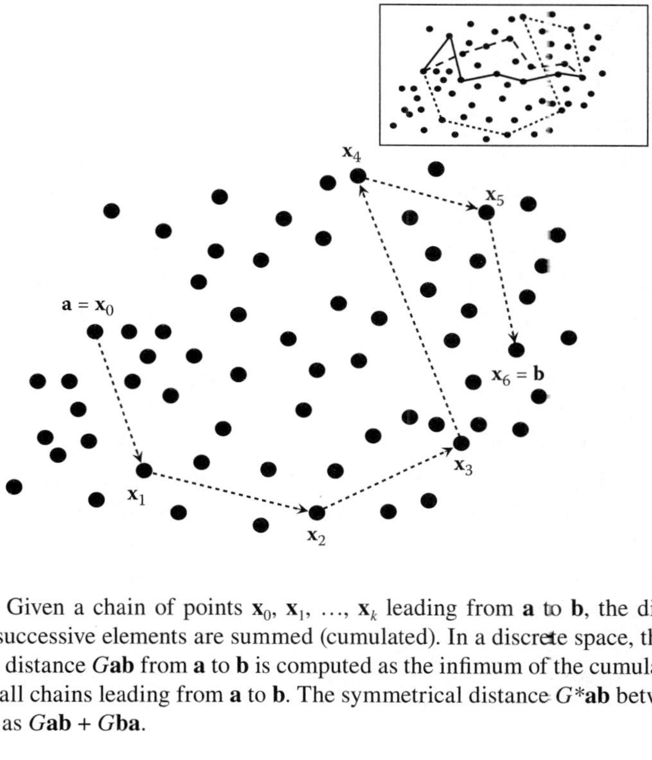


*Figure 9.3* Given a chain of points $\mathbf{x}_0, \mathbf{x}_1, \ldots, \mathbf{x}_k$ leading from **a** to **b**, the dissimilarities between its successive elements are summed (cumulated). In a discrete space, the (generally asymmetric) distance *G***ab** from **a** to **b** is computed as the infimum of the cumulated dissimilarities over all chains leading from **a** to **b**. The symmetrical distance *G****ab** between **a** and **b** is computed as *G***ab** + *G***ba**.

and the (asymmetric) Fechnerian distance $G(\mathbf{a}, \mathbf{b})$ is defined as the infimum of

$$\sum_{i=0}^{k} D\left(\mathbf{x}_i, \mathbf{x}_{i+1}\right)$$

computed across all possible finite chains of stimuli

$$\mathbf{a} = \mathbf{x}_0, \mathbf{x}_1, \ldots, \mathbf{x}_k, \mathbf{x}_{k+1} = \mathbf{b}$$

connecting **a** to **b**. Here the deviation from Fechner's original theory is greater than in the Multidimensional Fechnerian Scaling: we dispense not only with unidimensionality, but also with the "infinitesimality" of dissimilarities being cumulated. But the idea of computing dissimilarities from discrimination probabilities and obtaining distances by some form of dissimilarity cumulation is retained.

The purpose of this work is to present a sweeping generalization of Fechner's theory which is applicable to *all possible* stimulus spaces endowed with "same-different" discrimination probabilities. This theory, called *Universal Fechnerian Scaling* (UFS), is presented in the trilogy of papers Dzhafarov and Colonius (2007), Dzhafarov (2008a), and Dzhafarov (2008b). We follow these papers closely, but omit proofs, examples, and technical explanations. Our focus is on the mathematical foundations of UFS, which are formed by an abstract theory called *Dissimilarity Cumulation* (DC): it provides a general definition of a *dissimilarity function* and shows how this function is used to impose on stimulus sets topological and metric properties.

The potential sphere of applicability of UFS is virtually unlimited. The ability to decide whether two entities are the same or different is the most basic faculty of all living organisms and the most basic requirement of artificial perceiving systems, such as intelligent robots. The perceiving system may be anything from an organism to a person to a group of consumers or voters to an abstract computational procedure. The stimuli may be anything from letters of alphabet (from the point of view of grammar school children) to different lung dysfunctions represented by X-ray films (from the point of view of a physician) to brands of a certain product (from the point of view of a group of consumers) to political candidates or propositions (from the point of view of potential voters) to competing statistical models (from the point of view of a statistical fitting procedure). Thus, if stimuli are several lung dysfunctions each represented by a potentially infinite set of X-ray films, a physician or a group of physicians can be asked to tell if two randomly chosen X-ray films do or do not indicate one and the same dysfunction. As a result each pair of dysfunctions is assigned the probability with which their respective X-ray representations are judged to indicate different ailments. If stimuli are competing statistical models, the probability with which models **x** and **y** are "judged" to be different can be estimated by the probability with which a dataset generated by the model **x** allows one to reject the model **y** (see Dzhafarov & Colonius, 2006a, for details). The questions to the perceiving system can be formulated in a variety of forms: "Are **x** and **y** the same (overall)?" or "Do **x** and **y** differ in respect to *A*?" or "Do **x** and **y** differ if one ignores their difference in property *B*?" or "Do **x** and **y** belong to one and the same category (from a given list)?", and so on. Note the difference from the other known scaling procedure based on discrimination probabilities, Thurstonian Scaling (Thurstone, 1927a,b). This procedure only deals with the probabilities with which one stimulus is judged to have more of a particular property (such as attractiveness, brightness, loudness, etc.) than another stimulus. The use of these probabilities therefore requires that the investigator know in advance which properties are relevant, that these properties be semantically unidimensional (i.e., assessable in terms of "greater–less"), and that the perception of the stimuli be entirely determined by these properties. No such assumptions are needed in UFS. Moreover, in the concluding section of the chapter it is mentioned that the discrimination probabilities may very well be replaced with other pairwise judgments of "subjective difference" between two stimuli, and that the theory can even be applied beyond the context of pairwise judgments altogether, for example, to categorization judgments. It is also mentioned there that the dissimilarity cumulation procedure can be viewed as an alternative to the nonmetric versions of Multidimensional Scaling, applying therefore in all cases in which one can use the latter.*

## 9.2 Psychophysics of discrimination

We observe the following notation conventions. Boldface lowercase letters, **a**, **b′**, **x**, $\mathbf{y}_n$, ..., always denote elements of a set of stimuli. Stimuli are merely names (qualitative entities), with no algebraic operations defined on them. Real-valued functions of one or more arguments that are elements of a stimulus set are indicated by strings without parentheses:

$$\psi\mathbf{ab},\ D\mathbf{abc}, D\mathbf{X}_n,\ \Psi^{(1)}\mathbf{ab},\ \ldots.$$

### *9.2.1 Regular Minimality and canonical representations*

Here, we briefly recapitulate some of the basic concepts and assumptions underlying the theory of same–different discrimination probabilities. A toy example in Figure 9.4 provides an illustration. A detailed description and examples can be found in Dzhafarov (2002d, 2003a) and Dzhafarov and Colonius (2005a, 2006a).

The arguments **x** and **y** of the discrimination probability function

$$\psi^*\mathbf{xy} = \Pr\,[\mathbf{x} \text{ and } \mathbf{y} \text{ are judged to be different}]$$

* As a data-analytic procedure, UFS is implemented (as of September 2009) in three computer programs: the R-language package "fechner" described in Ünlü, Kiefer, and Dzhafarov (2009) and available at CRAN; a MATLAB-based program FSCAMDS developed at Purdue University and available at http://www1.psych.purdue.edu/~ehtibar/Links.html; and a MATLAB toolbox developed at Oldenburg University and available at http://www.psychologie.uni-oldenburg.de/stefan.rach/31856.html.

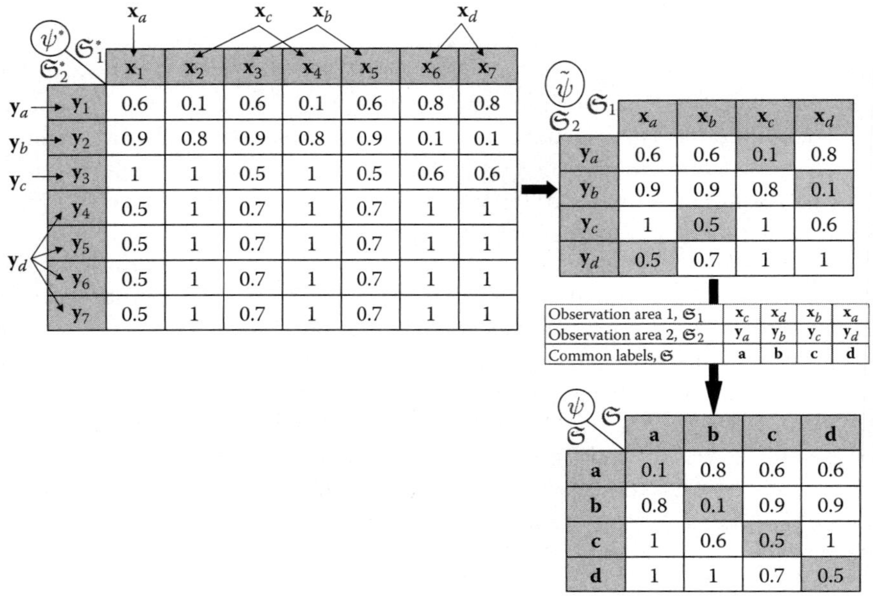


*Figure 9.4* A toy example used in Dzhafarov & Colonius (2006a). The transformation from $(\mathfrak{S}_1^*, \mathfrak{S}_2^*, \psi^*)$ to $(\mathfrak{S}_1, \mathfrak{S}_2, \tilde{\psi})$ is the result of "lumping together" psychologically equal stimuli (e.g., the stimuli $\mathbf{y}_4$, $\mathbf{y}_5$, $\mathbf{y}_6$, $\mathbf{y}_7$ are psychologically equal in $\mathfrak{S}_2^*$, stimuli $\mathbf{x}_2$ and $\mathbf{x}_4$ are psychologically equal in $\mathfrak{S}_1^*$). The space $(\mathfrak{S}_1, \mathfrak{S}_2, \tilde{\psi})$ satisfies the Regular Minimality condition (the minimum in each row is also the minimum in its column) because of which $(\mathfrak{S}_1, \mathfrak{S}_2, \tilde{\psi})$ can be canonically transformed into $(\mathfrak{S}, \psi)$, by means of the transformation table shown in between.

belong to two distinct observation areas,

$$\psi^*: \mathfrak{S}_1^* \times \mathfrak{S}_2^* \rightarrow [0, 1].$$

Thus, $\mathfrak{S}_1^*$ (the first observation area) may represent stimuli presented chronologically first or on the left, whereas $\mathfrak{S}_2^*$ (the second observation area) designates stimuli presented, respectively, chronologically second or on the right. The adjectives "first" and "second" refer to the ordinal positions of stimulus symbols within a pair $(\mathbf{x}, \mathbf{y})$.

For $\mathbf{x}, \mathbf{x}' \in \mathfrak{S}_1^*$, we say that the two stimuli are *psychologically equal* (or metameric) if $\psi^*\mathbf{xy} = \psi^*\mathbf{x}'\mathbf{y}$ for any $\mathbf{y} \in \mathfrak{S}_2^*$. Analogously, the psychological equality for $\mathbf{y}, \mathbf{y}' \in \mathfrak{S}_2^*$ is defined by $\psi^*\mathbf{xy} = \psi^*\mathbf{xy}'$, for any $\mathbf{x} \in \mathfrak{S}_1^*$. It is always possible to "*reduce*" the observation areas, that is, relabel their elements so that psychologically equal stimuli receive identical labels and are no longer distinguished. The discrimination probability function $\psi^*$ can then be redefined as

$$\tilde{\psi}: \mathfrak{S}_1 \times \mathfrak{S}_2 \rightarrow [0, 1].$$

The law of Regular Minimality is the statement that there are functions $\mathbf{h}: \mathfrak{S}_1 \rightarrow \mathfrak{S}_2$ and $\mathbf{g}: \mathfrak{S}_2 \rightarrow \mathfrak{S}_1$ such that

$$(P_1)\quad \tilde{\psi}\mathbf{x}[\mathbf{h}(\mathbf{x})] < \tilde{\psi}\mathbf{xy} \text{ for all } \mathbf{y} \neq \mathbf{h}(\mathbf{x})$$

$$(P_2)\quad \tilde{\psi}[\mathbf{g}(\mathbf{y})]\mathbf{y} < \tilde{\psi}\mathbf{xy} \text{ for all } \mathbf{x} \neq \mathbf{g}(\mathbf{y})$$

$$(P_3)\qquad \mathbf{h} \equiv \mathbf{g}^{-1}$$

Stimulus $\mathbf{y} = \mathbf{h}(\mathbf{x}) \in \mathfrak{S}_2$ is called the *Point of Subjective Equality* (PSE) for $\mathbf{x} \in \mathfrak{S}_1$; analogously, $\mathbf{x} = \mathbf{g}(\mathbf{y}) \in \mathfrak{S}_1$ is the PSE for $\mathbf{y} \in \mathfrak{S}_2$. The law of Regular Minimality states therefore that every stimulus in each of the (reduced) observation areas has a unique PSE in the other observation area, and that **y** is the PSE for **x** if and only if **x** is the PSE for **y**. In some contexts the law of regular minimality is an empirical assumption, but it can also serve as a criterion for a properly defined stimulus space. For a detailed discussion of the law and its critiques see Dzhafarov (2002d, 2003a, 2006), Dzhafarov and Colonius (2006a), and Ennis (2006).

Due to the law of Regular Minimality, one can always relabel the stimuli in $\mathfrak{S}_1$ or $\mathfrak{S}_2$ so that any two mutual PSEs receive one and the same label. In other words, one can always bijectively map $\mathfrak{S}_1 \to \mathfrak{S}$ and $\mathfrak{S}_2 \to \mathfrak{S}$ so that $\mathbf{x} \mapsto \mathbf{a}$ and $\mathbf{y} \mapsto \mathbf{a}$ if and only if $\mathbf{x} \in \mathfrak{S}_1$ and $\mathbf{y} \in \mathfrak{S}_2$ are mutual PSEs: $\mathbf{y} = \mathbf{h}(\mathbf{x})$, $\mathbf{x} = \mathbf{g}(\mathbf{y})$. The set of labels $\mathfrak{S}$ is called a *canonically transformed* stimulus set. Its elements too, for simplicity, are referred to as stimuli. The discrimination probability function $\tilde{\psi}$ can now be presented in a *canonical form*,

$$\psi : \mathfrak{S} \times \mathfrak{S} \to [0, 1],$$

with the property

$$\psi\mathbf{aa} < \min\{\psi\mathbf{ab}, \psi\mathbf{ba}\}$$

for any **a** and $\mathbf{b} \neq \mathbf{a}$. Note that the first and the second **a** in $\psi\mathbf{aa}$ may very well refer to physically different stimuli (equivalence classes of stimuli): hence one should exercise caution in referring to $\psi\mathbf{aa}$ as the probability with which **a** is discriminated from "itself."

## 9.2.2. From discrimination to dissimilarity

For the canonically transformed function $\psi$, the *psychometric increments of the first and second kind* are defined as, respectively,

$$\Psi^{(1)}\mathbf{ab} = \psi\mathbf{ab} - \psi\mathbf{aa}$$

and

$$\Psi^{(2)}\mathbf{ab} = \psi\mathbf{ba} - \psi\mathbf{aa}.$$

Due to the canonical form of $\psi$ these quantities are always positive for $\mathbf{b} \neq \mathbf{a}$.

The main assumption of UFS about these psychometric increments is that both of them are dissimilarity functions. The meaning of this statement becomes clear later, after a formal definition of a dissimilarity function is given.

Denoting by $D$ either $\Psi^{(1)}$ or $\Psi^{(2)}$ one can compute the (generally asymmetric) Fechnerian distance $G\mathbf{ab}$ by considering all possible finite chains of stimuli $\mathbf{x}_1 \ldots \mathbf{x}_k$ for all possible $k$ and putting

$$G\mathbf{ab} = \inf_{k, x_1 \ldots x_k} \left[ D\mathbf{a}\mathbf{x}_1 + D\mathbf{x}_1\mathbf{x}_2 + \ldots + D\mathbf{x}_k\mathbf{b} \right].$$

The overall Fechnerian distance is then computed as

$$G^*\mathbf{ab} = G_1\mathbf{ab} + G_1\mathbf{ba}.$$

This quantity can be interpreted as the infimum of $D$-lengths of all finite closed loops that contain points **a** and **b**. That is,

$$G^*\mathbf{ab} = \inf_{\substack{k, \mathbf{x}_1 \ldots \mathbf{x}_k \\ l, \mathbf{y}_1 \ldots \mathbf{y}_l}} \left[ D\mathbf{a}\mathbf{x}_1 + D\mathbf{x}_1\mathbf{x}_2 + \ldots + D\mathbf{x}_k\mathbf{b} + D\mathbf{b}\mathbf{y}_1 + D\mathbf{y}_1\mathbf{y}_2 + \ldots + D\mathbf{y}_l\mathbf{a} \right]$$

It is easy to see that the $D$-length of any given loop remains invariant if $D \equiv \Psi^{(1)}$ is replaced with $D \equiv \Psi^{(2)}$ and the loop is traversed in the opposite direction. The value of $G^*\mathbf{ab}$ therefore does not depend on which of the two psychometric increments is taken for $D$. Henceforth we tacitly assume that $D$ may be replaced with either $\Psi^{(1)}$ or $\Psi^{(2)}$, no matter which.

## 9.3 Dissimilarity Cumulation theory

### *9.3.1 Topology and uniformity*

To explain what it means for a function $D : \mathfrak{S} \times \mathfrak{S} \to \mathbb{R}$ to be a dissimilarity function, we begin with a more general concept. Function $D : \mathfrak{S} \times \mathfrak{S} \to \mathbb{R}$ is a (uniform) *deviation function* if it has the following properties: for any $\mathbf{a}, \mathbf{b} \in \mathfrak{S}$ and any sequences $\mathbf{a}_n$, $\mathbf{a}'_n$, $\mathbf{b}_n$, $\mathbf{b}'_n$ in $\mathfrak{S}$,

$[D1.]$ $\mathbf{a} \neq \mathbf{b} \Rightarrow D\mathbf{ab} > 0$;

$[D2.]$ $D\mathbf{aa} = 0$;

$[D3.]$ (Uniform Continuity) If $D\mathbf{a}_n\mathbf{a}'_n \to 0$ and $D\mathbf{b}_n\mathbf{b}'_n \to 0$, then $D\mathbf{a}'_n\mathbf{b}'_n - D\mathbf{a}_n\mathbf{b}_n \to 0$.

See Figure 9.5 for an illustration of Property $D3$. If $D$ is a symmetric metric, then it is a deviation function, with the uniform continuity property holding as a theorem.

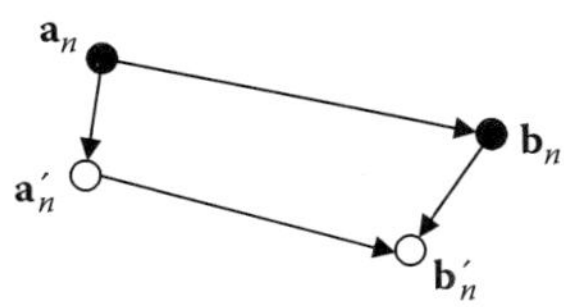


*Figure 9.5* An illustration for property *D*3 (uniform continuity). Consider an infinite sequence of quadrilaterals $\mathbf{a}_1\mathbf{a}'_1\mathbf{b}'_1\mathbf{b}_1$, $\mathbf{a}_2\mathbf{a}'_2\mathbf{b}'_2\mathbf{b}_2$, ..., such that the *D*-lengths of the sides $\mathbf{a}_n\mathbf{a}'_n$ and $\mathbf{b}_n\mathbf{b}'_n$ (directed as shown by the arrows) converge to zero. Then the difference between the *D*-lengths of the sides $\mathbf{a}_n\mathbf{b}_n$ and $\mathbf{a}'_n\mathbf{b}'_n$ (in the direction of the arrows) converges to zero.

If *D* is an asymmetric metric, then it is a deviation function if and only if it additionally satisfies the "invertibility in the small" condition,

$$D\mathbf{a}_n\mathbf{a}'_n \to 0 \Rightarrow D\mathbf{a}'_n\mathbf{a}_n \to 0.$$

In the following the term *metric* (or *distance*), unless specifically qualified as symmetric, always refers to an asymmetric metric (distance) invertible in the small.

*D* induces on $\mathfrak{S}$ the notion of convergence: we define $\mathbf{a}_n \leftrightarrow \mathbf{b}_n$ to mean $D\mathbf{a}_n\mathbf{b}_n \to 0$. The notation is unambiguous because convergence $\leftrightarrow$ is an equivalence relation (i.e.,it is reflexive, symmetric, and transitive). In particular, $\mathbf{a}_n \leftrightarrow \mathbf{a}$ means both $D\mathbf{a}\mathbf{a}_n$ 0 and $D\mathbf{a}_n\mathbf{a} \to 0$. The convergence $(\mathbf{a}^1_n, \ldots, \mathbf{a}^k_n) \leftrightarrow (\mathbf{b}^1_n, \ldots, \mathbf{b}^k_n)$ can be defined, e.g., by $\max_i D\mathbf{a}^i_n\mathbf{b}^i_n \to 0$.

A *topological basis* on $\mathfrak{S}$ is a family of subsets of $\mathfrak{S}$ covering $\mathfrak{S}$ and satisfying the following property (Kelly, 1955, p. 47): if $\mathfrak{a}$ and $\mathfrak{b}$ are within the basis, then for any $\mathbf{x} \in \mathfrak{a} \cap \mathfrak{b}$ the basis contains a set $\mathfrak{c}$ that contains $\mathbf{x}$. Given a topological basis on $\mathfrak{S}$, the *topology* on $\mathfrak{S}$ (a family of *open sets* "based" on this basis) is obtained by taking all possible unions of the subsets comprising the basis (including the empty set, which is the union of an empty class of such subsets). Deviation *D* induces on $\mathfrak{S}$ a topology based on

$$\mathfrak{B}_D(\mathbf{x},\varepsilon) = \{\mathbf{y} \in \mathfrak{S} : D\mathbf{x}\mathbf{y} < \varepsilon\}$$

taken for all $\mathbf{x} \in \mathfrak{S}$ and all real $\varepsilon > 0$. We call this topology (based on $\mathfrak{B}_D$-balls) the *D-topology.*

These topological considerations, as it turns out, can be strengthened: *D* induces on $\mathfrak{S}$ not only a topology but a more restrictive structure, called *uniformity.* Recall (Kelly, 1955, p. 177) that a family of subsets of $\mathfrak{S} \times \mathfrak{S}$ forms a *basis for a uniformity* on $\mathfrak{S}$ if it satisfies the following four properties: if $\mathfrak{A}$ and $\mathfrak{B}$ are members of the basis, then

1. $\mathfrak{A}$ includes as its subset $\Delta = \{(\mathbf{x}, \mathbf{x}) : \mathbf{x} \in \mathfrak{S}\}$.
2. $\mathfrak{A}^{-1} = \{(\mathbf{y}, \mathbf{x}) : (\mathbf{x}, \mathbf{y}) \in \mathfrak{A}\}$ includes as its subset a member of the basis.

3. For some member $\mathfrak{C}$ of the basis, $\{(\mathbf{x}, \mathbf{z}) \in \mathfrak{S}^2 : \text{for some } \mathbf{y}, (\mathbf{x}, \mathbf{y}) \in \mathfrak{C} \wedge (\mathbf{y}, \mathbf{z}) \in \mathfrak{C}\} \subset \mathfrak{A}$.
4. $\mathfrak{A} \cap \mathfrak{B}$ includes as its subset a member of the basis.

Given a uniformity basis on $\mathfrak{S}$, the uniformity on $\mathfrak{S}$ ("based" on this basis) is obtained by taking each member of the basis and forming its unions with all subsets of $\mathfrak{S} \times \mathfrak{S}$.A member of a uniformity is called an *entourage*. Deviation $D$ induces on $\mathfrak{S}$ a uniformity based on entourages

$$\mathfrak{U}_D(\varepsilon) = \{(\mathbf{x}, \mathbf{y}) \in \mathfrak{S}^2 : D\mathbf{x}\mathbf{y} < \varepsilon\}$$

taken for all real $\varepsilon > 0$. This uniformity satisfies the so-called separation axiom:

$$\cap_\varepsilon \mathfrak{U}_D(\varepsilon) = \{(\mathbf{x}, \mathbf{y}) \in \mathfrak{S}^2 : \mathbf{x} = \mathbf{y}\}.$$

We call this uniformity the *D-uniformity*. The $D$-topology is precisely the topology induced by the $D$-uniformity (Kelly, 1955, p. 178):

$$\mathfrak{B}_D(\mathbf{x}, \varepsilon) = \{\mathbf{y} \in \mathfrak{S} : (\mathbf{x}, \mathbf{y}) \in \mathfrak{U}_D(\varepsilon)\}$$

is the restriction of the basic entourage $\mathfrak{U}_D(\varepsilon)$ to the pairs ($\mathbf{x}$ = const, $\mathbf{y}$).

### *9.3.2 Chains and dissimilarity function*

Chains in space $\mathfrak{S}$ are finite sequences of elements, written as strings: **ab**, **abc**, $\mathbf{x}_1 \ldots \mathbf{x}_k$, etc. Note that the elements of a chain need not be pairwise distinct. A chain of *cardinality* $k$ (a $k$-chain) is the chain with $k$ elements (vertices), hence with $k-1$ links (edges). For completeness, we also admit an empty chain, of zero cardinality. We use the notation

$$D\mathbf{x}_1 \ldots \mathbf{x}_k = \sum_{i=1}^{k-1} D\mathbf{x}_i \mathbf{x}_{i+1},$$

and call it the $D$-length of the chain $\mathbf{x}_1 \ldots \mathbf{x}_k$.

If the elements of a chain are not of interest, it can be denoted by a boldface capital, such as **X**, with appropriate ornaments. Thus, **X** and **Y** are two chains, **XY** is their concatenation, **aXb** is a chain connecting **a** to **b**. The cardinality of chain **X** is denoted $|\mathbf{X}|$. Unless otherwise specified, within a sequence of chains, $\mathbf{X}_n$, the cardinality $|\mathbf{X}_n|$ generally varies: $\mathbf{X}_n = \mathbf{x}_1^n \ldots \mathbf{x}_{k_n}^n$.

A uniform deviation function $D$ on $\mathfrak{S}$ is a uniform dissimilarity (or, simply, dissimilarity) function on $\mathfrak{S}$ if it has the following property:

[$D$4.] for any sequence of chains $\mathbf{a}_n \mathbf{X}_n \mathbf{b}_n$,

$$D\mathbf{a}_n \mathbf{X}_n \mathbf{b}_n \to 0 \Rightarrow D\mathbf{a}_n \mathbf{b}_n \to 0.$$

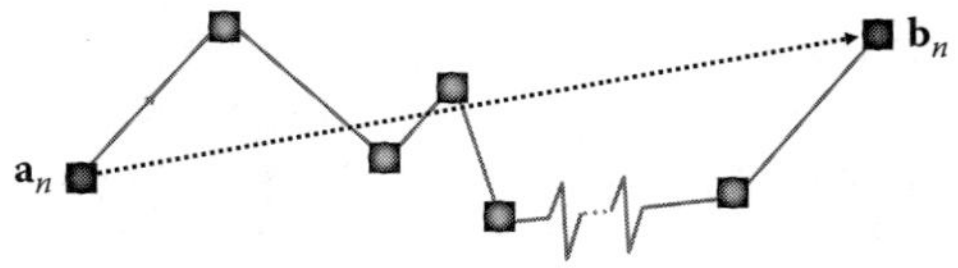


*Figure 9.6* An Illustration for Property $D4$ (chain property). Consider an infinite sequence of chains $\mathbf{a}_1\mathbf{X}_1\mathbf{b}_1, \mathbf{a}_2\mathbf{X}_2\mathbf{b}_2, \ldots$, such that $|\mathbf{X}_n|$ increases beyond bounds with $n \to \infty$, and $D\mathbf{a}_n\mathbf{X}_n\mathbf{b}_n$ converges to zero. Then $D\mathbf{a}_n\mathbf{b}_n$ (the $D$-length of the dotted arrow) converges to zero too.

See Figure 9.6 for an illustration. If $D$ is a metric, then $D$ is a dissimilarity function as a trivial consequence of the triangle inequality.

### 9.3.3 Fechnerian distance

The set of all possible chains in $\mathfrak{S}$ is denoted by $C_{\mathfrak{S}}$, or simply $C$. We define function $G\mathbf{ab}$ by

$$G\mathbf{ab} = \inf_{\mathbf{X}\in C} D\mathbf{aXb}.$$

$G\mathbf{ab}$ is a metric, and $G^*\mathbf{ab} = G\mathbf{ab} + G\mathbf{ba}$ is a symmetric metric (also called "overall"). We say that the metric $G$ and the overall metric $G^*$ are induced by the dissimilarity $D$. Clearly, $G^*\mathbf{ab}$ can also be defined by

$$G^*\mathbf{ab} = \inf_{(\mathbf{X},\mathbf{Y})\in C^2} D\mathbf{aXbYa} = \inf_{(\mathbf{X},\mathbf{Y})\in C^2} D\mathbf{bXaYb}.$$

### 9.3.4 Topology and uniformity on $(\mathfrak{S},G)$

It can be shown that

$$D\mathbf{a}_n\mathbf{b}_n \to 0 \Leftrightarrow G\mathbf{a}_n\mathbf{b}_n \to 0,$$

and

$$\mathbf{a}_n \leftrightarrow \mathbf{b}_n \Leftrightarrow G\mathbf{a}_n\mathbf{b}_n \to 0 \Leftrightarrow G\mathbf{b}_n\mathbf{a}_n \to 0 \Leftrightarrow G^*\mathbf{a}_n\mathbf{b}_n = G^*\mathbf{b}_n\mathbf{a}_n \to 0.$$

As a consequence, $G$ induces on $\mathfrak{S}$ a topology based on sets

$$\mathfrak{B}_G(\mathbf{x},\varepsilon) = \{\mathbf{y} \in \mathfrak{S} : G\mathbf{xy} < \varepsilon\}$$

taken for all $\mathbf{x} \in \mathfrak{S}$ and positive $\varepsilon$. This topology coincides with the $D$-topology. Analogously, $G$ induces on $\mathfrak{S}$ a uniformity based on the sets

$$\mathfrak{A}_G(\varepsilon) = \{(\mathbf{x}, \mathbf{y}) \in \mathfrak{S}^2 : G\mathbf{xy} < \varepsilon\}$$

taken for all positive $\varepsilon$. This uniformity coincides with the $D$-uniformity. The metric $G$ is uniformly continuous in $(\mathbf{x}, \mathbf{y})$, i.e., if $\mathbf{a}'_n \leftrightarrow \mathbf{a}_n$ and $\mathbf{b}'_n \leftrightarrow \mathbf{b}_n$, then

$$G\mathbf{a}'_n\mathbf{b}'_n - G\mathbf{a}_n\mathbf{b}_n \to 0.$$

The space $(\mathfrak{S},D)$ being uniform and metrizable, we get its standard topological characterization (see, e.g., Hocking & Young, 1961, p. 42): it is a *completely normal space*, meaning that its singletons are closed and any its two separated subsets $\mathfrak{A}$ and $\mathfrak{B}$ (i.e., such that $\overline{\mathfrak{A}} \cap \mathfrak{B} = \mathfrak{A} \cap \overline{\mathfrak{B}} = \emptyset$) are contained in two disjoint open subsets.

The following is an important fact which can be interpreted as that of internal consistency of the metric $G$ induced by means of dissimilarity cumulation: once $G\mathbf{ab}$ is computed as the infimum of the $D$-length across all chains from $\mathbf{a}$ to $\mathbf{b}$, the infimum of the $G$-length across all chains from $\mathbf{a}$ to $\mathbf{b}$ equals $G\mathbf{ab}$:

$$D\mathbf{a}\mathbf{X}_n\mathbf{b} \to G\mathbf{ab} \Rightarrow G\mathbf{a}\mathbf{X}_n\mathbf{b} \to G\mathbf{ab},$$

where we use the notation for cumulated $G$-length analogous to that for $D$-length,

$$G\mathbf{x}_1 \ldots \mathbf{x}_k = \sum_{i=1}^{k-1} G\mathbf{x}_i\mathbf{x}_{i+1}.$$

Extending the traditional usage of the term, one can say that $G$ is an *intrinsic metric*. This is an extension because traditionally the notion of intrinsic metric presupposes the existence of paths (continuous images of segments of reals) and their lengths. In subsequent sections we consider special cases of dissimilarity cumulation in which the intrinsicality of $G$ does acquire its traditional meaning.

## 9.4 Dissimilarity cumulation in arc-connected spaces

### *9.4.1 Path and their lengths*

Because the notion of uniform convergence in the space $(\mathfrak{S},D)$ is well-defined,

$$\mathbf{a}_n \leftrightarrow \mathbf{b}_n \Leftrightarrow D\mathbf{a}_n\mathbf{b}_n \to 0,$$

we can meaningfully speak of continuous and uniformly continuous functions from reals into $\mathfrak{S}$.

Let $\mathbf{f} : [a, b] \to \mathfrak{S}$, or $\mathbf{f}|[a, b]$, be some continuous (hence uniformly continuous) function with $\mathbf{f}(a) = \mathbf{a}$, $\mathbf{f}(b) = \mathbf{b}$, where $\mathbf{a}$ and $\mathbf{b}$ are not necessarily distinct. We call such a function a *path* connecting $\mathbf{a}$ to $\mathbf{b}$. A space is called *arc-connected* (or *path-connected*) if any two points in it can be connected by a path. Even though arcs have not yet been introduced, the terms "arc-connected" and "path-connected" are synonymous, because $(\mathfrak{S},D)$ is a Hausdorff space, so if two points in it are connected by a path they are also connected by an arc (see, e.g., Hocking & Young, 1961, pp. 116–117). Hereafter we assume that $(\mathfrak{S},D)$ is an arc-connected space.

Choose an arbitrary *net* on $[a, b]$,

$$\mu = (a = x_0 \le x_1 \le \ldots \le x_k \le x_{k+1} = b),$$

where the $x_i$'s need not be pairwise distinct. We call the quantity

$$\delta\mu = \max_{i=0,1,\ldots,k} (x_{i+1} - x_i)$$

the net's *mesh*. As $\delta\mu_n \to 0$, nets $\mu_n$ provide a progressively better approximation for $[a, b]$.

Given a net $\mu = (x_0, x_1, \ldots, x_k, x_{k+1})$, any chain $\mathbf{X} = \mathbf{x}_0\mathbf{x}_1 \ldots \mathbf{x}_k\mathbf{x}_{k+1}$ (with the elements not necessarily pairwise distinct, and $\mathbf{x}_0$ and $\mathbf{x}_{k+1}$ not necessarily equal to **a** and **b**) can be used to form a *chain-on-net*

$$\mathbf{X}^\mu = ((x_0, \mathbf{x}_0), (x_1, \mathbf{x}_1), \ldots, (x_k, \mathbf{x}_k), (x_{k+1}, \mathbf{x}_{k+1})).$$

Denote the class of all such chains-on-nets $\mathbf{X}^\mu$ (for all possible pairs of a chain $\mathbf{X}$ and a net $\mu$ of the same cardinality) by $\mathcal{M}_a^b$. Note that a chain-on-net is not a function from $\{x : x \text{ is an element of } \mu\}$ into $\mathfrak{S}$, for it may include pairs $(x_i = x, \mathbf{x}_i)$ and $(x_j = x, \mathbf{x}_j)$ with $\mathbf{x}_i \neq \mathbf{x}_j$. Note also that within a given context $\mathbf{X}^\mu$ and $\mathbf{X}^\nu$ denote one and the same chain on two nets, whereas $\mathbf{X}^\mu$, $\mathbf{Y}^\mu$ denote two chains on the same net.

We define the *separation* of the chain-on-net $\mathbf{X}^\mu = ((x_0, \mathbf{x}_0), \ldots, (x_{k+1}, \mathbf{x}_{k+1})) \in \mathcal{M}_a^b$ from a path $\mathbf{f}|\,[a, b]$ as

$$\sigma_\mathbf{f}\left(\mathbf{X}^\mu\right) = \max_{x_i \in \mu} D\mathbf{f}(x_i)\mathbf{x}_i.$$

For a sequence of paths $\mathbf{f}_n|\,[a, b]$, any sequence of chains-on-nets $\mathbf{X}_n^{\mu_n} \in \mathcal{M}_a^b$ with $\delta\mu_n \to 0$ and $\sigma_{\mathbf{f}_n}(\mathbf{X}_n^{\mu_n}) \to 0$ is referred to as a sequence *converging with* $\mathbf{f}_n$. We denote such convergence by $\mathbf{X}_n^{\mu_n} \to \mathbf{f}_n$. In particular, $\mathbf{X}_n^{\mu_n} \to \mathbf{f}$ for a fixed path $\mathbf{f}|\,[a, b]$ means that $\delta\mu_n \to 0$ and $\sigma_\mathbf{f}(\mathbf{X}_n^{\mu_n}) \to 0$: in this case we can say that $\mathbf{X}_n^{\mu_n}$ converges *to* $\mathbf{f}$. See Figure 9.7 for an illustration.

We define the *D-length* of $\mathbf{f}|\,[a, b]$ as

$$D\mathbf{f} = \liminf_{\mathbf{X}^\mu \to \mathbf{f}} D\mathbf{X} = \liminf_{\substack{\delta\mu \to 0 \\ \sigma_\mathbf{f}(\mathbf{X}^\mu) \to 0}} D\mathbf{X},$$

where all $\mathbf{X}^\mu \in \mathcal{M}_a^b$.

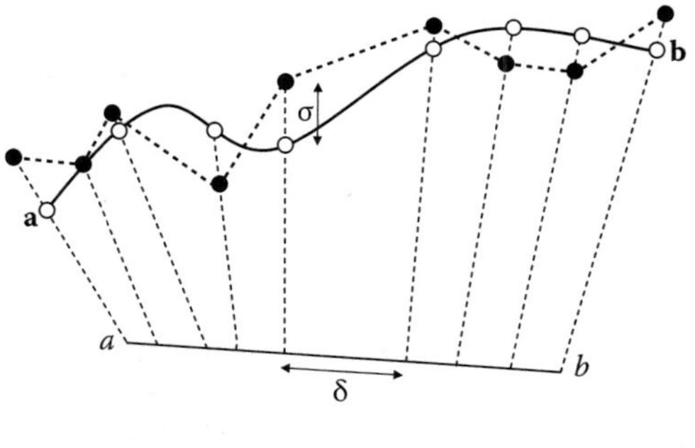


*Figure 9.7* A chain-on-net $\mathbf{X}^\mu$ is converging to a path $\mathbf{f}$ as $\sigma = \sigma_\mathbf{f}(\mathbf{X}^\mu) \to 0$ and $\delta = \delta\mu \to 0$.

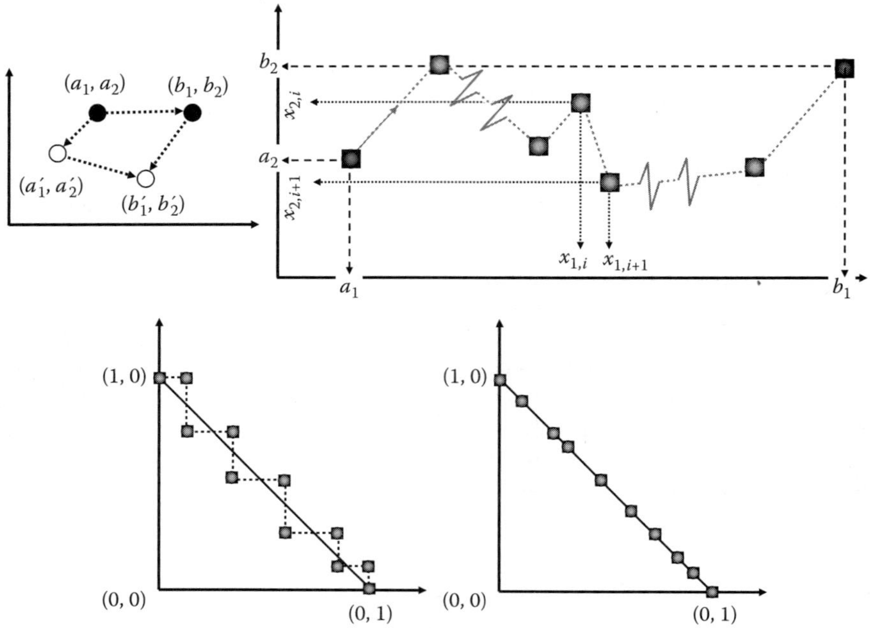


*Figure 9.8* A demonstration of the fact that inscribed chains are not suffcient for $D$-length computations. The $D$ from $(a_1,a_2)$ to $(b_1,b_2)$ is defined as $|a_1 - b_1| + |a_2 - b_2| + \min\{|a_1 - b_1|, |a_2 - b_2|\}$. It is a dissimilarity function, as illustrated in the top panels. Bottom left: the staircase chain has the cumulated dissimilarity 2, and 2 is the true $D$-length of the hypotenuse. Bottom right: the inscribed chain has the cumulated dissimilarity 3.

Given a path $\mathbf{f}|\,[a, b]$, the class of the chains-on-nets $\mathbf{X}^\mu$ such that $\delta\mu < \delta$ and $\sigma_\mathbf{f}(\mathbf{X}^\mu) < \varepsilon$ is nonempty for all positive $\delta$ and $\varepsilon$, because this class includes appropriately chosen *inscribed* chains-on-nets

$$((a, \mathbf{a}), (x_1, \mathbf{f}(x_1)), \ldots, (x_k, \mathbf{f}(x_k)), (b, \mathbf{b})).$$

Here, obviously, $\sigma_\mathbf{f}(\mathbf{X}^\mu)$ is identically zero. Note, however, that with our definition of $D$-length one generally cannot confine one's consideration to the inscribed chains-on-nets only (see Figure 9.8).

Let us consider some basic properties of paths. For any path $\mathbf{f}|\,[a, b]$ connecting $\mathbf{a}$ to $\mathbf{b}$,

$$D\mathbf{f} \geq G\mathbf{ab}.$$

That is, the $D$-length of a path is bounded from below by $G\mathbf{ab}$. There is no upper bound for $D\mathbf{f}$; this quantity need not be finite. Thus, it is shown below that when $D$ is a metric, the notion of $D\mathbf{f}$ coincides with the traditional notion of path length; and examples of paths whose length, in the traditional sense, is infinite, are well-known (see, e.g., Chapter 1 in Papadopoulos, 2005). We call a path *D-rectifiable* if its $D$-length is finite.

We next note the additivity property for path length. For any path $\mathbf{f}|\,[a, b]$ and any point $z \in [a, b]$,

$$D\mathbf{f}|\,[a,b] = D\mathbf{f}|\,[a,z] + D\mathbf{f}\,[z,b].$$

$D\mathbf{f}$ for any path $\mathbf{f}|\,[a, b]$ is nonnegative, and $D\mathbf{f} = 0$ if and only if $\mathbf{f}$ is constant (i.e., $\mathbf{f}\,([a, b])$ is a singleton).

The quantity

$$\sigma_{\mathbf{f}}(\mathbf{g}) = \max_{x\in[a,b]} D\mathbf{f}(x)\mathbf{g}(x)$$

is called the *separation* of path $\mathbf{g}|\,[a, b]$ from path $\mathbf{f}|\,[a, b]$. Two sequences of paths $\mathbf{f}_n$ and $\mathbf{g}_n$ are said to be *(uniformly) converging* to each other if $\sigma_{\mathbf{f}_n}(\mathbf{g}_n) \to 0$. Due to the symmetry of the convergence in $\mathfrak{S}$, this implies $\sigma_{\mathbf{g}_n}(\mathbf{f}_n) \to 0$, so the definition and terminology are well-formed. We symbolize this by $\mathbf{f}_n \to \mathbf{g}_n$. In particular, if $\mathbf{f}$ is fixed then a sequence $\mathbf{f}_n$ converges to $\mathbf{f}$ if $\sigma_{\mathbf{f}}(\mathbf{f}_n) \to 0$. We present this convergence as $\mathbf{f}_n \to \mathbf{f}$. Note that if $\mathbf{f}_n \to \mathbf{f}$, the endpoints $\mathbf{a}_n = \mathbf{f}_n(a)$ and $\mathbf{b}_n = \mathbf{f}_n(b)$ generally depend on $n$ and differ from, respectively $\mathbf{a} = \mathbf{f}(a)$ and $\mathbf{b} = \mathbf{f}(b)$.

The following very important property is called the *lower semicontinuity* of $D$-length (as a function of paths). For any sequence of paths $\mathbf{f}_n \to \mathbf{f}$,

$$\liminf_{n\to\infty} D\mathbf{f}_n \geq D\mathbf{f}.$$

### *9.4.2 G-lengths*

Because the metric $G$ induced by $D$ in accordance with

$$G\mathbf{ab} = \inf_{\mathbf{X}} D\mathbf{aXb}$$

is itself a dissimilarity function, the *G-length* of a path $\mathbf{f} : [a, b] \to \mathfrak{S}$ should be defined as

$$G\mathbf{f} = \liminf_{\substack{\mathbf{X}^{\mu}\in\mathcal{M}_a^b \\ \mathbf{X}^{\mu}\xrightarrow{G}\mathbf{f}}} G\mathbf{X},$$

where (putting $\mathbf{X} = \mathbf{x}_0\mathbf{x}_1 \ldots \mathbf{x}_k\mathbf{x}_{k+1}$),

$$G\mathbf{X} = \sum_{i=0}^{k} G\mathbf{x}_i\mathbf{x}_{i+1},$$

and the convergence $\mathbf{X}^{\mu} \xrightarrow{G} \mathbf{f}$ (where $\mu$ is the net $a = x_0, x_1, \ldots, x_k, x_{k+1} = b$ corresponding to $\mathbf{X}$) means the conjunction of $\delta\mu \to 0$ and

$$\sigma_{\mathbf{f}}^{*}\left(\mathbf{X}^{\mu}\right) = \max_{i=0,\ldots,k+1} G\mathbf{f}(x_i)\mathbf{x}_i \to 0 .$$

It is easy to see, however, that $\mathbf{X}^{\mu} \xrightarrow{G} \mathbf{f}$ and $\mathbf{X}^{\mu} \to \mathbf{f}$ are interchangeable:

$$\mathbf{X}^{\mu} \to \mathbf{f} \Leftrightarrow \mathbf{X}^{\mu} \xrightarrow{G} \mathbf{f} .$$

Because $G$ is a metric, we also have, by a trivial extension of the classical theory (e.g., Blumenthal, 1953),

$$G\mathbf{f} = \sup G\mathbf{Z}$$

with the supremum taken over all inscribed chains-on-nets $\mathbf{Z}^{\nu}$; moreover,

$$G\mathbf{f} = \lim_{n\to\infty} G\mathbf{Z}_n$$

for any sequence of inscribed chains-on-nets $\mathbf{Z}_n^{\nu_n}$ with $\delta\nu_n \to 0$.

As it turns out, these traditional definitions are equivalent to our definition of $G$-length. Moreover the $D$-length and $G$-length of a path are always equal: for any path $\mathbf{f}$,

$$D\mathbf{f} = G\mathbf{f}.$$

### *9.4.3 Other properties of D-length for paths and arcs*

The properties established in this section parallel the basic properties of path length in the traditional, metric-based theory (Blumenthal, 1953; Blumenthal & Menger, 1970; Busemann, 2005). We note first the uniform continuity of length traversed along a path: for any $D$-rectifiable path $\mathbf{f}|\,[a, b]$ and $[x, y] \subset [a, b]$, $D\mathbf{f}|\,[x, y]$ is uniformly continuous in $(x, y)$, nondecreasing in $y$ and nonincreasing in $x$ (see Figure 9.9).

The next issue we consider is the (in)dependence of the $D$-length of a path on the path's parametrization. The $D$-length of a path is not determined by its image $\mathbf{f}([a, b])$ alone but by the function $\mathbf{f} : [a, b] \to \mathfrak{S}$. Nevertheless two paths $\mathbf{f}|\,[a, b]$ and $\mathbf{g}|\,[c, d]$ with one and the same image do have the same $D$-length if they are related to each other in a certain way. Specifically, this happens if $\mathbf{f}$ and $\mathbf{g}$ are each others' reparametrizations, by which we mean that, for some nondecreasing and onto (hence continuous) mapping $\phi : [c, d] \to [a, b]$,

$$\mathbf{g}(x) = \mathbf{f}(\phi(x)),\ x \in [c, d].$$

Note that we use a "symmetrical" terminology (*each other's* reparametrizations) even though the mapping $\phi$ is not assumed to be invertible. If it is invertible, then it is an increasing homeomorphism, and then it is easy to see that $D\mathbf{f} = D\mathbf{g}$. This equality extends to the general case (see Figure 9.10).

We define an *arc* as a path that can be reparametrized into a homeomorphic path. In other words, $\mathbf{g}|\,[c, d]$ is an arc if one can find a nondecreasing and onto (hence

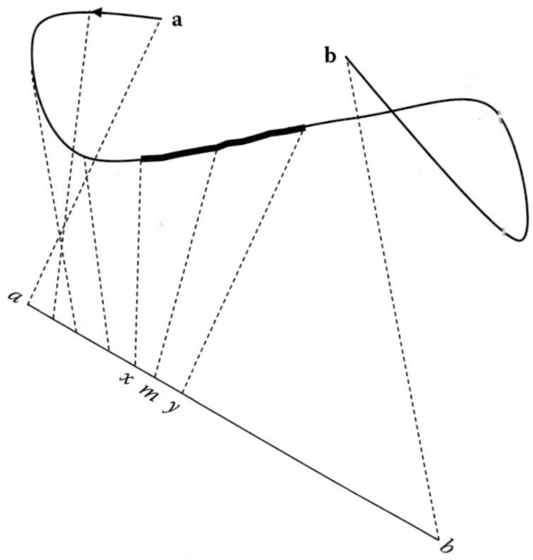


*Figure 9.9* Uniform continuity of length: as $x$ and $y$ get closer to each other, the length of the corresponding piece of the path converges to zero.

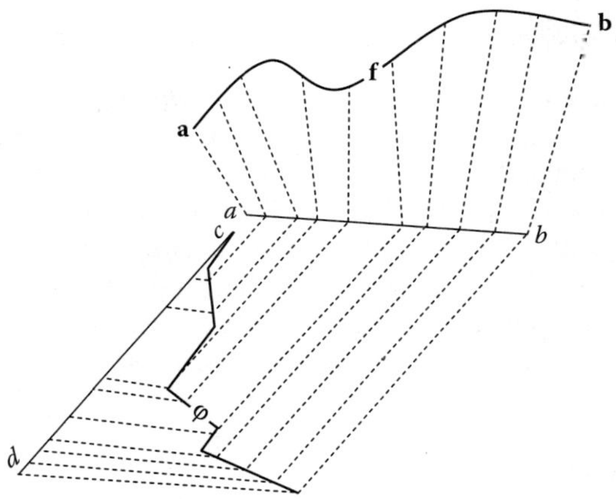


*Figure 9.10* The path **f** on $[a, b]$ can be reparametrized without its length affected into a path on $[c, d]$ mapped onto $[a, b]$ by a nondecreasing function $\phi$.

continuous) mapping $\phi : [c, d] \to [a, b]$, such that, for some one-to-one and continuous (hence homeomorphic) function $\mathbf{f} : [a, b] \to \mathfrak{S}$,

$$\mathbf{g}(x) = \mathbf{f}(\phi(x)),$$

for any $x \in [c, d]$. It can be shown (by a nontrivial argument) that any path contains an arc with the same endpoints and the $D$-length that cannot exceed the $D$-length of

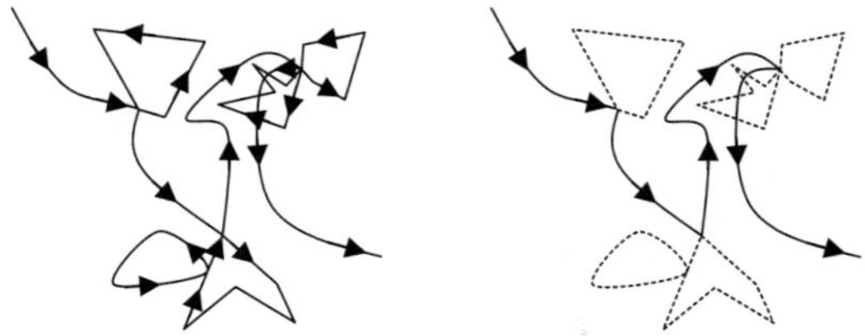

*Figure 9.11* One can remove closed loops from a path and be left with a shorter arc.

the path (see Figure 9.11). Stated rigorously, let $\mathbf{f}|[a,b]$ be a $D$-rectifiable path connecting **a** to **b**. Then there is an arc $\mathbf{g}|[a,b]$ connecting **a** to **b**, such that

$$\mathbf{g}([a,b]) \subset \mathbf{f}([a,b]),$$

and

$$D\mathbf{g}|[a,b] \le D\mathbf{f}|[a,b],$$

where the inequality is strict if $\mathbf{f}|[a,b]$ is not an arc. This result is important, in particular, in the context of searching for shortest paths connecting one point to another (Section 9.4.4): in the absence of additional constraints this search can be confined to arcs only.

### 9.4.4 Complete dissimilarity spaces with intermediate points

A dissimilarity space $(\mathfrak{S}, D)$ is said to be a space *with intermediate points* if for any distinct **a**, **b** one can find an **m** such that $\mathbf{m} \notin \{\mathbf{a}, \mathbf{b}\}$ and $D\mathbf{amb} \le D\mathbf{ab}$ (see Figure 9.12). This notion generalizes that of *Menger convexity* (Blumenthal, 1953, p. 41; the term itself is due to Papadopoulos, 2005). If $D$ is a metric, the space is Menger-convex if, for any distinct **a**, **b**, there is a point $\mathbf{m} \notin \{\mathbf{a}, \mathbf{b}\}$ with $D\mathbf{amb} = D\mathbf{ab}$. (The traditional definition is given for symmetric metrics but it can be easily extended.)

Recall that a space is called *complete* if every Cauchy sequence in it converges to a point. Adapted to $(\mathfrak{S}, D)$, the completeness means that given a sequence of points $\mathbf{x}_n$ such that

$$\lim_{\substack{k\to\infty \\ l\to\infty}} D\mathbf{x}_k\mathbf{x}_l = 0,$$

there is a point **x** in $\mathfrak{S}$ such that

$$\mathbf{x}_n \leftrightarrow \mathbf{x}.$$

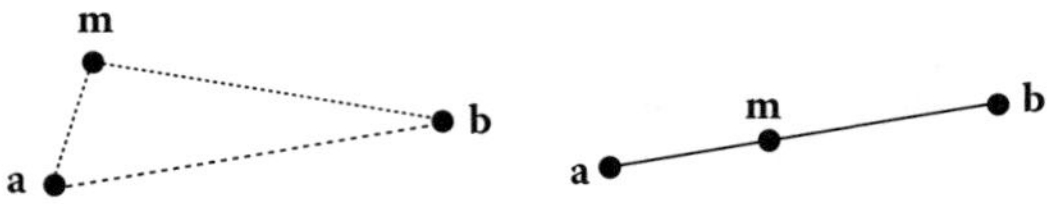


*Figure 9.12* Point **m** is intermediate to **a** and **b** if $D\mathbf{amb} \le D\mathbf{ab}$. E.g., if $D$ is Euclidean distance (right panel), any **m** on the straight line segment connecting **a** to **b** is intermediate to **a** and **b**.

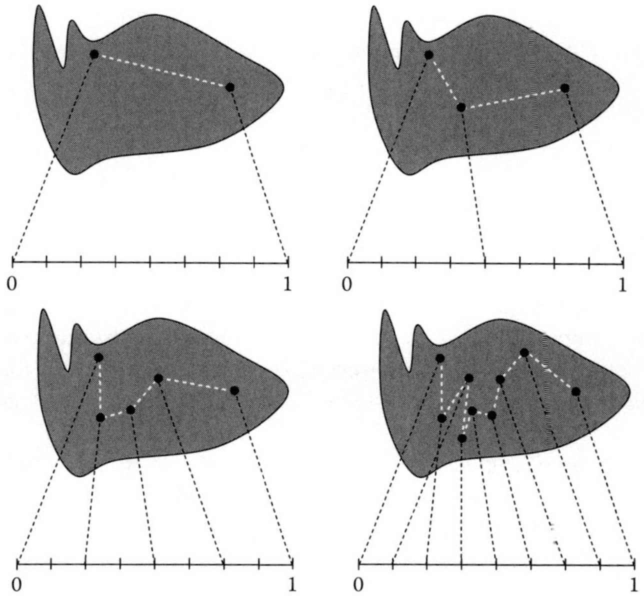


*Figure 9.13* In a complete space with intermediate points any points **a** and **b** can be connected by chains whose cardinality increases beyond bounds and the dissimilarity between successive elements converged to zero. As a result the chains converge, pointwise and in length, to an arc whose length is not greater than *D***ab**.

Blumenthal (1953, pp. 41–43) proved that if a Menger-convex space is complete then **a** can be connected to **b** by a *geodesic arc*, that is, an arc **h** with $D\mathbf{h} = D\mathbf{ab}$ (where $D$ is a symmetric metric). As it turns out, this result can be generalized to nonmetric dissimilarity functions, in the following sense: in a complete space with intermediate points, any **a** can be connected to any **b** by an arc **f** with

$$D\mathbf{f} \leq D\mathbf{ab}.$$

See Figure 9.13 for an illustration. It follows that $G\mathbf{ab}$ in such a space can be viewed as the infimum of lengths of all arcs connecting **a** to **b**. Put differently, in a complete space with intermediate points the metric $G$ induced by $D$ is intrinsic, in the traditional sense of the word.

## 9.5 Conclusion

Let us summarize. Universal Fechnerian Scaling is a theory dealing with the computation of subjective distances from pairwise discrimination probabilities. The theory is applicable to all possible stimulus spaces subject to the assumptions that (a) discrimination probabilities satisfy the law of Regular Minimality, and (b) the two canonical psychometric increments of the first and second kind, $\Psi^{(1)}$ and $\Psi^{(2)}$, are dissimilarity functions.

A dissimilarity function $D\mathbf{ab}$ (where $D$ can stand for either $\Psi^{(1)}$ or $\Psi^{(2)}$) for pairs of stimuli in a canonical representation is defined by the following properties:

$D1$. $\mathbf{a} \neq \mathbf{b} \Rightarrow D\mathbf{ab} > 0$;
$D2$. $D\mathbf{aa} = 0$;
$D3$. If $D\mathbf{a}_n\mathbf{a}'_n \to 0$ and $D\mathbf{b}_n\mathbf{b}'_n \to 0$, then $D\mathbf{a}'_n\mathbf{b}'_n - D\mathbf{a}_n\mathbf{b}_n \to 0$; and
$D4$. for any sequence $\mathbf{a}_n\mathbf{X}_n\mathbf{b}_n$, where $\mathbf{X}_n$ is a chain of stimuli, $D\mathbf{a}_n\mathbf{X}_n\mathbf{b}_n \to 0 \Rightarrow D\mathbf{a}_n\mathbf{b}_n \to 0$.

It allows us to impose on the stimulus space the (generally asymmetric) Fechnerian metric $G\mathbf{ab}$, computed as as the infimum of $D\mathbf{aXb}$ across all possible chains $\mathbf{X}$ inserted between $\mathbf{a}$ and $\mathbf{b}$. The overall (symmetric) Fechnerian distance $G^*\mathbf{ab}$ between $\mathbf{a}$ and $\mathbf{b}$ is defined as $G\mathbf{ab} + G\mathbf{ba}$. This quantity does not depend on whether one uses $\Psi^{(1)}$ or $\Psi^{(2)}$ in place of $D$.

The dissimilarity $D$ imposes on stimulus space a topology and a uniformity structure that coincide with the topology and uniformity induced by the Fechnerian metric $G$ (or $G^*$). The metric $G$ is uniformly continuous with respect to the uniformity just mentioned. Stimulus space is topologically characterized as a completely normal space.

The Dissimilarity Cumulation theory can be specialized to arc-connected spaces with no additional constraints imposed either on these spaces or on the type of paths. We have seen that the path length can be defined in terms of a dissimilarity function as the limit inferior of the lengths of appropriately chosen chains converging to paths. Unlike in the classical metric based theory of path length, the converging chains generally are not confined to inscribed chains only: the vertices of the converging chains are allowed to "jitter and meander" around the path to which they are converging. Given this difference, however, most of the basic results of the metric-based theory are shown to hold true in the dissimilarity-based theory.

The dissimilarity-based length theory properly specializes to the classical one when the dissimilarity in question is itself a metric (in fact without assuming that this metric is symmetric). In this case the limit inferior over all converging chains coincides with that computed over the inscribed chains only. It is also the case that the length of any path computed by means of a dissimilarity function remains the same if the dissimilarity function is replaced with the metric it induces.

We have considered a class of spaces in which the metrics induced by the dissimilarity functions defined on these spaces are intrinsic: which means that the distance between two given points can be computed as the infimum of the lengths of all arcs connecting these points. We call them spaces with intermediate points, the concept generalizing that of the metric-based theory's Menger convexity.

All of this shows that the properties $D3$ and $D4$ of a dissimilarity function rather than the symmetry and triangle inequality of a metric are essential in dealing with the notions of path length and intrinsic metrics.

In conclusion, it should be mentioned that the notion of dissimilarity and the theory of dissimilarity cumulation has a broader field of applicability than just discrimination functions. Thus, it seems plausible to assume that means or medians of direct *numerical estimates of pairwise dissimilarities*, of the kind used in Multidimensional Scaling (MDS, see, e.g., Borg & Groenen, 1997), can be viewed as dissimilarity values in the technical sense of the present theory. This creates the possibility of using the dissimilarity cumulation procedure as a data-analytic technique alternative to (and, in some sense, generalizing) MDS. Instead of nonlinearly transforming dissimilarity estimates $D\mathbf{ab}$ into distances of a preconceived kind (usually, Euclidean distances in a low-dimensional Euclidean space) one can use dissimilarity cumulation to compute distances $G^*\mathbf{ab}$ from untransformed $D\mathbf{ab}$ and then see if these stimuli are isometrically (i.e., without changing the distances $G^*\mathbf{ab}$ among them) embeddable in a low-dimensional Euclidean space (or another geometric structure with desirable properties). This approach can be used even if the dissimilarity estimates are nonsymmetric. A variety of modifications readily suggest themselves, such as taking into account only small dissimilarities in order to reduce the dimensionality of the resulting Euclidean representation.

Another line of research links the theory of dissimilarity cumulation with *information geometry* (see, e.g., Amari & Nagaoka, 2000) and applies to the categorization paradigm. Here, each stimulus **a** is characterized by a vector of probabilities $(a_1, \ldots, a_k)$,

$$\sum_{i=1}^{k} a_i = 1,$$

where $a_i$ indicates the probability with which **a** is classified (by an observer or a group of people) into the $i$th category among certain $k > 1$ mutually exclusive and collectively exhaustive categories. It can be shown, to mention one application, that the square root of the symmetrical version of the Kullback–Leibler divergence measure (Kullback & Leibler, 1951),

$$D\mathbf{ab} = \sqrt{\mathrm{Div}_{\mathrm{KL}}\mathbf{ab}} = \sqrt{\sum_{i=1}^{k} (a_i - b_i)\log\frac{a_i}{b_i}},$$

is a (symmetric) dissimilarity function on any closed subarea of the area

$$\left\{ \mathbf{x} = \left(x_1, \ldots, x_k\right) : x_1 > 0, \ldots, x_k > 0, \sum_{i=1}^{k} x_i = 1 \right\}.$$

The stimuli **x** can also be viewed as belonging to a $(k - 1)$-dimensional unit sphere, with coordinates $\sqrt{x_1}, \ldots, \sqrt{x_k}$. The cumulation of $D\mathbf{ab}$ leads to the classical for information geometry spherical metric in any spherically convex area of the stimulus space (i.e., an area which with any two stimuli it contains also contains the smaller arc of the great circle connecting them). In those cases where the spherical convexity is not satisfied (e.g., if the sphere has gaps with no stimuli, or stimuli form a discrete set), the computation of the distances along great circles has to be replaced with more general computations using finite chains of stimuli.

## Acknowledgment

This research has been supported by NSF grant SES 0620446 and AFOSR grants FA9550-06-1-0288 and FA9550-09-1-0252. I am grateful to my long-term collaborator Hans Colonius who, among other things, opened to me the wealth of the German-language literature on the subject. I am grateful to James T. Townsend and Devin Burns who critically read the first draft of the chapter and suggested improvements.

## References

Amari, S., & Nagaoka, H. (2000). *Methods of information geometry*. Providence, RI: American Mathematical Society.

Blumenthal, L. M. (1953). *Theory and applications of distance geometry*. London: Oxford University.

Blumenthal, L. M., & Menger, K. (1970). *Studies in geometry*. San Francisco: W.H. Freeman.

Borg, I., & Groenen, P. (1997). *Modern multidimensional scaling*. New York: Springer-Verlag.

Busemann, H. (2005). *The geometry of geodesics*. Mineola, NY: Dover.

Creelman, C. D. (1967). Empirical detectability scales without the jnd. *Perceptual & Motor Skills, 24,* 1079–1084.

Dzhafarov, E. N. (2001). Fechnerian psychophysics. In N. J. Smelser and P. B. Baltes (Eds.) *International encyclopedia of the social and behavioral sciences* (Vol. 8, pp. 5437–5440). New York: Pergamon Press.

Dzhafarov, E. N. (2002a). Multidimensional Fechnerian scaling: Regular variation version. *Journal of Mathematical Psychology, 46,* 226–244.

Dzhafarov, E. N. (2002b). Multidimensional Fechnerian scaling: Probability-distance hypothesis. *Journal of Mathematical Psychology, 46,* 352–374.

Dzhafarov, E. N. (2002c). Multidimensional Fechnerian scaling: Perceptual separability. *Journal of Mathematical Psychology*, *46*, 564-582.

Dzhafarov, E. N. (2002d). Multidimensional Fechnerian scaling: Pairwise comparisons, regular minimality, and nonconstant self-similarity. *Journal of Mathematical Psychology, 46,* 583–608.

Dzhafarov, E. N. (2003a). Thurstonian-type representations for "same–different" discriminations: Deterministic decisions and independent images. *Journal of Mathematical Psychology*, *47,* 208–228.

Dzhafarov, E. N. (2003b). Thurstonian-type representations for "same-different" discriminations: Probabilistic decisions and interdependent images. *Journal of Mathematical Psychology, 47,* 229–243. [see Dzhafarov, E. N. (2006). Corrigendum to "Thurstonian-type representations for 'same–different' discriminations: Probabilistic decisions and interdependent images." *Journal of Mathematical Psychology*, *50,* 511.]

Dzhafarov, E. N. (2004). Perceptual separability of stimulus dimensions: A Fechnerian approach. In C. Kaernbach, E. Schröger, & H. Müller (Eds.), *Psychophysics beyond sensation: Laws and invariants of human cognition* (pp. 9–26). Mahwah, NJ: Erlbaum.

Dzhafarov, E. N. (2006). On the law of regular minimality: Reply to Ennis. *Journal of Mathematical Psychology*, *50,* 74–93.

Dzhafarov, E. N. (2008a). Dissimilarity cumulation theory in arc-connected spaces. *Journal of Mathematical Psychology*, *52,* 73–92. [see Dzhafarov, E. N. (2009). Corrigendum to "Dissimilarity cumulation theory in arc-connected spaces". *Journal of Mathematical Psychology, 53,* 300.]

Dzhafarov, E. N. (2008b). Dissimilarity cumulation theory in smoothly connected spaces. *Journal of Mathematical Psychology*, *52,* 93–115.

Dzhafarov, E. N., & Colonius, H. (1999). Fechnerian metrics in unidimensional and multidimensional stimulus spaces. *Psychonomic Bulletin and Review*, *6,* 239–268.

Dzhafarov, E. N., & Colonius, H. (2001). Multidimensional Fechnerian scaling: Basics. *Journal of Mathematical Psychology*, *45,* 670–719.

Dzhafarov, E. N., & Colonius, H. (2005a). Psychophysics without physics: A purely psychological theory of Fechnerian scaling in continuous stimulus spaces. *Journal of Mathematical Psychology*, *49,* 1–50.

Dzhafarov, E. N., & Colonius, H. (2005b). Psychophysics without physics: Extension of Fechnerian scaling from continuous to discrete and discrete-continuous stimulus spaces. *Journal of Mathematical Psychology*, *49,* 125–141.

Dzhafarov, E. N., & Colonius, H. (2006a). Regular minimality: A fundamental law of discrimination. In H. Colonius & E. N. Dzhafarov (Eds.), *Measurement and representation of sensations* (pp. 1–46). Mahwah, NJ: Erlbaum.

Dzhafarov, E. N., & Colonius, H. (2006b). Generalized Fechnerian scaling. In H. Colonius & E. N. Dzhafarov (Eds.), *Measurement and representation of sensations* (pp. 47–88). Mahwah, NJ: Erlbaum.

Dzhafarov, E. N., & Colonius, H. (2006c). Reconstructing distances among objects from their discriminability. *Psychometrika*, *71,* 365–386.

Dzhafarov, E. N., & Colonius, H. (2007). Dissimilarity cumulation theory and subjective metrics. *Journal of Mathematical Psychology*, *51,* 290–304.

Falmagne, J. C. (1971). The generalized Fechner problem and discrimination. *Journal of Mathematical Psychology*, *8,* 22–43.

Fechner, G. T. (1860). *Elemente der psychophysik* [*Elements of Psychophysics*]. Leipzig: Breitkopf & Härtel.

Fechner, G. T. (1877). *In Sachen der psychophysik* [*In the matter of psychophysics*]. Leipzig: Breitkopf & Härtel.

Fechner, G. T. (1887). Über die psychischen massprinzipien und das Webersche gesetz [On the principles of mental measurement and Weber's law]. *Philosophische Studien*, *4,* 161–230.

Helmholtz, H. von. (1891). Versucheinererweiterten anwendungdes Fechnerschen gesetzes im farbensystem [An attempt at a generalized application of Fechner's Law to the color system]. *Zeitschrift für die Psychologie und die Physiologie der Sinnesorgane*, *2,* 1–30.

Hocking, J. H. & Young, G. S. (1961). *Topology*. Reading, MA: Addison-Wesley.

Kelly, J. L. (1955). *General topology*. Toronto: Van Nostrand.

Krantz, D. (1971). Integration of just-noticeable differences. *Journal of Mathematical Psychology, 8,* 591–599.

Kullback, S., & Leibler, R. A. (1951). On information and suffciency. *Annals of Mathematical Statistics*, *22,* 79–86.

Luce, R. D. (2002). A psychophysical theory of intensity proportions, joint presentations, and matches. *Psychological Review*, *109,* 520–532.

Luce, R. D. (2004). Symmetric and asymmetric matching of joint presentations. *Psychological Review*, *111,* 446–454.

Luce, R. D., & Edwards W. (1958). The derivation of subjective scales from just noticeable differences. *Psychological Review, 65,* 222–237.

Luce, R. D., & Galanter, E. (1963). Discrimination. In R. D. Luce, R. R. Bush, & E. Galanter (Eds.), *Handbook of mathematical psychology* (Vol. 1, 191–244). New York: Wiley.

Papadopoulos, A. (2005). *Metric spaces, convexity and nonpositive curvature*. Zurich, Switzerland: European Mathematical Society.

Pfanzagl, J. (1962). Über die stochastische Fundierung des psychophysischen Gesetzes [On stochastic foundations of the psychophysical law]. *Biometrische Zeitschrift, 4,* 1–14.

Riesz, R. R. (1933). The relationship between loudness and the minimum perceptible increment of intensity. *Journal of the Acoustical Society of America, 4,* 211–216.

Schrödinger, E. von. (1920). Farbenmetrik [Color metrics]. *Zeitschrift für Physik*, 12, 459– 466.

Schrödinger, E. von. (1920/1970). Outline of a theory of color measurement for daylight vision. In D. L. MacAdam (Ed.), *Sources of color science* (pp. 397–447, 481–520).Cambridge, MA: MIT Press.

Schrödinger, E. von. (1926/1970). Thresholds of color differences. In D. L. MacAdam (Ed.), *Sources of color science* (pp. 183–193). Cambridge, MA: MIT Press.

Stevens, S. S. (1975). Psychophysics: Introduction to its Perceptual, Neural, and Social Prospects. New York: Wiley.

Thurstone, L. L. (1927a). Psychophysical analysis. *American Journal of Psychology, 38,* 368–389.

Thurstone, L. L. (1927b). A law of comparative judgments. *Psychological Review, 34,* 273–286.

Ünlü, A., Kiefer, T., & Dzhafarov, E. N. (2009). Fechnerian scaling in R: The package Fechner. *Journal of Statistical Software, 31,* 1–24.

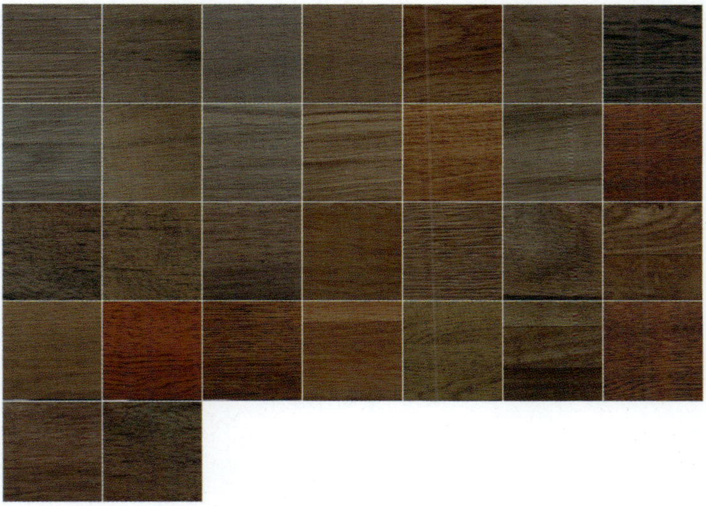

*Figure 6.1* An overview of the 30 wood samples used in the MONAT study. The first two rows are real wood. Row one contains tiger oak panels, of which the three left panels are untreated (raw, weathered, and sanded, respectively) and the other four are waxed, oiled, varnished, and manufactured, respectively. The second row is the same for cognac oak. The bottom three rows contain artificial wood panels (3 laminates, 1 veneer, 9 vinyl, 3 paper copy, respectively).

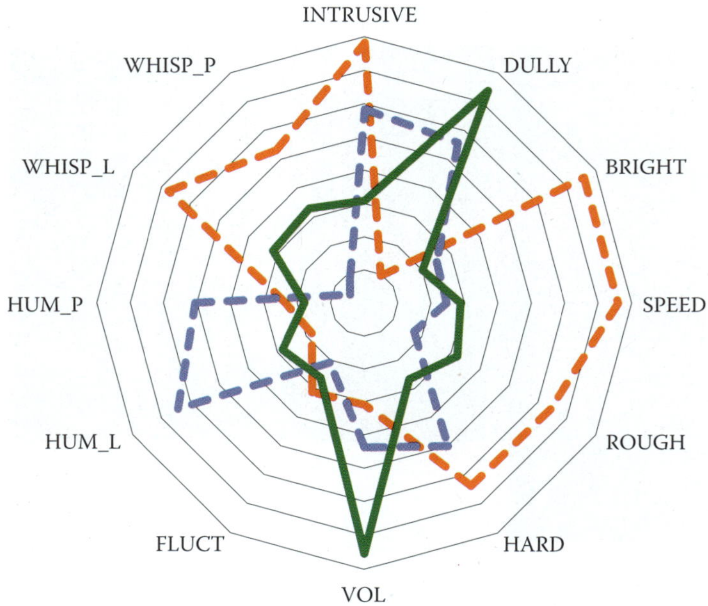


*Figure 11.1* Sensory profiles obtained for three air-conditioning noises from Siekierski, Derquenne, and Martin (2001). Labels of the *semantic descriptors* are Intrusive, Dully, Brightness, Speed, Roughness, Hardness, Voluminous, Fluctuation, Humming, Whispering. The letters L and P correspond to the Level and Pitch, respectively, of the whispering (noise) part and the humming (motor) part.

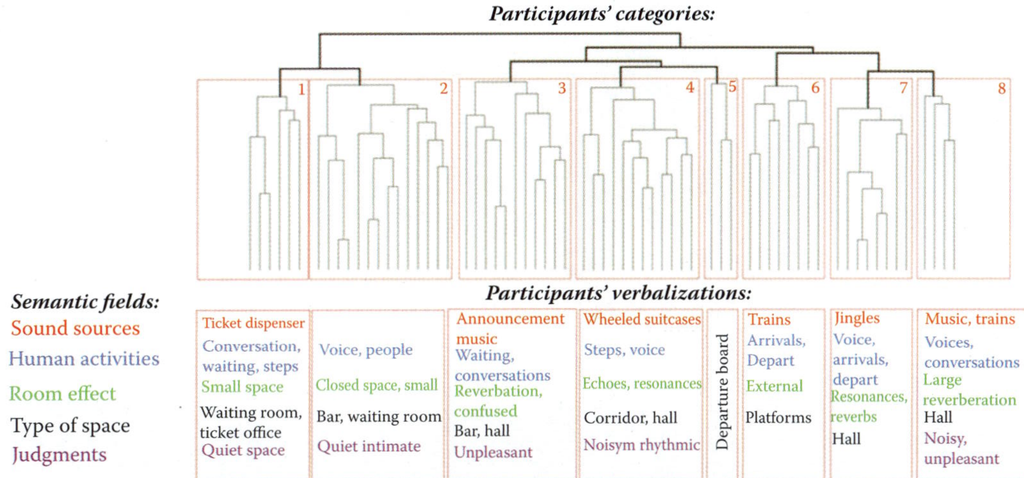


*Figure 11.2* Dendrogram representing the categories of train station soundscapes found in Tardieu et al. (2008). The descriptions of the categories provided by the participants are reported on the table below, grouped into five semantic fields. The most cited verbalizations are shown in a larger size font.

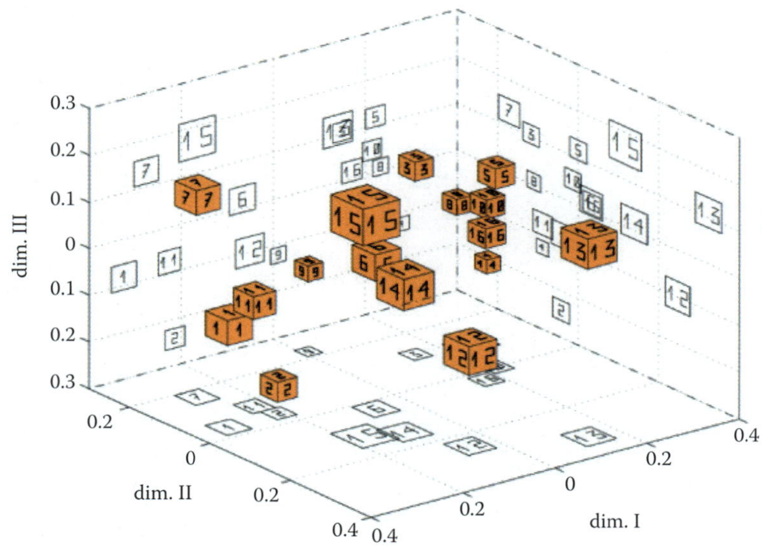


*Figure 11.3* Three-dimensional space for car sounds: dimension I is explained by the energy ratio between the harmonic and noisy parts, dimension II by the spectral centroid, and dimension III by the decrease in the spectral envelope.

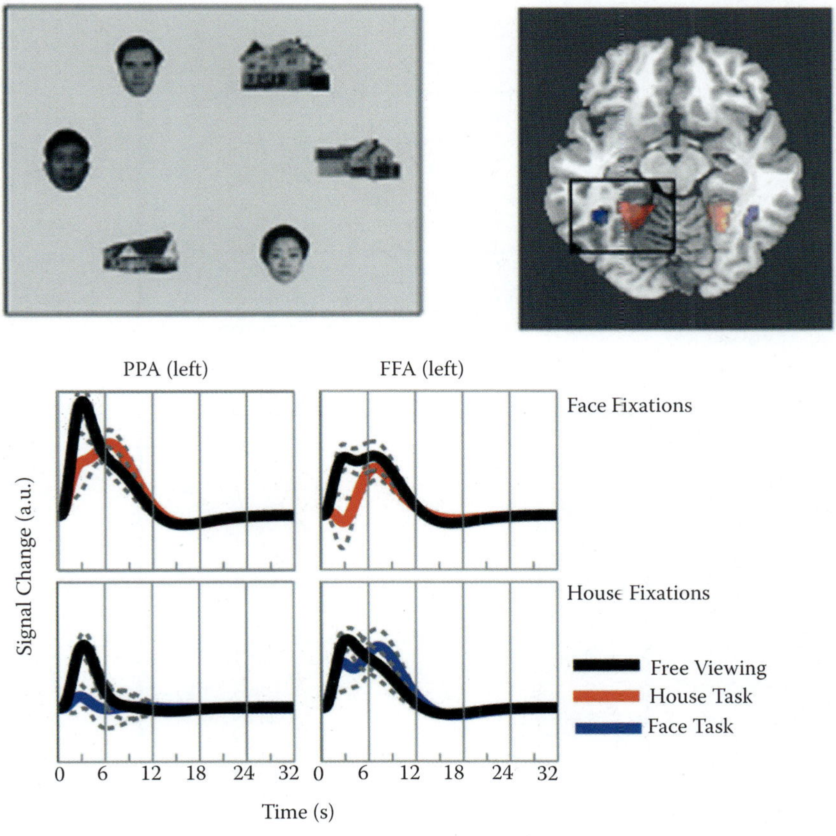


*Figure 13.6* Top left: Example stimulus. Top right: Investigated brain regions, FFA (blue) and PPA (red), left hemisphere activations are within the rectangle. Bottom: Estimated hemodynamic responses for fixations toward houses (upper row) and faces (underside row) in left FFA (left column) and left PPA (right column). Colors indicate task; dashed lines denote standard error of the mean. Vertical axes show percentages of the mean whole-brain signal.

(a)

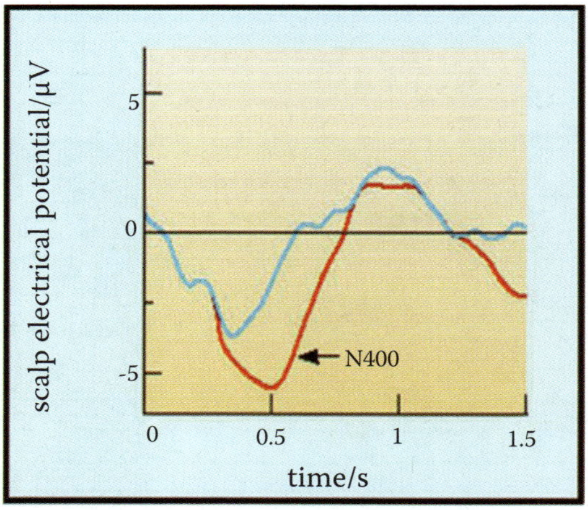


(b)

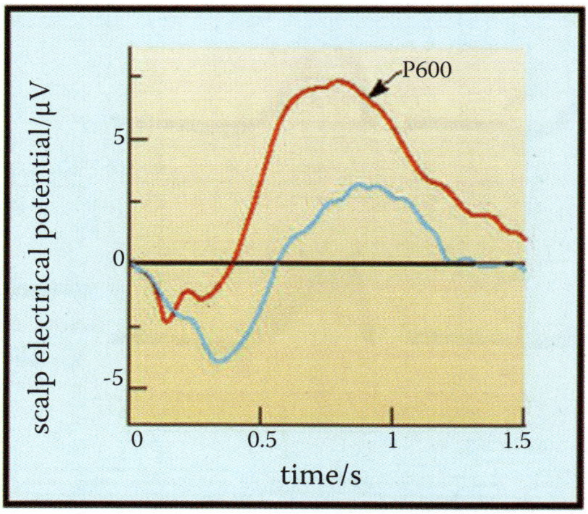


*Figure 14.3* (a) N400 component. This component has the form of a negative wave peaking about 400 ms after the onset of a semantically incongruent word. Event-related potential trace for "The shirt was ironed" (blue line) versus "The thunderstorm was **ironed**" (red line). The key word is ironed, and the deviation is called the N400. (Reprinted from Friederici, 2002.) (b) P600 component. The presentation of syntactic violations produces an increase in the positivity at around 600 ms after stimulus presentation. Posterior event-related potential trace for "The shirt was ironed" (blue line) versus "The shirt was **on** ironed" (red line). The key word is ironed, and the deviation is called the P600. (Reprinted from Friederici, 2002.)

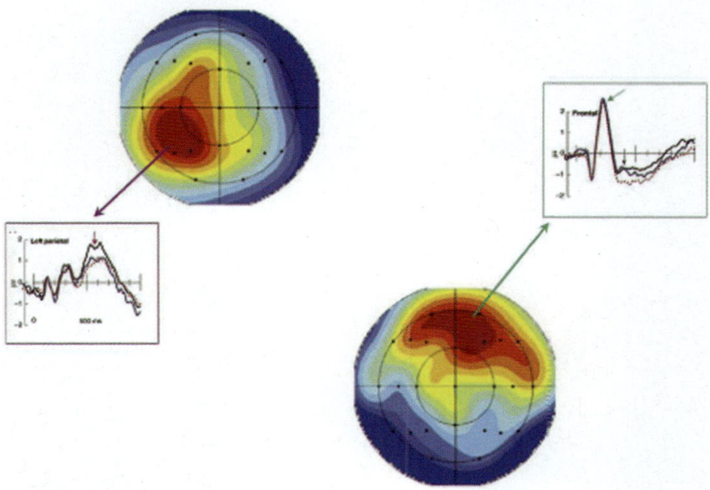


(a) (b)

*Figure 14.4* ERP old/new effects. (a) Grand-average ERPs from left parietal with the parietal old/new effect indicated by the purple arrow. (b) Grand-average ERPs from frontal electrodes with the mid-frontal old/new effect indicated by the green arrow. Repeated measures analyses of variance (ANOVAs) focused on mean amplitudes from 300 to 500 msec. Data adapted from Curran (2000).

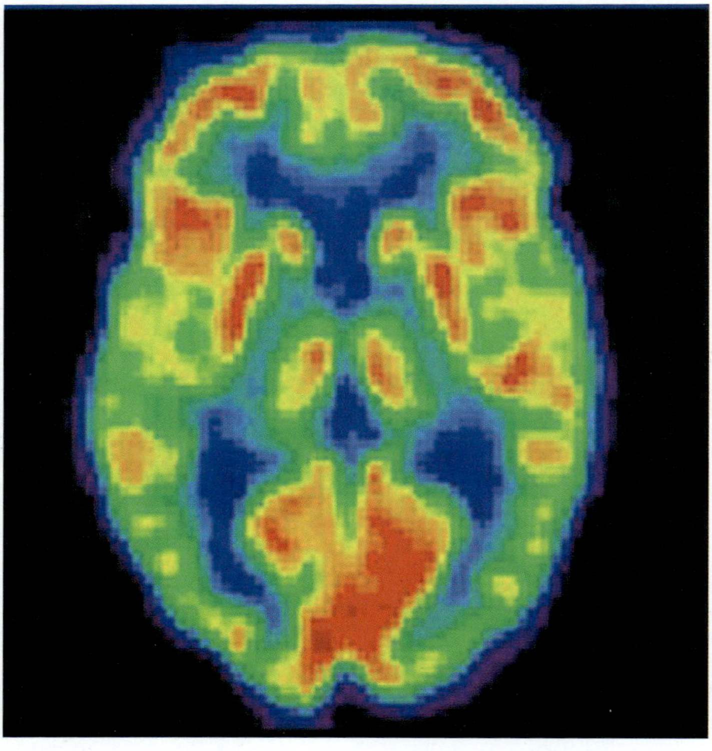

*Figure 14.7* Example of a PET image showing areas of different color tones, each shade representing different molecular parameters of the underlying brain structures.

# 10 Neural networks and fuzzy systems

*Christian Eitzinger and Wolfgang Heidl*
Profactor GmbH
Steyr-Gleink, Austria

## 10.1 Introduction

Neural networks and fuzzy systems both belong to the area of soft computing. They try to reproduce properties of human thinking and the neurobiology of the human brain to create new mathematical structures. This new way of looking at mathematics has led to developments in a range of fields such as modeling of human vision, control of complex dynamical systems, and even the prediction of financial markets.

For the purpose of "measurement with persons," neural networks and fuzzy systems are of high relevance, because they both consider the "human element" at different levels of abstraction. This specific property makes them interesting mathematical structures for modeling human judgment, behavior, or decisions.

Both neural networks and fuzzy systems have developed into huge fields of research and we are thus limited to only a brief introduction. We explain the basic elements that make up neural networks and fuzzy systems and then take a big step forward, by almost 40 years of research, to recent models of the human visual cortex.

## 10.2 Neural networks

The development of neural networks was initiated by the wish to reproduce the capability of the human brain to deal with complicated tasks such as understanding speech or identifying objects in an image. The observation was that the human brain was outperformed by even the simplest calculator in terms of precision and speed when doing basic calculations, but that artificial systems utterly failed in many tasks that would be considered straightforward by a human. It was soon understood that computing power alone would not solve the problem and that something more was needed to enhance the performance of artificial systems on complicated tasks. Consequently, the idea emerged to use the results of neurophysiology and to try to duplicate these in artificial systems, thus combining the precision and speed of computers with the flexibility and learning capabilities of the human brain. A good overview can be found in, for example, Lin and Lee (1995).

### *10.2.1 Properties of biological neural networks*

There are several features that made biological neural networks different from artificial systems at least by the time the idea of neural networks was created. Today we might look at these features slightly differently, in the presence of the Web 2.0 and GRID computing, but with respect to smaller entities the main issues are still valid:

*Adaptivity:* The human brain is dynamically changing and adapting to new inputs, which do not appear in a previously defined pattern. More recent inputs will be more relevant to the brain than inputs from the distant past. The brain is able to learn from examples by complicated reward and punishment processes.

*Interconnected structure*: The basic components of the brain—the neurons—make up a highly interconnected structure. The brain itself consists of approximately $10^{11}$ neurons, where each neuron is connected to another 10,000 neurons. It is in these connections that information is stored and learning takes place.

*Structural robustness*: As the number of neurons is very large, the functioning of the brain does not depend on a single neuron and not even on a large number of neurons. If many neurons cease to function, then the performance of the brain gradually decreases but does not deteriorate abruptly. We observe this as part of the aging process that is accompanied by a slow decay of the number of neurons. This robustness achieved by distributed storing of knowledge is a property of huge interest in artificial systems and in particular in military applications.

*Hierarchical structure*: The information processing from the sensors to the higher cortical regions is not a one-step process, but the brain is set up in the form of interconnected layers, where each layer fulfills specific tasks. Modern diagnostic technologies such as functional magnetic resonance imaging (fMRI) allow us to identify regions that become activated during various tasks. This technology is still in its early stages and much work needs to be done on refining experiments in order to provide more insight not only into the spatial organization of brain areas but also their temporal hierarchy.

*Size*: In terms of computing elements the human brain is huge. Even compared to high-performance computers, the number of neurons and their connections is still large. In addition to this the adult brain has had many years or decades to learn and it has a powerful sensory system at its disposal that provides input and positive or negative feedback. It thus creates the experience that makes each individual unique.

*Parallel computation*: Processing in the brain is massively parallel and asynchronous, which enables the brain to process large amounts of information in a comparatively short time. Even structures of sequential layers that were used in earlier models of the brain (e.g., in human decision making) are now being reviewed and replaced by highly interconnected structures that are assumed to be evaluated in parallel.

We now start to develop artificial neural networks and at the end of the "neural networks" section take a look back at their properties and compare them to those of biological neural networks.

### *10.2.2 Mathematical representation of artificial neural networks*

The basic biological computing elements of which the brain is built are the neurons. Each neuron consists of a cell body (soma), extensions that transfer incoming signals to the soma (dendrites), and a single output nerve fiber (axon) which sends signals to other neurons. The junction points that connect the axons to the dendrites of the next neuron are called synapses; this is the place were memory resides. In all of these parts complicated electrochemical processes generate the well-known electrical behavior of neurons (Gupta and Knopf, 1993).

In terms of information processing each neuron transforms the aggregation of the stimulus signals received by the dendrites into a sequence of frequency-modulated pulses called action potentials. Two important properties of the action potential are directly related to the encoding abilities of a neuron. The first one is the rise time (latency), which it takes for the resulting action potential to rise after the stimulus has been applied. This response time has been observed to decrease exponentially with the intensity of the stimulus. The second property is the minimum time that has to pass before another action potential can be generated by the axon. This time, which is the minimum time between two consecutive pulses, is called the refractory period. If a stimulus greater than a specific threshold value is applied, both the latency and the refractory period will control the frequency of the generated action potentials. A stimulus with high intensity will generate a short rise time and a short refractory period, thus producing a high pulse frequency. From experiments it has been found that the relationship between the intensity of the stimulus and the frequency of the action potentials is linear over a limited range with a saturation characteristic at high and low stimulus levels.

If the dynamical processes within the neuron are neglected, then it can be described as a function $f{:}R^N \rightarrow R$ that maps a vector of $N$ input variables (stimuli) to one output (frequency of action potentials). To resemble the biological concept of neurons this function is composed of a linear part, which is the aggregation of the incoming stimuli, where the inputs $x$ undergo some kind of linear transformation such as

$$a = w^T x \tag{10.1a}$$

to give the activation $a$ of this neuron. This also resembles the processing of the inputs in the synaptic connections, where connections with positive weights ($w_i > 0$) are considered to be excitatory and connections with negative weights ($w_i < 0$) are inhibitory. The output is then found by applying a usually nonlinear activation function, of which the step-function is the simplest:

$$y = step(a) = \begin{cases} 0 & \text{if} \quad a < 0 \\ 1 & \text{if} \quad a \geq 0 \end{cases} \tag{10.1b}$$

As said before, the neuron also includes some kind of threshold operation, where the activation has to rise above a specific value, before an output is produced. To integrate this behavior into our model, Equation (10.1a) will be modified to

$$a = w^T x + b, \tag{10.1c}$$

where $b$ is called bias or offset value. Depending on whether $w^T x$ is greater than $b$ an output of 1 or 0 is produced. The three formulas (10.1a–c) constituted the first model of a neuron developed around 1940. However, the discontinuous behavior of the step-function made it hard to analyze larger structures of such neurons, in particular given the limited computing power available at that time. About 30 years later research on artificial neurons and neural networks re-emerged and led to the field that we now know as artificial neural networks.

In addition to the development of computers, the most important structural modification was the replacement of the step-function with a continuous mapping of activations to the intervals [0,1] or [–1,1]. This has the computational advantage that the output is not limited to the values 0 and 1, and that the function is continuously differentiable, which gives rise to efficient training methods. Commonly used activation functions are shown in Figure 10.1.

Among them there are the unipolar sigmoid activation function

$$y = \frac{1}{1+e^{-a}}$$

and the bipolar sigmoid activation functions

$$y = \frac{2}{1+e^{-a}} - 1 \text{ or } y = \tanh(a).$$

Another activation function, which does not exactly fit into the scheme introduced above, is the radial basis function, where the outputs are found from

$$y = e^{\frac{1}{2}\sum (x_i - w_i)^2}.$$

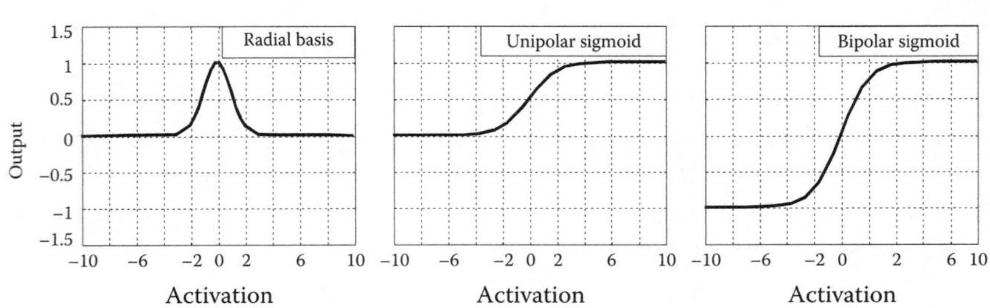


*Figure 10.1* Shapes of commonly used activation functions.

This function will generate greater outputs if the vector of inputs $x$ is similar to the vector of weights $w$ and the distance between the two vectors is small.

Independent of the specific activation function used, the neurons are set up in layers and the layers are then combined to form multilayer networks. This usually allows an efficient mathematical description in terms of matrix operations. For a layer of $N$ neurons and $M$ inputs the output of neuron $i$, $i = 1, 2, \ldots, N$ with activation function $f{:}R^M \rightarrow R$ can be found by

$$y_i = f(w_i^T x + b_i)$$

or for the whole layer $f{:}R^M \rightarrow R^N$

$$y = f(Wx + b),$$

where $W$ is the matrix of weights and $b$ is the vector of offset values. The activation function $f$ is applied to each element of the resulting vector of activations. Neural networks usually consist of an input layer, a number of hidden layers, and an output layer. For simple feed-forward networks each layer processes the outputs of the preceding layer and sends its own outputs to the following layer. When outputs are directed back to the same or preceding layers, then the network is a feedback network. Feedback networks, which have closed loops, are called recurrent networks. A typical structure of a feed-forward network is shown in Figure 10.2.

Learning in these networks is done almost exclusively by variants of the so-called backpropagation algorithm. The basic idea is very simple. The output of the network $y$ is compared to a target vector $t$, resulting in an error $e = t - y$. Based on this error changes for the weights $\Delta w$ are calculated so that the error decreases. An additional error signal is calculated for the inputs of the layer, and based on this error signal the weights of the upstream layer are modified. This process can be repeated recursively until we reach the input layer. Quite soon it was found that this procedure

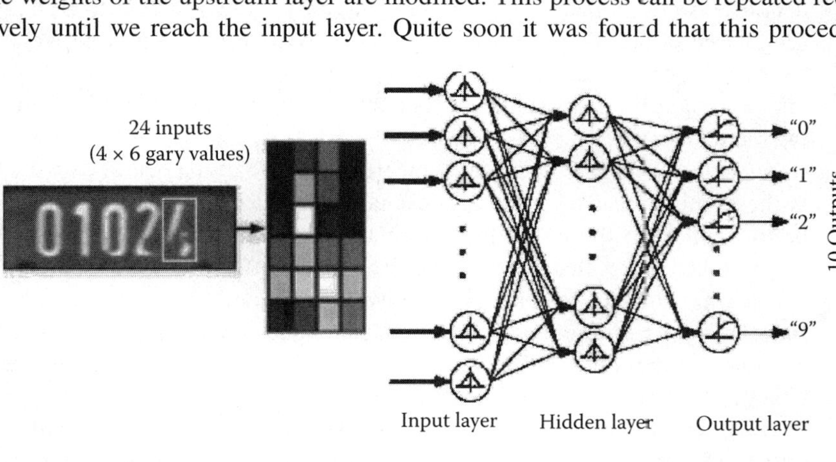


*Figure 10.2* Feed-forward network for optical character recognition with an input, a hidden, and an output layer.

is equivalent to a gradient descent method, where the changes for the weights are calculated so as to proceed in the direction of the error gradient, when minimizing the sum of squares error.

$$\Delta w_k = -\frac{\partial \frac{1}{2}(t - y_k)^2}{dw} \quad \textit{and} \quad w_{k+1} = w_k + \lambda \Delta w_k .$$

Repeated updating of the weights with an appropriate, small step size $\lambda$ finally leads to a local minimum of the error and the network has learned to reproduce the target vector $t$.

An example of a neural network for optical character recognition is shown in Figure 10.2. The input is a small image containing a character 0..9. The image is split into a $4 \times 6$ grid and the average gray value is calculated for each grid element. These 24 values constitute the input to the network, which consequently has a size of 24 neurons in the input layer. A small hidden layer with 8 neurons then feeds its outputs into an output layer with 10 neurons. Each output neuron represents one character from 0 to 9 and is trained to produce a value of 0.9 if the character shown in the bitmap is the one represented by this neuron. Otherwise the value is trained to be 0.1. This network is trained on 3,000 images, for 5,000 iterations using the back-propagation algorithm, and achieves an average recognition rate of 98%. It has to be noted that this example is just for demonstrating the use of neural networks; it does not represent the state of the art with respect to optical character recognition.

### *10.2.3 Properties of artificial neural networks*

*Adaptivity*: The adaptation of artificial neural networks has been achieved by the different learning schemes. It can be proven that a sufficiently large neural network is able to approximate any continuous function to a chosen degree of accuracy. Clearly, learning by backpropagation is not very strongly related to the natural learning process, but it has proved to be effective and different variants of backpropagation are still the main training methods used for neural networks.

*Interconnected structure*: The interconnected structure of the neural network is the property that most closely resembles the natural properties of the brain. Similar to the brain, the information is stored in the connections (the weights) rather than the neurons. The main difference between artificial neural networks and biological networks is the number of connections. In order for a neural network to be evaluated and trained in a reasonable amount of time, artificial networks are usually quite small compared to biological networks.

*Structural robustness*: Artificial neural networks in principle possess the property of structural robustness. Removing a neuron leads to a degradation in performance, but does not lead to total failure of the networks. This is sometimes used to reduce the size of networks.

*Hierarchical structure*: Artificial neural networks possess a layered structure of an input layer, a varying number of hidden layers, and an output layer. This layered structure proved to be useful in a wide range of applications; however, it does not have a very strong resemblance to biological neural networks. Recent developments of neural networks try to recreate the human brain's processing steps in a much more precise way than earlier designs (Riesenhuber & Poggio, 1999).

*Size*: The main difference between artificial networks and biological networks is size. The number of connections in the human brain is still unmatched by artificial networks and it still remains to be seen how such very large artificial networks behave. The second major difference is time and input used for learning. Biological networks have a very long time (decades) to learn and receive a rich spectrum of input and feedback, which is not present in any implementation of artificial neural networks.

*Parallel computation:* This is a well-known feature of artificial neural networks. Although the computations within each layer could be done in parallel and the evaluation of a whole network would then take only a few massively parallel computational steps, almost all neural networks are implemented on standard computers, where the evaluation is done sequentially. Thus the mathematical model has the ability of parallel computation, but the usual implementation does not.

### *10.2.4 Fuzzy systems*

Another major topic in the area of soft computing is fuzzy sets. The purpose of fuzzy sets is to capture the vagueness of linguistic expressions and make them mathematically accessible. The following sections describe only the basics of fuzzy sets; further information can be found for example, in Gebhart, Kruse, and Klawonn (1993).

The invention of fuzzy sets is attributed to Lotfi Zadeh and was published in a famous paper on "Fuzzy Sets" in 1965. The idea emerged from systems theory and was focused on capturing the inherent imprecision of biological or natural systems. The fundamental idea is that the membership of an element in a set is gradual rather than binary (crisp). This change gave rise to a whole new field of mathematics, creating fuzzy set theory, fuzzy numbers, fuzzy control, and a wide range of associated mathematical concepts such as triangular norms.

For a crisp set $A$ a unique characteristic function $\mu{:}U\rightarrow\{0,1\}$ can be defined, which divides the universe of discourse $U$ into a group of members and a group of nonmembers.

$$\mu_A(x) = \begin{cases} 0 & \text{if} \quad x \in A \\ 1 & \text{if} \quad x \notin A \end{cases}$$

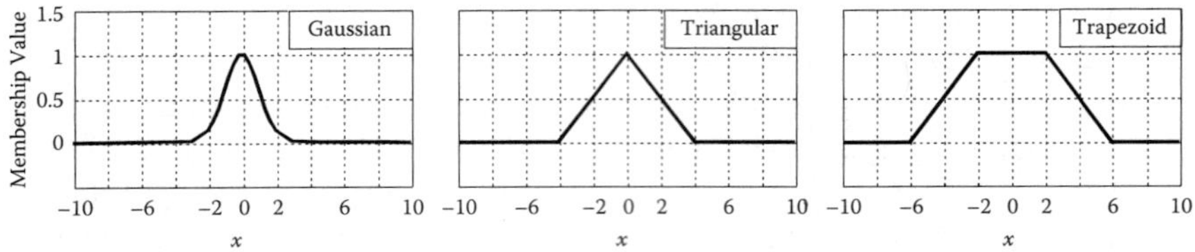


*Figure 10.3* Typical membership functions of fuzzy sets.

For a fuzzy set the membership function maps each element to a degree of membership in the interval [0, 1], such that $\mu_A(x) \in [0,1]$.

This gradual transition enables mathematicians to adequately describe objects that we use in our daily communication. An illustrative example is that of a "pile of sand." Starting from a large pile we remove the sand grain by grain. We find that there is no single moment in time when the pile of sand ceases to be a pile of sand according to the commonly accepted meaning. However, once there are only a few grains left, it will not be a pile any longer. Consequently, the object under consideration fulfills the property of being a pile of sand to a certain degree depending on how closely it matches our expectations in the current context.

Typical membership functions are shown in Figure 10.3. In theory membership functions have to fulfill only one very basic property: that they map the objects in the universe of discourse to membership values in the range of 0 to 1. In practice there are a few functions that are used in almost all applications, such as triangular-shaped functions, trapezoid functions, and monotone increasing functions. In some cases smooth approximations of these functions are used to avoid the problems associated with the differentiability of the corners.

### 10.2.5 *Fuzzy sets and rules*

Similar to concepts of classical set theory one can define intersections, unions, and other operations on fuzzy sets. Given two fuzzy sets represented by their membership function $\mu_A$ and $\mu_B$, defined on the same universe of discourse, we may, for example, define their intersection as

$$\mu_{A \cap B} = \mu_A \cdot \mu_B.$$

The product has a few properties that make it a plausible operation for calculating the intersection of $A$ and $B$; for example, it will be nonzero only if $\mu_A$ and $\mu_B$ are nonzero. However, this is not the only possibility. One could also define

$$\mu_{A \cap B} = \min(\mu_A, \mu_B),$$

which would lead to a slightly different result, but still preserve the most relevant properties of an intersection. In fact there is a whole class of functions that may serve as intersections; these are called *t*-norms (Klement, Mesiar, & Papp, 2000).

Similarly, we may consider the different options for calculating the union of two fuzzy sets *A* and *B*. Two such options would be

$$\mu_{A\cup B} = \mu_A + \mu_B - \mu_A\mu_B \text{ or } \mu_{A\cup B} = \max(\mu_A, \mu_B).$$

Again there is a whole class of such functions, which are called *t*-conorms.

It should be pointed out that there are significant theoretical challenges that have to be considered when dealing with intersections and unions of fuzzy sets. For nonfuzzy sets it is basic knowledge that the intersection of a set *A* with itself is again *A*. However, if we choose the product as our way of calculating the intersection of two fuzzy sets, then we find that the intersection of fuzzy set *A* with itself does not in general preserve its membership function, inasmuch as

$$\mu_{A\cap A} = \mu_A \cdot \mu_A \neq \mu_A.$$

On the other hand, if *min*(.,.) is chosen for the intersection, then we find that this property is preserved.

The big advantage of fuzzy methods that makes them different from all other mathematical concepts is the possibility to create rules in linguistic form. Such sets of rules are also called "fuzzy inference systems." The rules can be easily understood and interpreted by humans and allow the discovery of a priori unknown relationships. A wide range of methods exist to automatically extract such fuzzy rules from experimental datasets (Cox, 2005). If, for example, one would try to model relationships between physical properties and human perception of surfaces, one might end up with rules such as

(R1) IF surface is ROUGH and color is RED then PERCEPTION is VERY WARM.
(R2) IF surface is SMOOTH and color is DARK then PERCEPTION is COLD.

The capitalized words ("ROUGH", "DARK", "COLD", etc.) are fuzzy sets defined on appropriate universes of discourse. The input variables "surface" and "color" are nonfuzzy quantities usually represented by real numbers. The output "perception" is a fuzzy set, which for some applications has to be converted back into a real number. This process is called defuzzification and many different methods have been developed for this purpose. We just mention the center-of-gravity defuzzification that calculates the center of gravity of the resulting fuzzy membership function.

The procedure for evaluating such a rule system is shown in Figure 10.4 and is done as follows. First we need to determine the degree to which each rule is fulfilled by calculating the degree of membership for each input variable in their respective fuzzy sets. We may find, for example, that

$$\mu_{\mathrm{ROUGH}}(surface) = 0.8 \qquad \mu_{\mathrm{SMOOTH}}(surface) = 0.1$$

$$\mu_{\mathrm{RED}}(color) = 0.6 \qquad \mu_{\mathrm{DARK}}(color) = 0.5$$

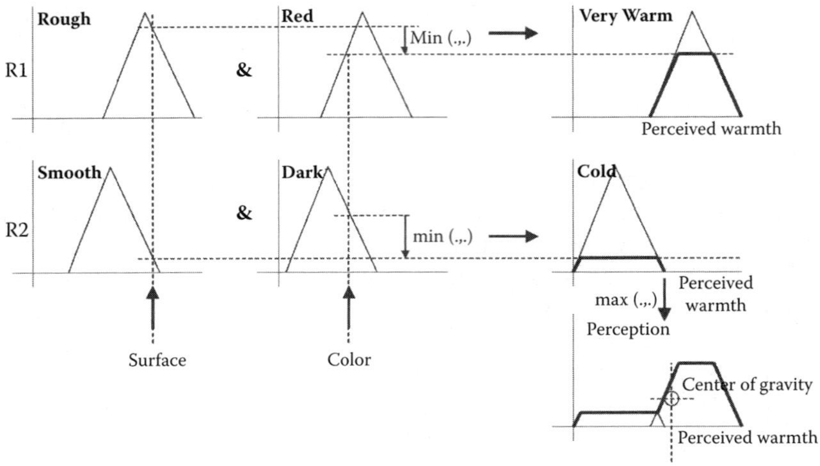


*Figure 10.4* Fuzzy inference with two rules, min/max aggregation and center-of-gravity defuzzification. Evaluation of the rules R1 and R2 for a surface that is quite rough and has a somewhat dark red color. Rule R1 applies to a degree of 0.6 and rule R2 applies to a degree of 0.1. By combining the results of both rules (bottom, right) we end up a with a fuzzy membership function that describes the perception of warmth of the surface. This fuzzy membership function may be defuzzified using the center-of-gravity method. See text for further explanation.

If we take *min*(.,.) as fuzzy "and", then we find that rule (R1) is fulfilled to a degree of min(0.8,0.6) = 0.6 and rule (R2) is fulfilled to a degree of min(0.5, 0.1) = 0.1. The output fuzzy set ("VERY WARM", "COLD") is then weighted according to the degree to which the respective rule is fulfilled. This weighting operation is usually done by applying a *t*-norm, such as min(0.6, $\mu_{\mathrm{VERY\_WARM}}(perception)$) and min(0.1, $\mu_{\mathrm{COLD}}(perception)$).

The second step is to aggregate all rules to obtain a single fuzzy output membership function for PERCEPTION. The aggregation operation is usually a *t*-conorm, such as max(.,.). The resulting membership function is thus

$$\mu_{\mathrm{PERCEPTION}}(perception) = \max(\min(0.6, \mu_{\mathrm{VERY\_WARM}}(perception)), \min(0.1, \mu_{\mathrm{COLD}}(perception)))$$

Occasionally, there is the need to convert the output into a nonfuzzy (crisp) real number, for example, if such rule systems are used in technical feedback control loops. Here we apply the center-of-gravity defuzzification, so that the final crisp output of the fuzzy rule system is obtained by

$$\frac{\int \mu(\text{perception}) \cdot \text{perception} \cdot d\text{perception}}{\int \mu(\text{perception}) \cdot d\text{perception}}.$$

### *10.2.6 Fuzziness versus probability*

It is important to distinguish between probability and fuzziness. Both try to capture a different type of uncertainty. Probability (at least the interpretation as relative frequence of occurrence) applies to the concept of large numbers of objects that do or do not possess a certain property. The uncertainty lies in the fact that we do not know which object is actually chosen. Once an object is selected from this large set, it can be determined with absolute certainty whether the object fulfills the property. The chance of choosing an object with the desired property is expressed by the probability distribution. Fuzziness does not need a large number of objects; it can be applied to a single object. However, given this single object, it is not fully clear whether the object fulfils the property under consideration. This fact is expressed by the value of the membership function for that object.

This difference is easily demonstrated by the example shown in Figure 10.5. The object shown in the image is somewhat close to a square. However, we would never say that "This is probably a square." For this particular object it can be easily determined, that—according to the mathematical definition—it is not a square. There is no probability involved.

On the other hand, aside from the exact mathematical definition, if we adopt a humanlike interpretation of "square," we would call this a "fuzzy square." To some degree it fulfils the most important properties. It has four corners, although not with an angle of exactly 90°, and edges of roughly the same length. One could, for example, say that this object fulfils the properties of a "square" to the degree of 0.75.

This raises the question of how the value of 0.75 is actually determined. The mainstream interpretation of fuzzy membership function is that of a statistical quantity. If, for example, one wants to determine the fuzzy membership function of the property "tall" (if applied to men), one could consider values in the range of 1.6 m to 2.3 m. An experimental procedure could obtain the opinions of a sufficiently large

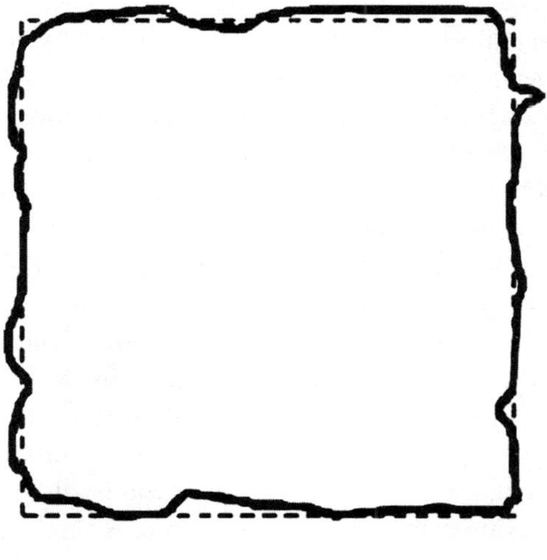

*Figure 10.5* A fuzzy square.

number of people about the meaning of "tall" in this context. Most people will agree that 1.6 m is not "tall," and there will also be an agreement that "2.3 m" is indeed "tall." Between these two extremes there will be a transition from "not tall" to "tall." A membership value 0.3 for the size of 1.8 m can thus be interpreted in a way that 30% of the participants in the experiment would call a man of 1.8 m "tall."

Clearly, such experimental procedures are not often used; however, in many technical applications it is surprisingly easy to find a good set of membership functions. Quite often the context and technical limitations provide important clues as to how a membership function should be chosen.

## 10.3 Recent models of object recognition in the visual cortex

In this section we take a big step forward, by almost 40 years of research in mathematical modeling of the human brain and artificial neural networks. The original concept of modeling the neuron as a nonlinear function of a linear combination of inputs has been substantially extended. Much more is now understood about the processing steps that go on in layers of neurons and this is particularly true for the layers that set up the human visual cortex. This part of the brain has received a great deal of attention in the past so that quite detailed and surprisingly precise models of the human visual system have now been developed. The original idea of having a layered structure of neurons, however, is still present in today's models. In the following we focus on artificial neural networks that model the task of object recognition and give an overview of recent results covering the steps from the perceived image through various brain areas to final recognition (Riesenhuber & Poggio, 1999). We first start with a description of the neurophysiological results and then give a mathematical representation of the whole model.

### *10.3.1 The visual cortex*

Processing of the retinal image is done along the ventral visual pathway, starting with the primary visual cortex (V1), followed by visual areas V2 and V4 and leading on to the inferotemporal cortex. The inferotemporal cortex is supposed to play an important role in object recognition and provides input to the prefrontal cortex that links perception and memory. The whole process is shown in Figure 10.6 and described in the following paragraphs.

The first processing step in the primary visual cortex (V1) is done by simple cells (S1) that are known to be orientation-sensitive. They respond to edges of high contrast in the image that are running in a certain direction. The activations of simple cells that respond to the same direction are aggregated by the complex cells (C1) over a certain small area. This aggregation over a small area leads to a slight invariance to position. In the next step, the aggregation is done over cells with similar position, but different orientation, which leads to so-called "composite feature" cells (S2). The following layer (C2) again combines the activation of S2 cells with similar features, but slightly different position. The assumption is that there is an alternating sequence

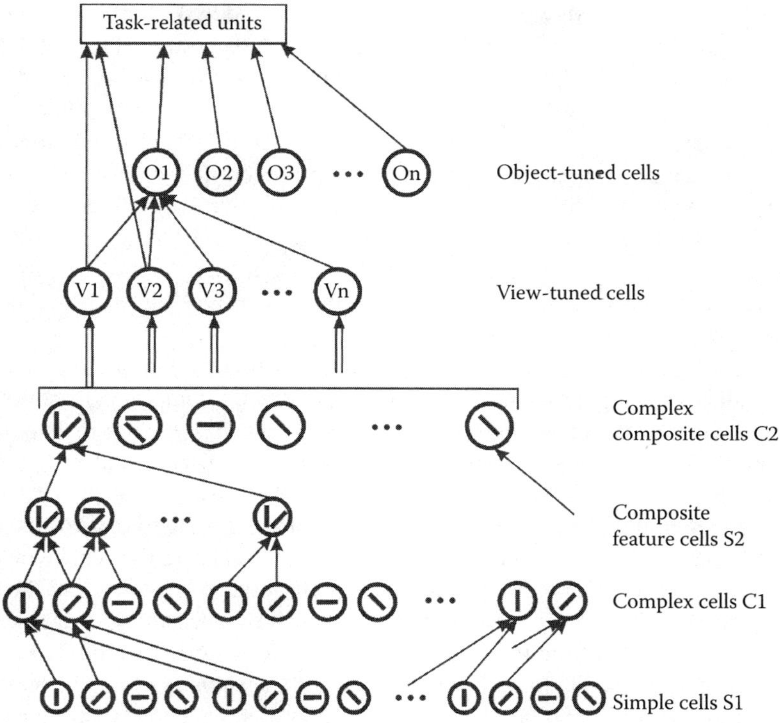


*Figure 10.6* The standard model of the human visual cortex.

of simple and complex cells, whose final output is sensitive to rotation in depth, to changes in illumination, and to any deformation of the object, but is invariant to translation and scale. The resulting units are thus tuned to a specific view of an object, which provides the selectivity required for object recognition.

In the second part of the model invariance with respect to rotation in depth is obtained by combining several different view-tuned units. The processing is supposed to take place in the anterior inferotemporal cortex. At this stage the processing steps become more complicated, with feedback loops involved and task-dependent units that perform visual tasks such as identification or classification. These higher-level functions take place in the inferotemporal cortex and the prefrontal cortex. Learning also takes place in these areas.

### *10.3.2 Computational model of the visual cortex*

The following description of a computational model of the object recognition capabilities of the visual cortex is taken from recent work by Serre, Wolf, Bileschi, Riesenhuber, and Poggio (2007). We do not reproduce the model in the full level of detail, but focus on the single neural mechanisms and their computational representation.

The function of the S1 simple cells is usually modeled by Gabor filters that prove to be very good at reproducing these cells on a range of experimental data. The Gabor filter depends on scale (frequency) and orientation. Usually a whole set of Gabor filters is considered with different scales and orientations, where 64 filters with 16 different scales and 4 different orientations (0°, 45°, 90°, 135°) are widely used. Each of these 64 images that result from the filtering process has high values on those areas that match to the direction and scale of the respective Gabor filters. Depending on the scale of the Gabor filter the images look blurred, with largest scales causing the strongest blurring effect. Another property of Gabor filters is that they also act as edge-detectors, causing low values in homogeneous areas and higher values on edges or regular patterns that match their frequency.

The first layer of complex cells (C1) performs an aggregation of the simple cells and introduces a slight invariance to position and scale. C1 complex cells cover about twice the size of a receptive field of simple cells. It thus makes sense to combine the 16 scales to 8 scale bands, each of which contains two adjacent scales. The aggregation is done by calculating the maximum over all activations of the S1 cells, in the scales belonging to the scale band. The size of the neighborhood for the maximum aggregation is determined by the average of the scales in the scale band. This aggregation over a neighborhood is not done at all possible locations, but the single neighborhoods only overlap by roughly half their size, such that a staggered grid is obtained. This aggregation is done independently for all orientations. The result is 32 images (8 scale bands times 4 orientations) with substantial blur. The maximum aggregation over a neighborhood and the reduction to 8 scale bands introduce a certain level of invariance to translation and scale.

The following S2 layer performs an aggregation over all orientations and also contains the first trainable components in the form of prototype image patches. The S2 cells are represented by Gaussian radial basis functions, similar to the one shown in Figure 10.1. The activation will be largest if the image patch matches the prototype patch. The prototypes are determined during the learning process. Such S2 maps are calculated for all of the 8 scale bands and for each prototype. Depending on the complexity of the task this may be several thousand maps.

The C2 units introduce a final shift and scale invariance by calculating the global maximum over all scales and positions and independently for all prototypes. The resulting maxima for all the prototypes are collected in a single vector that constitutes the output of our model. This vector is in turn input to a standard classifier, such as a linear classifier, a support vector machine, or a similar classifier, that finally performs the recognition by assigning the vector to a class of objects.

The learning process corresponds to the selection of the prototypes from the training images. In this model the selection is done by a sampling process, selecting patches at random positions and randomly chosen from a set of four different sizes.

This model was applied to a set of image databases of varying complexity, containing several thousand images. The main quality measure is the recognition rate, that is, the probability with which the model correctly recognizes the objects. The

*Table 10.1* The human cortex–based model achieves a significant improvement over benchmark methods for object recognition (Serre et al., 2007)

| *Object* | *Benchmark* | *New model* |
|---|---|---|
| Leaves | 84.0 | 97.0 |
| Cars | 84.8 | 99.8 |
| Faces | 96.4 | 98.2 |
| Airplanes | 94.0 | 96.7 |
| Motorcycles | 95.0 | 98.0 |
| Faces | 90.4 | 95.9 |
| Cars | 75.4 | 95.1 |

benchmarks for this assessment were standard approaches for object recognition (SIFT features). The recognition rates [%] are given in Table 10.1.

Clearly, for some types of objects this model shows a substantial improvement over existing methods. We consider this as one of the first powerful demonstrations of how biological models may achieve significant progress in areas that are currently dominated by engineered methods.

## References


Cox, E. (2005). *Fuzzy modeling and genetic algorithms for data mining and exploration*, Amsterdam: Elsevier.

Gebhart, J., Kruse, R., & Klawonn, F. (1993). *Fuzzy-systeme*. Stuttgart: B.G. Teubner.

Gupta, M. M., & Knopf, G. K., Eds. (1993). *Neuro-vision systems—Principles and applications*. Washington, DC: IEEE Press.

Klement, E. P., Mesiar, R., & Papp, E. (2000). *Triangular norms*. Dordrecht: Kluwer Academic.

Lin, C. T., & Lee, C. S. G. (1995). *Neural fuzzy systems: A neuro-fuzzy synergism to intelligent systems*, Englewood Cliffs, NJ: Prentice Hall.

Riesenhuber, M., & Poggio, T. (1999). Hierarchical models of object recognition in cortex. *Nature Neuroscience, 2,* 1019–1025.

Serre, T., Wolf, L., Bileschi, S., Riesenhuber, M., & Poggio, T. (2007) Robust object recognition with cortex-like mechanisms. *IEEE Transactions on Pattern Analysis and Machine Intelligence, 29*(3), 411–426.

Zadeh, L.A. (1965). Fuzzy sets. *Information and Control, 8*, 338–353.

# 11 Psychological measurement for sound description and evaluation

*Patrick Susini,*[1] *Guillaume Lemaitre,*[1] *and Stephen McAdams*[2]

[1]Institut de Recherche et de Coordination Acoustique/Musique
Paris, France

[2]CIRMMT
Schulich School of Music
McGill University
Montréal, Québec, Canada

## 11.1 Introduction

Several domains of application require one to measure quantities that are representative of what a human listener perceives. *Sound quality evaluation*, for instance, studies how users perceive the quality of the sounds of industrial objects (cars, electrical appliances, electronic devices, etc.), and establishes specifications for the design of these sounds. It refers to the fact that the sounds produced by an object or product are not only evaluated in terms of annoyance or pleasantness, but are also important in people's interactions with the object. Practitioners of sound quality evaluation therefore need methods to assess experimentally, or automatic tools to predict, what users perceive and how they evaluate the sounds. There are other applications requiring such measurement: evaluation of the quality of audio algorithms, management (organization, retrieval) of sound databases, and so on. For example, sound-database retrieval systems often require measurements of relevant perceptual qualities; the searching process is performed automatically using similarity metrics based on relevant descriptors stored as metadata with the sounds in the database.

The "perceptual" qualities of the sounds are called the *auditory attributes*, which are defined as percepts that can be ordered on a magnitude scale. Historically, the notion of auditory attribute is grounded in the framework of psychoacoustics. Psychoacoustical research aims to establish quantitative relationships between the physical properties of a sound (i.e., the properties measured by the methods and instruments of the natural sciences) and the perceived properties of the sounds, the auditory attributes. The physical properties of a sound that are related to the auditory attributes can be computed from the sound signal. These values therefore predict the auditory attributes from the sound signal alone and once well understood can be substituted for experimental measurements. They are called *psychoacoustical descriptors*. Psychoacoustical research has isolated several auditory attributes: loudness, pitch, duration, and sharpness, among others. Methods have been developed to measure these attributes experimentally, and algorithms have been devised to compute corresponding psychoacoustical descriptors.

Here we use the term "auditory attribute" in a slightly broader sense than the psychoacoustical definition. Indeed, listeners can recover many kinds of information from a sound. Not only do they perceive percepts that can be directly mapped to the physical properties of the sound, but most of the time they also recognize the source that caused the sound and identify its properties. Gaver (1993a, 1993b) initially formalized this idea by introducing the concepts of *musical listening* (focus on the sound itself) and *everyday listening* (focus on the properties of the source). By *measuring auditory attributes*, we therefore mean here "providing quantities representative of what a user perceives."

The purpose of this chapter is to present the measurement of these auditory attributes from an applied perspective. Some of these attributes are easily understood (and have a name) and have been studied in depth. For instance, loudness, pitch, and duration are auditory attributes for which experimental methods, and even mathematical predictive models, are easily accessible. Section 11.1 briefly summarizes some of the results and methods associated with these attributes. Other attributes are less easily specified and often require metaphors from other sensory modalities to be described: brightness (or sharpness), roughness, fluctuation strength, and so on. In Section 11.2, we present more specifically the methods used to explore these attributes. Because they cannot be easily and unequivocally specified to a listener, these attributes require indirect and multidimensional methods that allow exploration of sound perception. Section 11.2 presents several families of methods: semantic scales, similarity judgments and multidimensional scaling, sorting tasks, and cluster analyses. Section 11.3 presents examples of applications in sound quality. Finally, perspectives in the realm of sonic interaction design are briefly introduced.

## 11.1 Basic knowledge and methods

### *11.1.1 Peripheral auditory system*

We provide here a broad overview of the peripheral auditory system.* For a more complete description, interested readers should refer to Moore (2003).

#### *11.1.1.1 Description*

The human peripheral auditory system is composed of three parts: the outer ear, the middle ear, and the inner ear. The *outer ear* is mainly composed of the pinna and the auditory canal between the pinna and the eardrum. The outer ear amplifies the sound level at the eardrum for frequencies around 3 kHz. The *middle ear*, composed of three

* Animations by Prof. Herbert Hudde from Bochum University can be found at the following URL: http://www.ruhr-unibochum.de/ika/ika/forschung/gruppe_hudde/bohear_en.htm

very small ossicles, matches impedance between the air in the auditory canal (outer ear) and the fluids in the cochlea (inner ear). It also improves sound transmission for frequencies in the range of 0.5–4 kHz. From a psychoacoustical point of view, the most important part of the *inner ear* is the basilar membrane (BM) that can be considered as a "frequency analyzer." An incoming sound sets in motion the BM with a maximum displacement at a certain position that differs according to the frequency of the sound; the position of the maximum varies from the beginning (base) of the BM (oval window) for high frequencies to the end (apex) of the BM for low frequencies. The frequency producing a maximum of displacement on the BM is the center frequency of a bandpass filter for that position. Because different fibers of the auditory nerve are connected to different positions along the basilar membrane, the frequency selectivity of the basilar membrane results in a frequency decomposition of the sounds in the auditory nerve. The frequency selectivity of the auditory system has very important consequences for audition. Particularly, the "masking" phenomenon has introduced the concepts of critical bands (CB) and auditory filters and has resulted in a model that is the basis for the computation of psychoacoustical descriptors.

### *11.1.1.2 Masking, critical bands, and models*

Fletcher (1940) introduced the concept of critical bands to account for masking phenomena. For very narrow bands, he showed that the threshold of detection for a pure tone increases as the noise bandwidth increases. After a certain bandwidth, increasing the noise bandwidth no longer changes the tone threshold. Fletcher assumed that only an effective part of the noise masker, close to the frequency of the tone, has the power to mask the tone. The corresponding frequency region is the *critical band.* Further investigations showed that a model consisting of a bank of bandpass filters, the bandwidth of which increases with the center frequency, could account for masking (Zwicker, 1961; Zwicker & Fastl, 1972; Moore & Glasberg, 1983, 1990). The shape of each filter is asymmetric: roll-off is sharp for frequencies below the center frequency (100 dB/octave) and smooth for frequencies above the center frequencies. The steepness of the roll-off decreases as the level of the stimulus increases.

There are several models of these filters. Third-octave bandpass filters can roughly model the auditory filters. Fourth-octave bandpass filters have also been proposed and shown to approximate fairly well the auditory filters except for low frequencies (Hartmann, 1997). A more complex model uses the Gammatone filters (Patterson & Holdsworth, 1991). Finally, based on this concept of critical bands, several scales have been proposed: the *Bark scale* (Zwicker & Terhardt, 1980) and the *Equivalent Rectangular Bandwidth (ERB) scale* (Moore & Glasberg, 1983).

### *11.1.1.3 Psychoacoustical descriptors*

Models of the auditory system based on critical bands are used to compute psychoacoustical descriptors. The classical psychoacoustical descriptors are summarized in Zwicker and Fastl (1999) and Moore (2003).

The descriptor of loudness is widespread. Models have been standardized: ISO 532-A (Stevens' model); ISO 532-B for (Zwicker's model). A BASIC program is also available in Zwicker (1984). ANSI S3.4-2005 is a revision proposed by Moore and Glasberg (1996) and Moore, Glasberg, and Baer (1997). Corrections of this model have also been proposed allowing a better account of impulsive sounds in a background masking noise (Vos, 1998) and of time-varying sounds (Glasberg & Moore, 2002). Another descriptor of loudness (Meunier, Boulet, & Rabau, 2001) has been proposed for environmental and synthesized impulsive sounds. The loudness is well explained by a combination between the logarithm of the release time and the energy.

Psychoacoustical descriptors corresponding to other auditory attributes are also commonly used: spectral centroid and sharpness, roughness (Daniel and Weber, 1997), and so on (see Zwicker & Fastl, 1999, and Fastl, 1997, for summaries). They have also been implemented in several commercial software packages: BAS and ArtemiS by Head Acoustics, dBSonic by 01dB-Metravib, PULSE by Brüel & Kjaer, and LEA by Genesis. The available descriptors that have been implemented are based on experimental results using abstract sounds, thus these psychoacoustical descriptors sometimes need to be adapted for real sounds (see the work by Misdariis et al., 2010, on this question). Only the loudness descriptors have been standardized. They provide reliable results for stationary sounds, but further development is needed for nonstationary sounds.

### *11.1.2 Classical psychoacoustical methods*

The traditional psychoacoustical approach is unidimensional: it aims to establish a quantitative relationship between a single auditory attribute and a physical property of the sound.

#### *11.1.2.1 Indirect methods*

*11.1.2.1.1 Thresholds.* The indirect method is based on the measurement of thresholds. The *absolute threshold* is the minimum detectable level of a sound. For instance, for a pure tone it depends on the frequency of the tone. Under normal conditions, a young listener can hear frequencies between 20 Hz and 20 kHz. For most adults, the threshold increases rapidly above about 15 kHz. The *differential threshold* or *difference limen* (DL) is the smallest change in a sound to produce a *just-noticeable difference* (jnd) in the related auditory attribute.

*11.1.2.1.2 Confusion scaling.* By varying a physical parameter and measuring the DL for a given auditory attribute, a confusion scale for this attribute can be set. Assuming that all DLs correspond to equal changes of the auditory attribute (jnd), Fechner's law (1860, published in English in 1966) can be determined:

$$\psi = k \log(\phi)$$

where $\psi$ is the magnitude of the auditory attribute, $\phi$ is the physical parameter, and $k$ is a constant specific to each auditory attribute.

### *11.1.2.2 Direct methods*

*Ratio scaling* is a direct method relying on the ability of participants to make numerical judgments of the ratio between the magnitudes of their sensations. The usual methods are *magnitude estimation* and *production*. For magnitude estimation, the participants are required to assign a number proportional to their sensation (e.g., loudness) of the intensity for sounds presented at different levels. For the magnitude production method, the participant is required in this case to adjust the level of a test sound to a specified number proportional to its loudness The relation between the expressed sensation (e.g., loudness) using such methods and the corresponding acoustical values (e.g., sound pressure level) leads to the well-known psychophysical law, Steven's law:

$$\psi = k\,\phi^{\alpha}$$

where $\psi$ is the magnitude of the auditory attribute, $\phi$ is the physical parameter, and $k$ and $\alpha$ are constants specific to each auditory attribute. For instance, for the loudness of a 1-kHz tone, the exponent is 0.6: a 10-dB increase leads to a 2-sone increase. For a 3-kHz tone, the exponent is 0.67. Steven's law for loudness has led to the derivation of the sone scale.

The *cross-modal matching* method was proposed by S. S. Stevens (1959). The task consists in matching two sensations (e.g., loudness and muscular force sensation), one of which has been calibrated beforehand by a direct estimation method (Stevens, 1959). The matching function between the sensations is known or experimentally obtained. Then ratings related to the other sensation are directly deduced by way of the matching function. This method can be used to scale the loudness of time-varying sounds (see the next section).

## *11.1.3 Perspectives: Loudness of time-varying sounds*

The classical psychoacoustical methods have been broadly used to study the perception of short and stationary sounds. Everyday sound events and musical pieces, however, are usually nonstationary. The temporal fluctuations and durations (up to 20 minutes) of such nonstationary sounds do not allow the use of classical methods, but require continuous ratings of the sounds. The participant must in this case respond instantaneously to any variation of the sound. The methods and the devices usually proposed can be sorted into five categories.

1. The *method of continuous judgment using categories* was proposed by Kuwano and Namba (1978, 1985) with the aim of studying temporal fluctuations of the level of urban sounds. In this procedure, participants judge

the loudness at each instant using a response box with seven buttons corresponding to seven categories: very, very loud–very loud–loud–medium–soft–very soft–very, very soft. This process is applicable to long-duration stimuli, because the task is not difficult and participants experience little fatigue. The participants modify their judgment as soon as they perceive a change equivalent to the distance between two categories. The main disadvantage of the continuous category judgment method is that it does not allow one to obtain analogical responses as a function of the signal contour.

2. The *audiovisual adjustment method* was developed by Kuwano and Namba (1990). In this method, participants express their judgment by continuously adjusting the length of a line with a cursor so that the length is proportional to the auditory sensation. The main problem with this method comes from the clipping or ceiling effect at the top end of the judgment scale, because the length of the line is limited (computer screen, sheet of paper, etc.). To get around this limitation, Kuwano and Namba (1990) elaborated a device with which the line presented on the terminal screen is projected on a large screen with an overhead projector. In a similar manner, Fastl (1989, 1991) performed an experiment in which the participant judged the instantaneous loudness by associating in real time the displacement of a potentiometer on a mixing table. However, this device provides little feedback (aside from hand/arm position) to the user.
3. The *continuous cross-modal matching method* proposed by Susini, McAdams, and Smith (2002) is based on the cross-modal matching method with a force-feedback device. The participant has to adjust a muscular force sensation to the perceived loudness. This device was used to assess 1-kHz pure tones (Susini, McAdams, & Smith, 2002), urban sound sequences (Susini & Maffiolo, 1999), and sounds of accelerating cars (Susini & McAdams, 2008). The method has proved to be a flexible experimental procedure allowing an individual calibration of the device as a function of each participant's perceptual scale, with the aim of avoiding compression or saturation effects in the responses.
4. The *analog categorical scaling* proposed by Weber (1991) combines the categorical and analogical methods. Participants can slide a cursor continuously along five discrete categories labeled (for example): very loud–loud–medium–soft–very soft. The distance between each category is considered as equivalent. This method has been widely used: for loudness evaluation of variable-amplitude sinusoidal sounds (Susini, McAdams, & Smith, 2002, 2007), for assessing speech quality (Hansen & Kollmeier, 1999; Gros & Chateau, 2001), for assessing the comfort of an urban sequence of a running bus (Parizet, Hamzaoui, Segaud, & Koch, 2003), and for brightness ratings of various sounds (Hedberg & Jansson, 1998).
5. The *semantic scale used in real-time* was introduced by several authors to study more complex auditory attributes than loudness, and more specifically to study real-time emotional response to music. The continuous response digital interface (CRDI) developed by Madsen (1996) allows a

continuous tracking of temporal variations of musical works, as does the two-dimensional emotional space (2DES) proposed by Schubert (1996) with which musically evoked emotions are evaluated in real time in a two-dimensional semantic space. Several authors used continuous rating to measure emotional force in music pieces (Sloboda & Lehmann, 2001; McAdams, Vines, Vieillard, Smith, & Reynolds, 2004).

## 11.2 Multidimensional and exploratory methods

It is not always easy to specify an auditory attribute a priori. Apart from pitch and loudness, very few words are specific to sound or easily understood by nonspecialists. Therefore, unidimensional techniques such as described above cannot be used to measure auditory attributes not easily communicated to participants, or those that are simply unknown to the experimenter. This section reports methods to explore or measure unspecified auditory attributes and more generally to determine the psychological aspects of sound perceived by listeners.

### *11.2.1 Judgments on multiple semantic scales*

The use of multiple semantic scales is a fruitful technique to assess different psychological aspects of sounds: auditory attributes (e.g., loudness, roughness), appraisal (e.g., preference), emotional response (e.g., beauty, arousal), and connotative dimensions of the sound source (e.g., the power of a sports car).

Semantic scales are category scales defined either by a single semantic descriptor (unipolar scale) or by a pair of antonymic descriptors (bipolar scale). The scales usually have between three and seven categories. It is usually preferred to use an odd number of intervals to include the middle point of the scale.

#### *11.2.1.1 Method and analysis*

The most used technique is the semantic differential (SD). Participants are asked to judge each stimulus directly along a set of scales labeled with two opposed semantic descriptors. Usually true antonym labels are used (e.g., good–bad, pure–rich, etc.), but alternatives have been proposed (e.g., good–not good).

The labels of the scales are called *semantic descriptors*. The ratings of a stimulus on the different semantic scales yield a multidimensional representation called the *semantic profile*; an example is presented in Figure 11.1. A factor analysis can combine semantic scales into main factors. A multiple regression analysis can highlight relationships between factors corresponding to cognitive aspects (e.g., preference) and factors corresponding to auditory attributes (e.g., loudness, roughness). The latter factors are interpreted by looking for acoustical or psychoacoustical descriptors that are correlated with them. Each semantic descriptor is hypothesized to be psychologically relevant to the whole set of stimuli under examination. On the other hand, it has to be understood by the participants of the experiment.

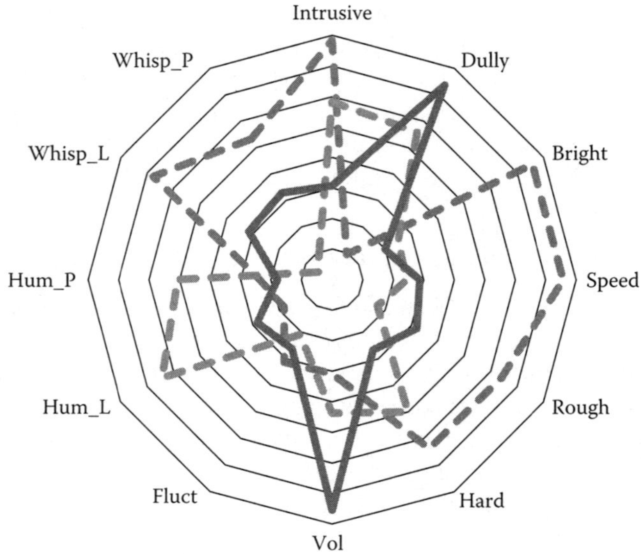


*Figure 11.1 (See color insert.)* Sensory profiles obtained for three air-conditioning noises from Siekierski, Derquenne, and Martin (2001). Labels of the *semantic descriptors* are Intrusive, Dully, Brightness, Speed, Roughness, Hardness, Voluminous, Fluctuation, Humming, Whispering. The letters L and P correspond to the Level and Pitch, respectively, of the whispering (noise) part and the humming (motor) part.

### *11.2.1.2 Examples of semantic scales used to describe sounds*

Since Solomon (1958) and von Bismarck (1974), the semantic differential technique proposed by Osgood (1952) has been widely used in the realm of sound perception to describe the multidimensional character of the timbre of musical instruments (Wedin & Goude, 1972; Pratt & Doak, 1976; Kendall & Carterette, 1992; Stepánek, 2006), environmental sounds (Björk, 1985; Zeitler & Hellbrück, 2001), and sound products, such as cars, vacuum cleaners, air conditioning noises, or refrigerators (Chouard & Hempel; 1999; Kyncl & Jiricek, 2001; Siekiersky, Derquenne, & Martin, 2001; Jeon, 2006).

Typically, results from the different studies have shown that the set of semantic differentials can be combined into three or four main factors that account for a great deal of the variance in the judgments. For instance, in von Bismarck's study on the timbre of synthetic sounds, results revealed four independent scales: "dull–sharp" (44% of the variance explained), "compact–scattered" (26%), "full–empty" (9%), and "colorful–colorless" (2%). Only the scales referring to sharpness were considered as candidates for a generally usable scale for the measurement of timbre. In Pratt and Doak (1976), three scales ("dull–bright", "pure–rich", "cold–warm") were selected to be the more significant descriptors for instrumental timbres. In summary, results from different studies revealed that descriptors related to sharpness ("sharp," "bright," "metallic," or at the opposite, "dull," "muffled," "round") are appropriate to describe the most salient aspect of timbre.

Kuwano and Namba (2001) report three main factors ("powerful," "metallic," and "pleasant") that had consistently been extracted in most of their former studies of sound quality. Furthermore, the semantic descriptor "powerful" was usually well correlated with computed loudness (Zwicker's loudness level based on ISO 532B), and the semantic descriptor "metallic" was well correlated with computed sharpness. The "pleasant" factor was related to cognitive and cultural factors as well as to physical properties of sounds. In Zeitler and Hellbrück's study (2001) on environmental sounds, four factors were linked, respectively, to a hedonic aspect ("ugly"–"beautiful"), timbre ("dark–light"), power ("weak–strong"), and rapid temporal variations ("unstable–stable"). The three latter factors were well correlated with three calculated descriptors, sharpness, loudness, and roughness, respectively. Results from other studies on sounds (speech or sonar sounds) are quite similar: the most important factors were generally interpreted as representing loudness, timbre (sharpness) or pitch, and an overall subjective impression.

### *11.2.1.3 Prerequisites to use semantic scales*

*11.2.1.3.1 Controlling loudness, pitch, and duration.* First, acoustical parameters such as loudness and pitch, as well as variations over time, strongly affect the perception of timbre. To study auditory attributes independently of those obvious parameters, it is therefore recommended to control them and to use steady-state sounds, equalized in loudness, pitch* and duration. This statement is in agreement with the current ANSI definition and summarized by Krumhansl (1989, p. 44): timbre is "the way in which musical sounds differ once they have been equated for pitch, loudness and duration." Otherwise, it is recommended to ask participants to ignore these parameters, following the proposal by Pratt and Doak (1976), who define timbre as "that attribute of auditory sensation whereby a listener can judge that two sounds are dissimilar using any criteria other than pitch, loudness or duration."

*11.2.1.3.2 Selecting an appropriate number of semantic scales.* Second, a restricted number of semantic pairs suitable for describing timbre have to be selected. Indeed, the preselection of semantic descriptors by the experimenter may strongly affect the results, for these descriptors may not necessarily conform with those a participant would use spontaneously. For instance, Pratt and Doak (1976) investigated (by a questionnaire) what were the most appropriate adjectives for describing timbre of instruments among a list of 19 commonly used terms. Seven words emerged as favorites: rich, mellow, colorful, brilliant, penetrating, bright, and warm. Similarly,

* For pitch, this can be done as for loudness by an adjustment procedure using the real-time SuperVP software program based on the phase vocoder technique; it is then possible to transpose, stretch, or shorten sounds in real-time.

in von Bismark (1974), participants were asked to rate each of 69 semantic scales in terms of their suitability for describing timbre. Finally, 28 scales were considered as representative. However, it should be noted that in von Bismarck's study, the 69 scales were rated independently of the sound selected for the study and thus may not be relevant for describing the perceptual dimensions of these sounds.

*11.2.1.3.3 Selecting relevant descriptors.* The third prerequisite consists in asking participants to judge the relevance of the semantic descriptors concerning the sounds used in the study. Faure (2010) gathered a set of semantic descriptors from a free verbalization experiment on 12 musical sounds. They were used to build semantic scales. The relevance of these scales was then judged for the same set of sounds. Comparison between the relevance judgments of the scales and the vocabulary produced spontaneously showed that several semantic descriptors that were spontaneously produced (such as "strong", "loud", etc.) were not considered as relevant when presented with the scales, even by the participants who produced them. Inversely, several semantic descriptors that were rarely used spontaneously were judged to be globally relevant by the majority of participants (e.g., "soft," "muffled/dull sounding," "metallic," "nasal"). In another study (Kyncl & Jiricek, 2001), participants freely described six vacuum cleaner sounds. Among the 33 pairs of semantic oppositions obtained from the vocabulary spontaneously produced, only 5 were consistently judged as relevant for describing the sounds ("fuzziness," "atypicality," "inefficiency," "loudness," and "pleasantness"). These studies highlight the importance of judging the relevance of descriptors used in SD-scales for a specific corpus of sounds.

*11.2.1.3.4 Defining the meaning of the scales.* The fourth prerequisite concerns the definition of the scales. Indeed, it is crucial that the participants correctly understand the meaning of the labels. For instance, in Faure (2010), the stimuli were equalized in loudness. Surprisingly, the participants spontaneously used the word "loud" to describe the sounds. Actually, the participants' comments revealed that they used "loud" to describe different perceptions: "strong in sonic presence, the attack," "evokes the power and persistence of the sound." Similarly, in von Bismarck (1974), although the sounds were equalized in loudness, participants used the scale "soft–loud" to describe attributes other than loudness, such as "unpleasant." Therefore, the experiment must clearly define the meaning of the semantic scales to eliminate any risk of semantic ambiguity. Presenting them in a sentence can help define the meaning of the descriptors. For instance Parizet and Nosulenko (1999) showed that ratings of internal noises of vehicles were more reliable when the semantic descriptors were presented in a sentence than when presented in isolation. Susini, Houix, Misdariis, Smith, and Langlois (2009) introduced the semantic descriptor "loud" by the sentence "The TV is too loud, we can't have a discussion." This sentence aimed at clearly indicating that "loud" referred to the sound level and not the unpleasantness.

In addition to the several prerequisites presented above, other recommendations should be taken into consideration when using the SD-scale technique to rate a corpus of sounds.

- Several studies have shown that subjects feel uncertain in giving ratings unless they can refer them to the whole sample of sounds. Thus the entire range of sounds has to be presented before the main experiment, and participants must be instructed to use the full range of the scale. In addition, it is recommended that the range of sensitivity corresponding to each semantic descriptor of the selected set of sounds be broad enough.
- Many studies on timbre have used the traditional semantic differential paradigm (e.g., dull–sharp). Bipolar adjective pairs raise the question of presenting the right antonym labels (is *dull* the opposite of *sharp* when used to describe sounds?). In Chouard and Hempel (1999), clear antonyms were found in about 23% of the cases for a list of 242 adjectives produced by the participants to describe interior car sounds. Thus an important problem in the use of bipolar opposites is that the "opposite" is sometimes unobtainable or not always a good antipode. To solve this problem, Kendall and Carterette (1992) proposed using a scale bounded by an attribute and its negation (e.g., sharp–not sharp) to rate the timbre of musical sounds. The authors termed this method *verbal attribute magnitude estimation* (VAME), because the task for the participant is to rate the degree to which an attribute is possessed by a stimulus.
- Finally, we recommend presenting the whole set of sounds for each semantic descriptor instead of the classical way consisting in presenting one sound to the participant, who has to evaluate it on the whole set of semantic descriptors. In a study by Parizet and colleagues (1999, 2005), the comparison of the two methods showed that the former proved to be more accurate and with a shorter duration than the classical one, because listeners were focused on one semantic descriptor at a time while hearing a new stimulus. In addition, to measure subject reliability or accuracy, random presentation of the stimuli can be repeated. Cross-correlation coefficients are calculated between the data from both presentations of the repeated stimuli to compute subject reliability.

### *11.2.2 Dissimilarity judgments and multidimensional scaling technique*

Semantic scales compare stimuli along dimensions directly described semantically. It is therefore possible to assess various psychological aspects of a corpus of sounds, ranging from elementary auditory attributes to cognitive and emotional aspects. The disadvantage is that the number of scales is often too high and, with the exception of a few studies mentioned in the previous section, some of the selected semantic descriptors are not perceptually relevant to the corpus studied and are sometimes redundant in relation to each other. However, this approach is appropriate to study the perception of various environmental sounds, as long as several prerequisites are taken into account.

In contrast, the multidimensional scaling technique (MDS) is based on dissimilarity ratings and thus does not require a priori assumptions concerning the number of perceptual dimensions or their nature, unlike the methods that use ratings along specified dimensions.

### *11.2.2.1 MDS and auditory perception*

The multidimensional scaling technique is a fruitful tool for studying perceptual relations among stimuli and for analyzing the underlying auditory attributes used by the participants to rate the perceived similarity between two sounds. MDS represents the perceived similarities in a low-dimensional Euclidean space (so-called *perceptual space*), so that the distances among the stimuli reflect the perceived similarities (see McAdams, Winsberg, Donnadieu, Soete, & Krimphoff, 1995, for a review of the different MDS algorithms). Each dimension of the space (so-called *perceptual dimension*) is assumed to correspond to a perceptual continuum that is common to the whole set of sounds. It is also assumed that each dimension can be well explained by an acoustic parameter or a psychoacoustical descriptor. In other words, the MDS technique is appropriate for describing sounds that are comparable along continuous auditory attributes, which means that it is appropriate for studying homogeneous corpora of sounds, that is, those made of sounds produced by the same type of source.

### *11.2.2.2 Method and analysis*

Participants rate the perceived dissimilarity between each pair of sounds under consideration, that is, $N(N - 1)/2$ ratings for $N$ stimuli, on a continuous scale labeled "Very Similar" at the left end and "Very Dissimilar" at the right end. Then, the dissimilarities are modeled as distances in a Euclidean space of $R$ dimensions expected to be the most relevant perceptual dimensions shared by the sounds. In the perceptual space, a large dissimilarity is represented by a large distance. The final and the most difficult part of this approach lies in matching perceptual dimensions to acoustical or psychoacoustical descriptors.

### *11.2.2.3 Example of MDS studies to describe timbre of musical sounds*

Many researchers have applied the MDS technique to characterize the perceptual dimensions of sounds, since the seminal studies by Peters (1960) and Plomp (1970). Peters (1960) started to apply the MDS technique to a corpus of sounds with a known dimensionality (16 pure tones composed of 4 frequencies at 4 sound pressure levels: the acoustical dimensionality is therefore 2). The analysis of the dissimilarity judgments from 39 participants successfully highlighted the two expected auditory attributes: pitch and loudness. He therefore concluded that the MDS technique might be useful to explore sets of sounds the auditory attributes of which would be unknown. To test this idea, he applied the technique to other corpora of sounds, for which the salient auditory attributes were unknown (synthetic complex sounds and speech sounds). The results were less easily interpretable (he found between three and six dimensions for the complex sounds). But compared to what he obtained with more traditional approaches (free verbal description, partition scaling, magnitude estimation), he concluded that "the most promising approach for the isolation and definition of perceptual dimensions of complex sounds was the MDS model" (p. 52). Plomp (1970) applied MDS to sets of musical sounds, which yielded three orthogonal dimensions.

Since then, several psychoacoustical studies using MDS have shown clearly that musical timbre is a multidimensional attribute. Grey (1977) identified three salient dimensions shared by a corpus of musical sounds. Using a refinement of the classical MDS technique (EXSCAL, developed by Winsberg & Carroll, 1989), Krumhansl (1989) also found a space with three dimensions shared by a corpus of synthesized musical sounds (winds, bowed string, plucked strings, mallet percussion). The same set of sounds was analyzed by McAdams, Winsberg, Donnadieu, Soete, and Krimphoff (1995), who also found a 3-D space. The first dimension of the perceptual space was correlated with the centroid of the amplitude spectrum. It has generally been reported to correspond to the semantic descriptors "metallic," "sharp," or "brilliant." The second dimension was correlated with the logarithm of the attack time of the amplitude envelope, and corresponds to the semantic descriptors "fast-slow attack," "resonant," or "dry." The third dimension was correlated with the spectral irregularity (logarithm of the spectral deviation of component amplitudes from a global spectral envelope derived from a running mean of the amplitudes of three adjacent harmonics) or the spectral flux (average of the correlations between amplitude spectra in adjacent time windows).

### *11.2.2.4 Prerequisites for using MDS to study auditory perception*

*11.2.2.4.1 Controlling loudness, pitch, and duration.* It is important to emphasize that the musical sounds used in the studies previously mentioned were equalized in pitch, subjective duration, and loudness, so that ratings would only concern the differences in timbre. Indeed, certain auditory attributes, such as loudness, might dominate and overpower less salient ones, as mentioned in Section 11.2.1.3 for semantic scales. Two sounds that differ mainly in terms of loudness will be judged obviously different according to this dimension, with little contribution from other dimensions of variation being taken into account.

*11.2.2.4.2 Selecting a homogeneous corpus of sounds.* As mentioned earlier, MDS is hypothesized to represent a corpus of sounds by a limited number of continuous auditory dimensions that are common to all the sounds. That means the corpus has to be composed of homogeneous sound objects (sounds produced by the same type of object or stimuli that sound rather similar, e.g., a class of car sounds) in order to avoid a perceptual structure that is strongly categorical for which the MDS approach is not adapted (see next section). A cluster analysis on the similarity ratings can reveal the degree of homogeneity of the sound corpus. If the tree structure obtained reveals a strong categorization of the corpus, it is advisable to determine which categories best represent the objectives of the study in order to obtain appropriate stimuli.

*11.2.2.4.3 Limiting the number of sounds.* As participants may become fatigued or lose motivation over time, application of the MDS technique is restricted to a rather small number of sounds (more or less 20 well-chosen sounds), because the number of pairs ($N(N-1)/2$) grows rapidly with the number of sounds ($N$). Thus a preliminary categorization experiment may be advisable in order to select the most representative sounds (see Susini, McAdams, Winsberg, Perry, Vieillard, & Rodet, 2004). Another possibility to avoid being confined to a small number of stimuli is to use sorting tasks. Indeed, the validity of using sorting tasks for sounds instead of paired comparisons has been tested and shown to be effective with two different sets of auditory stimuli (Bonebright, 1996). However, further tests have to be performed in order to confirm the validity for collecting data using sorting tasks.

*11.2.2.4.4 Collecting information from participants.* Once the perceptual configuration is obtained, it is important to identify the perceptual meaning of each dimension or even to label the dimensions using semantic descriptors, and also, to give a physical interpretation by establishing systematic relations between the stimulus characteristics and their locations in the space. Knowledge and familiarity with the sound corpus and perceptually relevant acoustic parameters are thus necessary in order to characterize the dimensions of the space objectively. Another option is to directly ask the participants to describe which sensation they attended to while judging the dissimilarities.

### *11.2.3 Sorting tasks*

The MDS technique is not appropriate for sets of sounds caused by very different and obviously identified sources. For instance, Susini, Misdariis, McAdams, & Winsberg (1998) applied an MDS analysis to an extremely heterogeneous set of environmental sounds (trains, cars, and planes). The analysis yielded a strongly categorical perceptual structure: listeners identified the sound sources rather than comparing them along continuous dimensions. Therefore, this predominant cognitive factor—recognition, classification, and identification of the sound source (see McAdams, 1993)—violated the assumption of underlying continuous dimensions required by the MDS technique. In this case, other experimental approaches are needed and, particularly, the sorting tasks.

#### *11.2.3.1 Sorting task, categorization, and auditory cognition*

Sorting tasks are very commonly used in cognitive psychology to address the questions of identification and categorization of sound sources. These questions are tightly bound: identifying the source of sound can be viewed as connecting auditory perception to concepts, and concepts to language, in a bidirectional relationship (McAdams, 1993; Goldstone & Kersten, 2003). Several approaches to the organization and processing of concepts and categories have been developed (see Goldstone & Kersten, 2003, or Komatsu, 1992 for a review). Before presenting the technical procedure of sorting tasks, we briefly recall the general principles of the prototypical approach to categorization developed by Rosch (1978), which is very often used as an underlying framework in sorting tasks. This approach is based on the notion of similarity and is therefore well adapted to account for perceptual concepts such as those used to describe sounds.

Rosch's approach to categorization relies on two principles. First categorization is based on the *cognitive economy* principle: categories allow organisms to handle the infinite number of stimuli by treating them as equivalent when the differentiation is irrelevant for the purpose at hand. The second principle is that *the world has structure*. Categorization of the world is thus not arbitrary, but relies on its perceived structure (Rosch, Mervis, Gray, Johnson, & Boyes-Braem, 1976).

Two concepts are often borrowed from Rosch's work: first, Rosch and her colleagues have experimentally identified three *levels* in taxonomies of objects:

- The base level: items in these categories share many elements in common.
- The superordinate level: this level is more inclusive than the base level, but items in the categories at this level share fewer elements in common.
- The subordinate level: items in the categories at this level share many elements in common, but the classes are less inclusive.

Second, Rosch has introduced the notion of analog category membership: categories are internally structured into a *prototype* and nonprototype members. For these latter members, there is a gradient of *category membership* (Rosch, 1978).

### *11.2.3.2 Method and analysis*

In a *sorting task*, listeners are required to sort a set of sounds and to group them into classes. When the experimenter does not specify any specific criteria that the listeners have to use, the task is called a *free-sorting task*. Usually, the listeners are also required to indicate the meaning of each class.* Sometimes, the listeners also have to select a prototype in each category (the most representative member).

Technically, because personal computers are widespread in the lab,† the procedure amounts to providing the listeners with an interface allowing them to listen to the sounds by clicking on icons and moving the icons so as to form groups.

To analyze the results, the partition of the sounds created by each listener is coded in an *incidence matrix* (in the matrix, 0 indicates that two sounds were in separate groups and 1 that they were in the same group). A *co-occurrence* matrix is then obtained by summing the incidence matrices, which can be interpreted as a proximity matrix (Kruskal & Wish, 1978). Therefore, as with dissimilarity ratings, sorting tasks result in estimating similarities between the sounds. However, the structure of these data might be different depending on the procedure. For instance, Aldrich,

---

* A *classification* of the sounds is the result of a sorting task. "Categories are equivalence classes of different (i.e., discriminable) entities and categorization is the ability to form such categories and treat discriminable entities as members of an equivalence class" (Sloutsky, 2003, p. 246).

† Things were rather more complicated without computers; see Vanderveer (1979).

Hellier, and Edworthy (2009) showed that dissimilarity ratings encouraged participants to use acoustical information, whereas a free-sorting procedure emphasized categorical information. Different techniques are available to visualize the proximity data. When the data follow the triangular inequality, but not the ultrametric inequality,* they are best represented in a low-dimensional geometrical space (e.g., by using MDS). When they also follow the ultrametric inequality, they are best represented in a tree representation (Legendre & Legendre, 1998). Cluster analyses create such representations. The most popular tree representation is the *dendrogram*. It consists in representing the data in a hierarchical tree. In such a tree, the leaves represent the sounds, and the height of the node that links two leaves represents the distance between the two sounds. The representation is hierarchical, well suited to represent class inclusion, and therefore fits well with Rosch's framework.

### *11.2.3.3 Examples of urban soundscape categorization*

Sorting tasks have been largely used to study the categorization of everyday sounds and soundscapes† (Guyot, 1996; Guyot, Castellengo, & Fabre, 1997; Vogel, 1999; Maffiolo, Dubois, David, Castellengo, & Polack, 1998; Guastavino, 2007; see Schulte-Fortkamp & Dubois, 2006, for a review of recent advances).

More recently, Tardieu, Susini, Poisson, Lazareff, and McAdams (2008) conducted an experiment that aimed to highlight the different types of auditory information that are perceived in the soundscapes of train stations. The goal was also to determine the information that participants used in the recognition of the space typology. Sixty-six soundscape samples were presented to participants in a free-categorization task with verbalization. The results showed that the listeners grouped together the samples into eight global categories. Further analysis aimed to explain the categories on the basis of the free verbalizations. Each verbalization was reduced to the words that contained a descriptive meaning. For example, the text "I have grouped here the sequences that took place in a ticket office. We clearly hear people talking about price and ticket" is reduced to the words "ticket office, clearly hear, people, talking about price." This reduction was made with the help of the software LEXICO (2003), which automatically counts every word in a text. Then, words are grouped into semantic fields that are deduced from the verbal descriptions. Five semantic fields were deduced (Figure 11.2): sound sources (e.g., trains, departure boards, ticket-punching machines, whistle, etc.), human activities (e.g., conversations, steps,

* The triangular inequality states that for any three points $A$, $B$, and $C$, $d(A,C) \geq d(A,B) + d(B,C)$, where $d$ is the distance between the two points. In a Euclidean space, the length of any side of a triangle cannot be greater than the sum of the other two sides. In an ultrametric space, this inequality is replaced by $d(A,C) \leq \max\{d(A, B), d(B, C)\}$. In this kind of space, any given side must be less than or equal to the longer of the other two sides. Note that this is less constraining than the Euclidean case. The ultrametric inequality is to most forms of hierarchical clustering what the triangle inequality is to two-way multidimensional scaling.

† The term "soundscape" was introduced in the late 1970s by the Canadian composer R. Murray Schafer (1977), who defined soundscape as the auditory equivalent to landscape. Beside Schafer's project, the term soundscape perception is used in a scientific context to characterize how inhabitants perceive, experience, and appraise their sonic environment.

***Participants' Categories:***

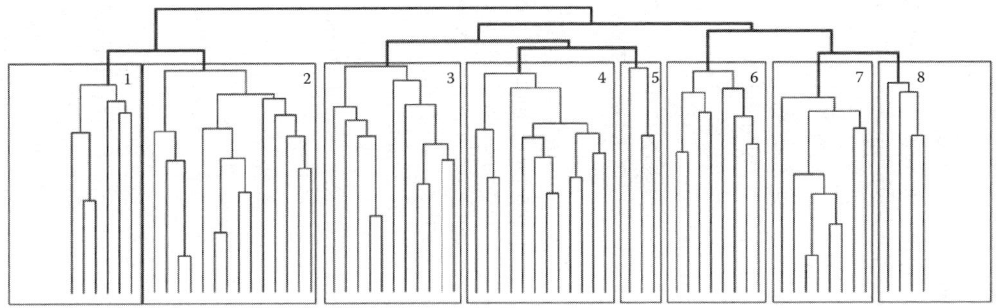


***Participants' Verbalizations:***

| ***Semantic Fields:*** | 1 | 2 | 3 | 4 | 5 | 6 | 7 | 8 |
|---|---|---|---|---|---|---|---|---|
| Sound sources | Ticket dispenser | – | Announcement music | Wheeled suitcases | Departure board | Trains | Jingles | Music, trains |
| Human activities | Conversation, waiting, steps | Voice, people | Waiting conversations | Steps, voice | | Arrivals, departures | Voice, arrivals, departures | Voices, conversations |
| Room effect | Small space | Closed space, small | Reverberation, confused | Echoes, resonances | | External | Resonances, reverbs. | Large reverberation |
| Type of space | Waiting room, ticket office | Bar, waiting room | Bar, hall | Corridor, hall | | Platforms | Hall | Hall |
| Judgments | Quiet space | Quiet, intimate | Unpleasant | Noisy, rhythmic | | – | – | Noisy, unpleasant |

*Figure 11.2* *(See color insert.)* Dendrogram representing the categories of train station soundscapes found in Tardieu et al. (2008). The descriptions of the categories provided by the participants are reported on the table below, grouped into five semantic fields. The most cited verbalizations are shown in a larger size font.

transaction, departure, etc.), room effect (e.g., reverberation, confined, exterior/interior, etc.), type of space (e.g., waiting room, platforms, halls, etc.), and personal judgment (e.g., annoying, pleasant, beautiful, musical, etc.).

#### *11.2.3.4 Prerequisites for using sorting tasks*

The sorting task is very intuitive for the listeners, and, in the case of the free-sorting task, has the great advantage of leaving the listeners free to arrange the sounds as they wish. Contrary to dissimilarity ratings, a large number of the sounds can be handled by the listeners in a session.

*11.2.3.4.1 Considering a large number of existing sounds.* It is possible with sorting tasks to test many existing sounds that are representative of the variety of sounds under consideration. For instance 74 environmental sounds were presented in Bonebright's study (2001), 150 recorded sound effects in Scavone, Lakatos, and Harbke's study (2002), 48 alarm sounds in Susini, Gaudibert, Deruty, and Dandrel's study (2003), and 66 train station soundscapes in Tardieu et al.'s study (2008).

*11.2.3.4.2 Collecting information on the type of similarities used for each category.* From a practical point of view, contrary to the MDS approach, categorization tasks are well adapted to describe perceptually heterogeneous corpora of sounds and to reveal different levels of similarities between the sounds. However, great care has to be taken when analyzing the categories because the type of similarities used by the participants may vary from one category to another, depending on the difficulty in identifying the sounds and on the expertise of the participants (more or less skill with sound evaluation). Indeed, three types of similarities have been identified (Lemaitre et al., 2010), based on acoustical properties (loudness, roughness, intensity fluctuations, etc.), identified physical interactions causing the sound (impact sound on glass, rattle sound on metal, sound effect, etc.) and meanings associated with the identified sound sources (sounds of breakfast, sounds that remind one of childhood, etc.).

*11.2.3.4.3 Selecting the type of similarities.* Semantic analyses of the verbal descriptions of the categories provide rich insights that reveal, on the one hand, the strategy used by the participants to form the categories, and on the other hand, the type of information used. However, semantic analyses are often time consuming and have to be done rigorously by experts. Lemaitre et al. (2010) proposed an alternative, which consists of asking the participants to rate for each category which type of similarity (acoustical, causal, semantic) they had used. The results may help the experimenter to understand the level of the perceptual structures underlying each category.

## 11.3 Application: Sound quality of environmental sounds

The quality of the acoustic environment is currently an important issue. Efforts are being made to account for the annoyance caused by noises (Guski, 1997). At the same time, designers are seeking to improve the sound quality of industrial products.

The idea of sound quality has emerged relatively recently. It refers to the fact that the sounds produced by an object or product are not only annoying or unpleasant, but are also a way for people to interact with an object. In the case of industrial products, it is therefore of major importance to design sounds to meet consumer expectations.

Since the beginning of the 1990s, sound quality has been conceived of mainly in the paradigm of psychoacoustics. This has led to the design of experimental methods and auditory descriptors relevant to sound quality. For instance, Zwicker and Fastl (1999) asked participants to rate *pleasantness* on a unidimensional scale (e.g., ratio scale). Then the pleasantness scores were correlated with psychoacoustical descriptors. Ellermeier, Mader, and Daniel (2004) gathered preference judgments of environmental sounds using a 2AFC (two alternative forced choice) procedure and analyzed them using the BTL technique (Bradley–Terry–Luce). This technique represented the perceived unpleasantness on a ratio scale. The unpleasantness scores were then predicted by a linear combination of psychoacoustic descriptors (roughness and sharpness). The semantic differential technique is also used to evaluate sound quality. It has been largely used for cars (Bisping, 1997; Chouard & Hemepl, 1999), vacuum cleaners (Ih et al., 2002), and refrigerators (Jeon, 2006). However, as noted in Section 11.2.3.1, defining the appropriate semantic descriptors of the scales must be done carefully.

Most of the studies use psychoacoustical descriptors (loudness, roughness, etc.) to explain unpleasantness scores or semantic ratings. These descriptors are currently included in most sound quality software packages, yet they are not always adapted to describing all kinds of everyday sounds. Indeed, it appears that relevant perceptual dimensions are different from one study to another according to the corpus of sounds under consideration. Therefore, there are no "universal" acoustical or psychoacoustical descriptors that can be used to measure relevant auditory attributes for all categories of environmental sounds, and which would thus provide the same effect on the sound quality of any product.

### *11.3.1 Application of the MDS technique to describe environmental sounds*

A crucial aspect for the research in sound quality is to determine the relevant auditory attributes related to a specific family of environmental sounds. The MDS technique has been shown to be a fruitful tool for revealing and characterizing the unknown perceptual dimensions underlying the timbre of musical sounds. During the last decade, the MDS technique has been successfully applied to different kinds of environmental sounds: everyday sounds (Bonebright, 2001), interior car sounds (Susini, McAdams, and Smith, 1997), air-conditioning noises (Susini et al., 2004), car door closing sounds (Parizet, Guyader, and Nosulenko, 2006), and car horn sounds (Lemaitre, Susini, Winsberg, McAdams, and Letinturier, 2007). For all the mentioned studies, MDS analyses led to 3-D perceptual spaces (Figure 11.3 presents the 3-D space obtained for car sounds) and all the dimensions except one were described by different acoustical parameters.

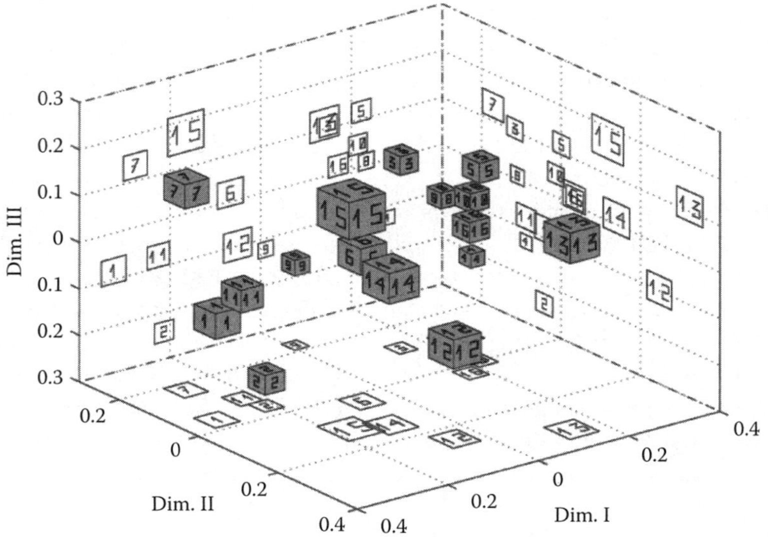


*Figure 11.3* *(See color insert.)* Three-dimensional space for car sounds: dimension I is explained by the energy ratio between the harmonic and noisy parts, dimension II by the spectral centroid, and dimension III by the decrease in the spectral envelope.

The spectral centroid* is the acoustical descriptor shared by all the perceptual spaces related to environmental sounds. Therefore, this descriptor appears to describe musical sounds as well as environmental sounds and is related to the semantic descriptors "metallic," "sharp," or "brilliant." Aside from the spectral centroid, no universal auditory attributes exist to characterize the timbre of any sound, and an inventory of the different salient auditory attributes to describe the different family of sounds is needed. A meta-analysis of 10 published timbre spaces conducted by McAdams, Giordano, Susini, Peeters, and Rioux (2006) using multidimensional scaling analyses (CLASCAL) of dissimilarity ratings on recorded, resynthesized or synthesized musical instrument tones, revealed four primary classes of descriptors: spectral centroid, spectral spread, spectral deviation, and temporal envelope (effective duration/attack time).

* The spectral centroid is the weighted mean frequency of the spectrum of the signal; each partial tone is weighted by its corresponding amplitude. The calculation of this feature can be more or less complex (see the work by Misdariis et al., 2010), but the basic expression is:

$$SC = \frac{\sum_i A_i \times f_i}{\sum_i A_i}$$

where $A_i$ and $f_i$ are the amplitude and frequency of the corresponding partial.

### *11.3.2 A general framework for sound quality*

In a more general framework, the MDS technique may be combined with another approach based on a semantic study of the corpus of sounds under consideration, in order to map preference judgments onto both relevant objective descriptors and appropriate semantic descriptors. Figure 11.4 presents the framework of the different stages of these related approaches. This general framework was applied using air-conditioning noises as an example in a three-part study by Susini, Perry, Winsberg, Vieillard, McAdams, and Winsberg (2001), Siekierski et al. (2001), and Junker, Susini, and Cellard (2001).

The first step consists in determining the perceptual space using the MDS technique. Then, in a second step, the acoustical descriptors that are correlated with the positions of the sounds along the perceptual dimensions are determined. In a parallel third step, the sounds are verbally described through a descriptive analysis that involves a small number of trained listeners. This step provides a list of selected semantic descriptors—which will be used to define relevant semantic scales—and a verbal description of the auditory cues used by the participants to compare the sounds in order to guide the research of the objective descriptors correlated with the auditory dimensions obtained in the previous stage. In the last step, participants rate their preference (or annoyance) of the sounds. The degree of preference (or, inversely, annoyance) associated with each sound is related to a function of the significant objective descriptors on the one hand, and the semantic descriptors on the other. The advantage of this global approach is that it does not limit the exploration and characterization of the components of sound quality to acoustical and semantic descriptors that are already known. It provides a method for finding new objective

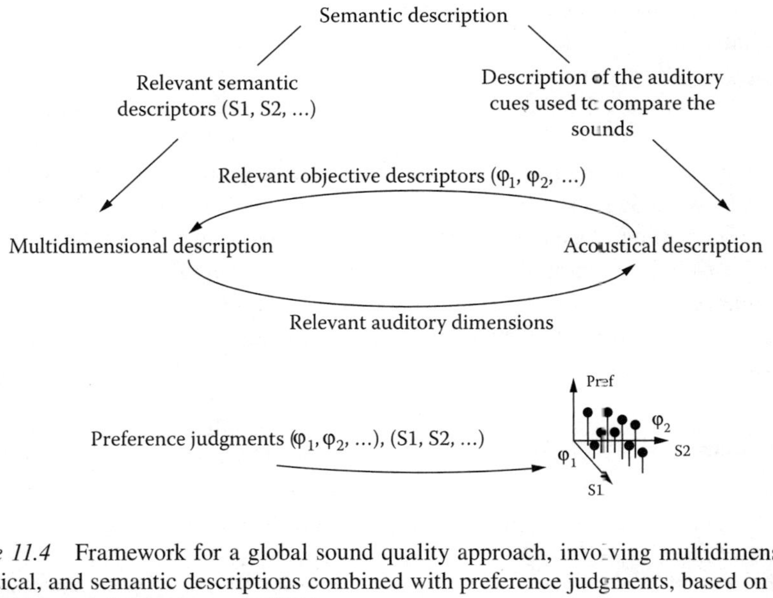


*Figure 11.4* Framework for a global sound quality approach, involving multidimensional, acoustical, and semantic descriptions combined with preference judgments, based on Susini et al. (2001) and Siekiersky et al. (2001).

and semantic descriptors that are perceptually relevant for describing and evaluating a sound object in the design process.

## 11.4 Perspectives: Sounds in continuous interactions

The methods reported in this chapter all address the measurement of quantities representative of what a human listener perceives. The evaluation of the perceived *sound quality* of industrial objects is a very important domain in which these methods are applied. Traditionally, the paradigm of sound quality evaluation considers a listener passively receiving information from the sounds of the product. Such evaluations would, for instance, study the acoustical properties of a car engine roar that a user prefers (aesthetics) and that are representative of a sports car (functionality).

New technologies for sensing and embedded computation, however, have made it possible for designers to consider sonic augmentations of a much wider array of everyday objects that incorporate electronic sensing and computational capabilities. Where continuous auditory feedback is concerned, the sound is no longer produced in a static or isolated way, but is rather coupled to human action in real time. This new domain of applications is called *sonic interaction design*.

From the standpoint of perception, the level of dynamical interactivity embodied by such artifacts is very different from the situation of passive listening in which most of the methods reported are carried out. In sonic interactions, participants are not listening to sequences of static sounds selected by an experimenter, but instead dynamically explore the sounds of an interactive object. This context may be thought to be more closely allied with enactive views of perception (e.g., Bruner, 1966) than with some of the more traditional approaches found in experimental auditory psychology.

The study of sonic interaction entails an understanding of perceptual–motor behavior, because these processes underlie any form of human interaction. New methods may therefore be required. Such methods experimentally study how users perform when required to do a task involving sonic interaction. An interesting example is provided in work by Rath (Rath & Rocchesso, 2005; Rath, 2006, 2007; Rath & Schleicher, 2008). They describe the Ballancer, a tangible interface consisting of a wooden plank that may be tilted by its user in order to drive a virtual ball rolling along the plank. The authors used this interface to study participants' abilities to use this auditory feedback in a task involving guiding the ball to a target region along the length of the plank, depending on the kind of sound used. Lemaitre et al. (2009) used another tangible interface (the Spinotron) implementing the metaphor of a child's spinning top to study how continuous sonic interactions guide the user in making a precise gesture.

## References

Aldrich, K. M., Hellier, E. J., & Edworthy, J. (2009), What determines auditory similarity? The effect of stimulus group and methodology, *Quarterly Journal of Experimental Psychology, 62*(1), 63–83.

Bisping, R. (1997). Car interior sound quality: Experimental analysis by synthesis, *Acta Acustica United with Acustica, 83,* 813–818.

Björk, E. A. (1985). The perceived quality of natural sounds, *Acustica, 57,* 185–188.

Bonebright, T. L. (1996). *Vocal affect expression: A comparison of multidimensional scaling solutions for paired comparisons and computer sorting tasks using perceptual and acoustic measures*, Doctoral dissertation, University of Nebraska.

Bonebright, T. L. (2001). Perceptual structure of everyday sounds: A multidimensional scaling approach. In *ICAD*, Helsinki, Finland.

Brunner, J. (1966). *Toward a theory of instruction*. Cambridge, MA: Harvard University Press.

Chouard, N., & Hempel, T. (1999). A semantic differential design especially developed for the evaluation of interior car sounds. In *Joint Meeting: ASA/EAA/DEGA* (*JASA* (105), Berlin), p. 1280.

Daniel, P., & Weber, R. (1997). Psychoacoustical roughness: Implementation of an optimized model," *Acta Acustica United with Acustica, 83*, 113–123.

Ellermeier, W., Mader, M., & Daniel, P. (2004). Scaling the unpleasantness of sounds according to the BTL model: Ratio-scale representation and psychoacoustical analysis, *Acta Acustica United with Acustica, 90,* 101–107.

Fastl, H. (1989). Average loudness of road traffic noise. In *InterNoise 89*, Newport Beach, CA.

Fastl, H. (1991). Evaluation and measurement of perceived average loudness. In A. Schick, J. Hellbrück, and R. Weber (Eds.), *Fifth Oldenburg Symposium on Psychological Acoustics* (BIS, Oldenburg), 205–216.

Fastl, H. (1997). The psychoacoustics of sound-quality evaluation, *Acta Acustica United with Acustica, 83,* 754–764.

Faure, A. (2010). Des sons aux mots, comment parle-t-on du timbre musical? Editions Edilivre—APARIS, Paris.

Fechner, G. T. (1966). *Elements of psychophysics*. New York: Holt, Rinehart and Winston (Original 1860).

Fletcher, H. (1940). Auditory patterns, *Review of Modern Physics*, *12*, 47–65.

Gaver, W. W. (1993a). What do we hear in the world? An ecological approach to auditory event perception. *Ecological Psychology*, *5,* 1–29.

Gaver, W. W. (1993b). How do we hear in the world? Explorations in ecological acoustics. *Ecological Psychology*, *5,* 285–313.

Glasberg, B. R., & Moore, B. C. J. (2002). A model of loudness applicable to time-varying sounds, *Journal of Audio Engineering Society, 50,* 331–342.

Goldstone, R. L., & Kersten, A. (2003). Concepts and categorization. In A. F. Healy & R. W. Proctor (Eds.), *Comprehensive handbook of psychology, Vol. 4: Experimental psychology*, chapter 22, pp. 599–621. New York: Wiley.

Grey, J. M. (1977). Multidimensional perceptual scaling of musical timbres, *Journal of the Acoustical Society of America, 61*, 1270–1277.

Gros, L., & Chateau, N. (2001). Instantaneous and overall judgments for time-varying speech quality: Assessments and relationships, *Acta Acustica United with Acustica, 87,* 367–377.

Guastavino, C. (2007). Catagorisation of environmental sounds, *Canadian Journal of Experimental Psychology, 61,* 54–63.

Guski, R. (1997). Psychophysical methods for evaluating sound quality and assessing acoustic information, *Acta Acustica United with Acustica, 83,* 765–774.

Guyot, F. (1996). Etude de la perception sonore en termes de reconnaissance et d'appréciation qualitative: Une approche par la catégorisation. Doctoral dissertation, Université du Maine.

Guyot, F., Castellengo, M., & Fabre, B. (1997). Etude de la catégorisation d'un corpus de bruits domestiques. In D. Dubois (Ed.), *Catégorisation et cognition,* Paris: Kimé.

Hansen, M., & Kollmeier, B. (1999). Continuous assessment of time-varying speech quality. *Journal of the Acoustical Society of America 106,* 2888–2899.

Hartmann, W. H. (1997). *Signals, sound, and sensation.* New York: AIP Press.

Hedberg, D., & Jansson, C. (1998). *Continuous rating of sound quality.* Stockholm: Karolinska Institutet.

Ih, J.-G., Lim D.-H., Jeong H., & Shin, S.-H. (2002) Investigation on the correlation between sound quality and spectral composition vacuum cleaner sound by using the orthogonal array. In *Sound Quality Symposium*, Dearborn, MI.

Jeon, J. Y. (2006). Sound radiation and sound quality characteristics of refrigerator noise in real living environments, *Applied Acoustics, 68,* 1118–1134.

Junker, F., Susini, P., & Cellard, P. (2001). Sensory evaluation of air-conditioning noise: Comparative analysis of two methods. In *ICA,* Rome, Italy, p. 342.

Kendall, R. A., & Carterette, E. C. (1992). Verbal attributes of simultaneous wind instrument timbres. I. von Bismarck's adjectives. *Music Perception, 4,* 185–214.

Komatsu, L. K. (1992). Recent views of conceptual structure. *Psychological Bulletin, 112*(3), 500–526.

Krumhansl, C. L. (1989). Why is musical timbre so hard to understand? In S. Nielsen, and O. Olsson (Eds.), *Structure and perception of electrostatic sound and music* (pp. 43–53). Amsterdam: Elsevier.

Kruskal, J. B., & Wish, M. (1978). *Multidimensional scaling.* Beverly Hills, CA: Sage.

Kuwano, S., & Namba, S. (1978). On the loudness of road traffic noise of longer duration (20 min) in relation to instantaneous judgment. In *ASA & ASJ* joint meeting. *(Journal of the Acoustical Society of America),* Berlin, *64,* 127–128.

Kuwano, S., & Namba, S. (1985). Continuous judgement of level-fluctuating sounds and the relationship between overall loudness and instantaneous loudness. *Psychology Research, 47,* 27–37.

Kuwano, S., & Namba, S. (1990). Continuous judgement of loudness and annoyance. In F. Müller (Ed.), *Fechner Day, Proceedings of the 6th Annual Meeting of the International Society for Psychophysics*, Würzburg, Germany, pp. 129–134.

Kuwano, S., & Namba, S. (2001). Dimensions of sound quality and their measurement. In *ICA,* Rome, Italy, p. 56.

Kyncl, L., & Jiricek, O. (2001). Psychoacoustic product sound quality evaluation. In *ICA,* Rome, Italy, p. 90.

Lamalle, C., Martinez, W., Fleury, S., Salem, A., Fracchiolla, B., Kuncova, A., & Maisondieu, A. (2003). *LEXICO 3, Outils de statistique textuelle—Manuel d'utilisation*, SYLED-CLA2T (Paris 3).

Legendre, P., & Legendre, L. (1998). *Numerical ecology.* Amsterdam: Elsevier.

Lemaitre, G., Houix, O., Misdariis, M., & Susini, P. (2010). Listener expertise and sound identification influence the categorization of environmental sounds, *Journal of Experimental Psychology: Applied, 16,* 16–32.

Lemaitre, G., Houix, O., Visell, Y., Franinovic, K., Misdariis, N., & Susini, P. (2009) Toward the design and evaluation of continuous sound in tangible interfaces: The spinotron. *International Journal of Human Computer Studies*, *67*, 976–993.

Lemaitre, G., Susini, P., Winsberg, S., McAdams, S., & Leteinturier, B. (2007). The sound quality of car horns: A psychoacoustical study of timbre, *Acta Acustica United with Acustica, 93,* 457–468.

Madsen, C. K. (1996). Empirical investigation of the "aesthetic response" to music: Musicians and nonmusicians. In *4th International Conference on Music Perception and Cognition,* Montreal, Canada, pp. 103–110.

Maffiolo, V., Dubois, D., David, S., Castellengo, M., & Polack, J. D. (1998). Loudness and pleasantness in structuration of urban soundscapes. In *InterNoise,* Christchurch, New Zealand.

McAdams, S., & Bigand, E. (Eds.). (1993). *Thinking in sound—The cognitive psychology of human audition,* Oxford: University Press.

McAdams, S., Giordano, B., Susini, P., Peeters, G., & Rioux, V. (2006). A meta-analysis of acoustic correlates of timbre dimensions. In *ASA,* Hawaii.

McAdams, S., Vines, B. W., Vieillard, S., Smith, B., & Reynolds, S. (2004). Influences of large-scale form on continuous ratings in response to a contemporary piece in a live concert setting. *Music Perception, 22,* 297–350.

McAdams, S., Winsberg, S., Donnadieu, S., Soete, G. D., & Krimphoff, J. (1995). Perceptual scaling of synthesized musical timbres: Common dimensions, specificities, and latent subject classes. *Psychological Research, 58,* 177–192.

Meunier, S., Boullet, I., & Rabau, G. (2001). Loudness of impulsive environmental sounds. In *ICA,* Rome, Italy, p. 91.

Misdariis, N., Minard, A., Susini, P., Lemaitre, G., McAdams, S., & Parizet, E., (2010). Environmental sound perception: Metadescription and modeling based on independent primary studies. *Journal on Audio, Speech, and Music Processing.* doi:10.1155/2010/362013.

Moore, B. C. J. (2003). *An introduction to the psychology of hearing* (5th ed.). New York: Academic Press.

Moore, B. C. J., & Glasberg, B. R. (1983). Suggested formulae for calculating auditory-filter bandwidths and excitation patterns. *Journal of the Acoustical Society of America, 74 (3),* 750–753.

Moore, B. C. J., & Glasberg, B. R. (1990). Derivation of auditory filter shapes from notched-noise data. *Hearing Research, 47,* 103–138.

Moore, B. C. J., & Glasberg, B. R. (1996). A revision of Zwicker's loudness model. *Acta Acustica United with Acustica, 82,* 335–345.

Moore, B. C. J., Glasberg, B. R., & Baer, T. (1997). A model for the prediction of thresholds, loudness and partial loudness. *Journal of the Audio Engineering Society, 45,* 224–240.

Osgood, C. E. (1952). The nature and measurement of meaning. *Psychological Bulletin, 49,* 197–237.

Parizet, E. (1999). Comparison of two semantic-differential test methods. In *EAA & ASA joint meeting. Journal of the Acoustical Society of America,* Berlin, p. 1189.

Parizet, E., Guyader, E., & Nosulenko, V. (2006). Analysis of car door closing sound quality. *Applied Acoustics, 69,* 12–22.

Parizet, E., Hamzaoui, N., and Sabatié, G. (2005). Comparison of some listening test methods: A case study. *Acta Acustica United with Acustica, 91,* 356–364.

Parizet, E., Hamzaoui, N., Segaud, L., & Koch J.-R. (2003). Continuous evaluation of noise discomfort in a bus. *Acta Acustica United with Acustica, 89,* 900–907.

Parizet, E., & Nosulenko, V. N. (1999). Multi-dimensional listening test: Selection of sound descriptors and design of the experiment. *Noise Control Engineering Journal, 47,* 1–6.

Patterson, R. D., & Holdsworth, J. (1991). A functional model of neural activity patterns and auditory images. *Advances in speech, hearing and language processing, Vol. 3.* London: JAI Press.

Peters, R. W. (1960). *Research on psychological parameters of sound,* (pp. 60–249). Hattiesburg: Mississippi Southern College.

Plomp, R. (1970). Timbre as a multidimensional attribute of complex tones. In R. Plomp & G. P. Smoorenburg (Eds.), *Frequency anaysis and periodicity detection in hearing* (pp. 397–414). Leiden: A. W. Sijthoff.

Pratt, R. L., & Doak, P. E. (1976). A subjective rating scale for timbre. *Journal of Sound and Vibration, 45,* 317–328.

Rath, M. (2006). On the relevance of auditory feedback for subjective and objective quality of control in a balancing task. In *Proceedings of the 2nd ISCA/DEGA Tutorial and Research Workshop on Perceptual Quality of Systems*, Berlin, pp. 85–88.

Rath, M. (2007). Auditory velocity information in a balancing task. In *ICAD*, Montréal, Canada, pp. 372–379.

Rath, M., & Rocchesso, D. (2005). Continuous sonic feedback from a rolling ball. *IEEE MultiMedia, 12*, 60–69.

Rath, M., & Schleicher, D. R. (2008). On the relevance of auditory feedback for quality of control in a balancing task. *Acta Acustica United with Acustica, 94*, 12–20.

Robinson, D. W., & Dadson, R. S. (1956). A re-determination of the equal-loudness relations for pure tones. *British Journal of Applied Physics, 7,* 166–181.

Rosch, E. (1978). Principles of categorisation. In E. Rosch and B. B. Lloyd (Eds.), *Cognition and categorization,* (pp. 27–47). Hillsdale, NJ: Lawrence Erlbaum Associates.

Rosch, E., Mervis, C. B., Gray, W. D, Johnson, D. M., & Boyes-Braem, P. (1976). Basic objects in natural categories. *Cognitive Psychology, 8*, 382–443.

Scavone, G. P., Lakatos, S., & Harbke, C. R. (2002). The sonic mapper: An interactive program for obtaining similarity ratings with auditory stimuli. In *ICAD,* Kyoto.

Schafer, R. M. (1977). *The tuning of the world.* New York: Random House.

Schubert, E. (1996). Continuous response to music using the two dimensional emotion space. In *ICMPC,* Montreal, Canada, pp. 263–268.

Schulte-Fortkamp, B., & Dubois, D. (2006). Recent advances in soundscape research. *Acta Acustica United with Acustica, 92*(6), 5–6.

Siekierski, E., Derquenne, C., & Martin, N. (2001). Sensory evaluation of air-conditioning noise: Sensory profiles and hedonic tests. In *ICA,* Rome, Italy, 326.

Sloboda, J. A., & Lehmann, A. C. (2001). Tracking performance correlates of changes in perceived intensity of emotion during different interpretations of a Chopin piano prelude. *Music Perception, 19,* 87–120.

Sloutsky, V. M. (2003) The role of similarity in the development of categorization. *Trends in Cognitive Science, 7,* 246–251.

Solomon, L. N. (1958), Semantic approach to the perception of complex sounds. *Journal of the Acoustical Society of America, 30*(5), 421–425.

Stepánek, J. (2006). Musical sound timbre: Verbal description and dimensions. In *DAFx-06,* Montréal.

Stevens, J. C., & Tulving, E. (1957). Estimations of loudness by a group of untrained observers, *American Journal of Psychology, 70,* 600–605.

Stevens, S. S. (1959). Cross-modality validations of subjective scales for loudness, vibrations, and electric shock. *Journal of Experimental Psychology, 57,* 201–209.

Susini, P., Gaudibert, P., Deruty, E., & Dandrel, L. (2003). Perceptive study and recommendation for sonification categories. In *ICAD*, Boston.

Susini, P., Houix, O., Misdariis, N., Smith, B., & Langlois, S. (2009.) Instruction's effect on semantic scale ratings of interior car sounds. *Applied Acoustics, 70*(3), 389–403.

Susini, P., & Maffiolo, V. (1999). Loudness evaluation of urban soundscapes by a cross-modal matching method. In *EAA & ASA joint meeting, Journal of the Acoustical Society of America*, Berlin, p. 943.

Susini, P., & McAdams, S. (1998). Global and continuous judgements of sounds with time-varying intensity: Cross-modal matching with a proprioceptive input device. In *ICA & ASA joint meeting*, *Journal of the Acoustical Society of America,* Seattle, p. 2812.

Susini, P., & McAdams, S. (2008). Loudness asymmetry ratings between accelerating and decelerating car sounds, in *Acoustics'08, ASA-EAA Joint Conference,* Paris.

Susini, P., McAdams, S., & Smith, B. (2002). Global and continuous loudness estimation of time-varying levels. *Acta Acustica United with Acustica, 88,* 536–548.

Susini, P., McAdams, S., & Smith, B. (2007). Loudness asymmetries for tones with increasing and decreasing levels using continuous and global ratings. *Acta Acustica United with Acustica, 93,* 623–631.

Susini, P., McAdams, S., and Winsberg, S. (1997). Perceptual characterisation of vehicle noises. In *EEA Symposium: Psychoacoustic, in industry and universities,* Eindhoven, The Netherlands.

Susini, P., McAdams, S., Winsberg, S., Perry, I., Vieillard, S., & Rodet, X. (2004). Characterizing the sound quality of air-conditioning noise. *Applied Acoustics, 65*(8), 763–790.

Susini, P., Misdariis, N., McAdams, S., & Winsberg, S. (1998). Caractérisation perceptive de bruits. *Acoustique et Techniques, 13,* 11–15.

Susini, P., Perry, I., Winsberg, S., Vieillard, S., McAdams, S., & Winsberg, S. (2001). Sensory evaluation of air-conditioning noise: Sound design and psychoacoutic evaluation. In *ICA,* Rome, Italy, p. 342.

Tardieu, J., Susini, P., Poisson, F., Lazareff, P., & McAdams, S. (2008). Perceptual study of soundscapes in train stations, *Applied Acoustics, 69,* 1224–1239.

Vanderveer, N. J. (1979) *Ecological acoustics: Human perception of environmental sounds.* Unpublished doctoral dissertation, Cornell University, Ithaca, NY.

Vogel, C. (1999). *Etude sémiotique et acoustique de l'identification des signaux sonores d'avertissement en contexte urbain.* Doctoral dissertation, Université Paris 6.

von Bismarck, G. (1974). Timbre of steady sounds: A factorial investigation of its verbal attributes, *Acustica, 30,* 146–158.

Vos, J. (1998). The loudness of impulse and road-traffic sounds in the presence of masking background noise, *Acta Acustica United with Acustica, 84,* 1119–1130.

Wedin, L., & Goude, G. (1972). Dimension analysis of the perception of timbres. *Scandinavian Journal of Psychology, 13,* 228–240.

Weber, R. (1991). The continuous loudness judgement of temporally variable sounds with an "analog" category procedure. In A. Schick, J. Hellbrück and R. Weber (Eds.), *Fifth Oldenburg Symposium on Psychological Acoustics,* (pp. 267–294) Oldenburg: BIS.

Winsberg, S., & Carroll, D. (1989). A quasi non-metric method for multidimal scaling via an extended Euclidian model. *Psychometrika, 54,* 217–229.

Zeitler, A., & Hellbrück, J. (2001). Semantic attributes of environmental sounds and their correlations with psychoacoustic magnitude. In *ICA,* Rome, Italy, p. 114.

Zwicker, E. (1961). Subdivision of the audible frequency range into critical bands, *Journal of the Acoustical Society of America, 33,* 248.

Zwicker, E. (1984). BASIC-Program for calculating the loudness of sounds from their 1/3-oct band spectra according to ISO 532-B, *Acustica, 55,* 63–67.

Zwicker, E., & Fastl, H. (1972). On the development of the critical band, *Journal of the Acoustical Society of America, 52,* 699–702.

Zwicker, E., & Fastl, H. (1999). *Psychoacoustics: Facts and models* (2nd ed.). Heidelberg: Spinger-Verlag.

Zwicker, R., and Terhardt, E. (1980). Analytical expressions for critical band rate and critical bandwidth as a function of frequency, *Journal of the Acoustical Society of America, 68,* 1523–1525.

# 12 Nociception and pain in thermal skin sensitivity

*Dieter Kleinböhl,[1] Rupert Hölzl,[1] and Jörg Trojan[2]*

[1]Otto–Selz-Institute for Applied Psychology
University of Mannheim
Mannheim, Germany

[2]Central Institute of Mental Health
Department of Cognitive and Clinical Neuroscience
Mannheim, Germany

## 12.1 Introduction

Body perception, or *interoception*, is made up of a multitude of sensory systems, coarsely sorted by functional aspects into *proprioception*, *visceroception*, and *nociception* (Sherrington, 1906). Proprioception, in its modern interpretation, includes the haptic-somatic sensitivity, with tactile and thermal submodalities of the skin senses, as well as the sensitivity for movement and position of the joints and the limbs and for body posture. Visceroception relates to the perception of signals from the intestines, originating from receptors in the hollow organs, which are sensitive for pressure and distension (Hölzl, Erasmus, & Möltner, 1996). *Nociception*, finally, is the processing of intense, noxious stimuli that may originate from all parts of the body, thus encompassing aspects of somatic-haptic sensitivity and visceroception.

A modern view of interoceptive sensitivity is given by Craig (2003a, 2002), who postulates from neurophysiologic criteria the existence of a phylogenetic ancient "homeostatic" system of small nerve fibers, including nociception, temperature sensitivity, and other interoceptive receptor systems maintaining bodily functions. This neurophysiologic coherent system of "homoeostatic afferents" is related to limbic brain areas involved in affective processing (e.g., anterior cingulate cortex, insula), and with brain areas modulating affect (e.g., amygdala, orbitofrontal cortex). The anterior insula is assumed to be central for the integration of body perception in the sense of an "interoceptive cortex" (Craig, 2003b). This brain area mediates homeostatic emotions, where pleasant bodily feelings indicate homeostasis and unpleasant feelings indicate a disturbance of homeostasis. In this view of a homeostatic small fiber system, nociceptive and thermoceptive sensitivity play a central role, being at the core of body perception itself. Another central feature of nociception is its plasticity: nociception includes a multitude of dynamic mechanisms on peripheral and central levels of processing that are capable of changing nociceptive transmission and pain perception. This feature is not always adaptive for the organism, and maladaption may lead to hyperalgesia and chronic pain under conditions not yet fully understood.

This chapter focuses on nociception, thermoception, and the pain experience, being a central component of body perception. It is organized in three parts: the first part sketches the neurophysiology of nociception and the physical conditions activating nociception. The second part focuses on mechanisms of dynamic change over time in nociception and pain. Dynamic change in nociception and pain is exemplified by three mechanisms on different levels of processing: neuronal plasticity on a cellular level, automatic processes in perception, leading to sensitization and habituation, and associative learning of altered pain perception. The third part presents three psychophysical procedures, based on experimental contact heat pain stimulation, for the assessment of the three selected mechanisms of dynamic change in nociception and pain.

## 12.2 Neurophysiology of nociception

The neuronal structures involved in the processing of nociceptive information are explained here. Together with the description of the specific physical stimuli eliciting nociception, this is part of the objective physiology of the senses. The neurophysiology of nociception is described for three levels of the nervous system which are organized in ascending order. Each level depends on the lower one and provides more complex capabilities of adaptive processing: first, peripheral nociception deals with the transmission from the receptor via afferent nerve fibers to the first central neuron in the spinal cord; second, spinal nociception relates to the neurons and nervous tracts within the spinal cord ascending to the brain stem and the brain; and third, the structures of the brain that are involved in pain processing. The relationship of the neurophysiological aspects of nociception with qualities of pain perception is also presented.

### *12.2.1 Peripheral nociception*

The term *nociception* was introduced to differentiate the "neural processes of encoding and processing noxious stimuli" from "the perception of pain" (Loeser & Treede, 2008). Peripheral nociception comprises the neuronal transmission from the peripheral receptor to the presynaptic endings of the peripheral nerve fiber on the first central neuron in the spinal cord.

Noxious events are detected and coded in the nervous system by a specific type of receptor, the *nociceptor*. Nociceptors are described as sensitive nerve endings whose morphology is not yet completely clarified. Nociceptors are found mainly in the skin, in the entire musculature of the body, and in the joints, as well as in internal organs and the intestines. Specific stimuli for nociceptors are strong thermal, mechanical, or chemical stimuli that might cause damage to the organism (Torebjörk, 1994). The majority of nociceptors are simultaneously responsive to mechanical, thermal, and chemical stimuli. For their multisensitivity these nociceptors are termed *polymodal nociceptors*. To a much lesser degree, there are also unimodal mechano- or thermosensitive nociceptors (Heppelmann, Messlinger, Schaible, & Schmidt, 1991; Zimmermann & Handwerker, 1984).

Activation of nociceptors is not solely due to exogenous stimulation. Noxious events might damage tissue and in this line trigger inflammation, with chemical mediators acting as algetic substances in the surrounding tissue (e.g., histamine, prostaglandine, bradykinin, and serotonin). These proinflammatory and algetic substances are synthesized in the organism and can be considered as endogenous noxious events, which are capable of triggering action potentials in nociceptive fibers. This might occur with, but also without additional exogenous noxious stimulation (Heppelmann et al., 1991; Mense, Hoheisel, Kaske, and Reinert, 1997).

The most common class of nociceptors consists of the polymodal C-fiber nociceptors sensible for mechanical and thermal stimuli (C-fiber mechano-heat nociceptors, CMHs; Raja, Meyer, & Campbell, 1990). The threshold of their neuronal response to contact heat stimulation, as measured by microneurography, lies in a wide physical temperature range of 38–50°C. This means that these nociceptors might be active at nonpainful temperatures normally not even perceived as hot. Therefore it requires considerable spatial and temporal summation of afferent influx for perception of thermal pain to occur (Nielsen & Arendt-Nielsen, 1998).

The second common class of nociceptive fibers is among the Aδ-fibers, covering the high intensity range of noxious temperatures. The polymodal Aδ-fiber nociceptors (A-fiber mechano-heat nociceptors, AMHs) will respond only above temperatures of 48°C. These fibers are further subdivided in two classes of AMH fibers, according to their temporal response properties: Type I AMH fibers will characteristically respond (within 600 ms) and adapt slowly to an intensive nociceptive stimulus. In type I AMHs, an increased sensitivity is observed after repeated noxious stimulation, which mediates at least in part the hyperalgesia and sensitization observed after such stimulus series (Meyer & Campbell, 1981; Raja et al., 1990). Type II AMHs, on the contrary, respond fast (<200 ms) and adapt quickly (Raja et al., 1990), thus mediating the characteristic pinpricking or stinging quality of “first pain.”

The specific nociceptive fibers innervating nociceptors belong to the group of so-called *small nerve fibers*, constituting the homeostatic small fiber system postulated by Craig (2003a). Small nerve fibers comprise the fast conducting myelinated Aδ-fibers and slow conducting unmyelinated C-fibers (Figure 12.1). In humans, 50% of all Aδ-fibers are estimated to be nociceptive, whereas for C-fibers, a much higher proportion of 90% is assumed to be nociceptive.

Aside from signaling physiological information for maintaining homeostasis (e.g., blood pressure, $O_2$ saturation), small fibers also innervate nonnoxious warm- and cold receptors in the skin: warm receptors respond via afferent C-fibers, and cold receptors via afferent Aδ-fibers (Darian-Smith, 1984). Small fibers therefore mediate the perception of a wide temperature range one might experience on the skin, ranging from noxious cold over nonnoxious cold to warmth, heat, painful heat, and noxious heat.

There is considerable overlap of the physical response properties of the contributing receptors (Figure 12.1) and also highly integrative processing of the afferent activation pattern in the different receptor/fiber systems subserving temperature and pain perception. The basic properties of the small fiber subsystems are therefore

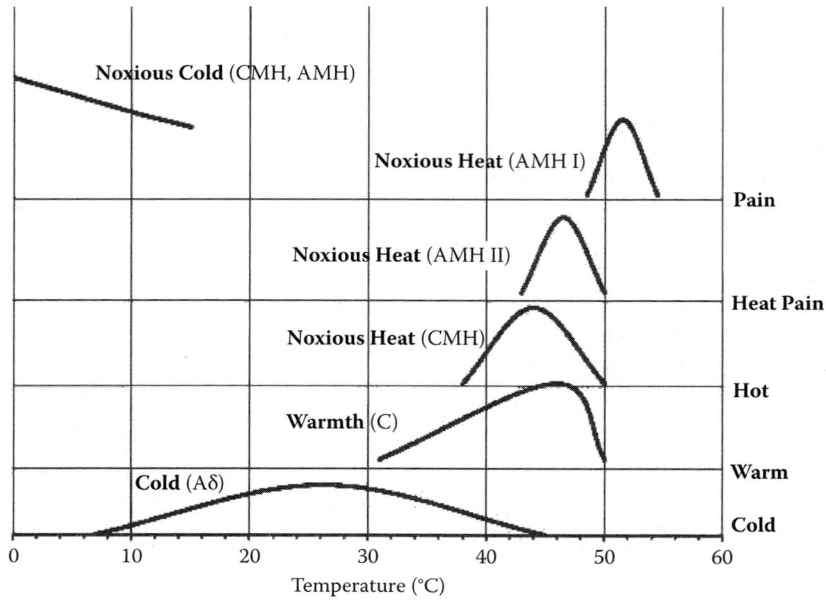


*Figure 12.1* Response properties of thermo-nociceptive small fiber receptors over temperature. Single curves indicate cumulated receptor activity dependent on temperature. Sensitivity curves are stacked in ascending order corresponding to the perceptual qualities on the right ordinate, indicating warm, hot, or painful sensations. There is considerable overlap of sensitivity ranges for the different receptor classes, especially in the noxious temperature range, starting approximately around 45°C (Data sources: Kleinböhl, 1996; Treede et al., 1998; Raja et al., 1990).

classified by the sensory modality and by the intensity range to which they respond. Another criterion for classification is the conduction velocity of the afferent fiber and its response properties (Raja et al., 1990; Table 12.1).

### *12.2.2 Spinal nociception*

The peripheral nociceptive nerve fibers enter the spinal cord via the dorsal root ganglion and the dorsal horn of the spinal cord, where they have presynaptic endings on central transmission neurons. Within the spinal cord, 10 histologically different cell layers (laminae) are described which differ, among other characteristics, by the proportion of afferent influx (Rexed, 1952). The nociceptive neurons of the dorsal horn lie in the superficial layers of the spinal cord, mainly in layers I and II, and also partially in the deep lamina V of the spinal cord (Cervero, 1986; Millan, 1999). The dorsal horn transmission neurons are subdivided in classes, according to their sensory properties (Mendell, 1966; Cervero, 1986):

*Class 1 of spinal transmission neurons* receives input from low-threshold mechanoceptive neurons, but shows no nociceptive responses.

*Table 12.1* Properties of peripheral nociceptive nerve fibers

| *Property* | *AMH[1]-type I* | *AMH[1]-type II* | *CMH[2]* |
|---|---|---|---|
| Conduction velocity [m/s] | 15.2 ± 9.9 | 31.1 ± 1.5 | 0.8 ± 0.1 |
| Thermal threshold [°C] | > 49 | 43 | 43.6 ± 0.6 |
| Mechanical threshold [bar] | 3.5 ± 0.3 | 1.7 | 6.0 ± 0.6 |
| Rise-time receptor [ms] | Slow: > 600 | Fast: < 200 | > 50 |
| Skin type | Hairy, glabrous | Hairy only | Hairy, glabrous |
| Perceptual qualities | Primary hyperalgesia | First pain | Second pain |

*Note:* Overview compiled by Kleinböhl (1996), based on a table from Raja et al. (1990).

[1] AMH: A-fiber-mechano-heat, a nerve fiber with a myelin sheath, allowing for fast-action potential conduction velocities.

[2] CMH: C-fiber-mechano-heat, an unmyelinated nerve fiber, and therefore allowing only for slow conduction velocities.

*Class 2 of spinal transmission neurons* receives convergent afferent influx from nociceptors and from low-threshold mechanoreceptors. These multireceptive neurons, also termed "low threshold" or "wide dynamic range" (WDR), may increase their sensitivity under certain stimulus conditions and, therefore, have been discussed as candidate mediators for hyperalgesia and chronic pain. Class 2 neurons are found in laminae II and V, the afferent influx to lamina II (also termed the "substantia gelatinosa") originating particularly from C-fibers of the skin (Cervero, 1986).

*Class 3 spinal transmission* neurons are innervated exclusively from high-threshold nociceptors, either purely mechanosensitive (class 3a) or mechano- and thermosensitive (class 3b). These neurons transfer information about intense noxious stimuli only. Therefore, they are also called "nociceptive specific" (NS) neurons. They are mostly, but not exclusively, located in lamina I and receive predominantly afferent influx from Aδ-fibers (Hylden, Hayashi, Bennett, & Dubner, 1985).

Nociceptive information is already processed on the level of the spinal cord, allowing an immediate response of the organism to noxious stimuli. Response channels for the release of sympathetic and nocifensive motor reflexes are activated via interneurons. The latter allow a quick motor response such as pulling away of the hand from a hot plate. Vegetative responses to noxious stimuli such as acceleration of breathing and heartbeat or an increase in blood pressure are modulated by a small part of the ascending nociceptive fibers, joining the medulla oblongata (Droste, 1988). Finally, vigilance and awareness are modulated by nociceptive input via the ascending reticular activating system (ARAS) in the formatio reticularis of the brain stem (Zimmermann, 1993).

### *12.2.2.1 Ascending nociceptive pathways*

The transmission of nociceptive information from the spinal cord to the brain is performed by two functionally and anatomically distinct pathways (lat. "tractus"), which are termed medial and lateral system according to their target nuclei in the thalamus. In the evolutionary older medial system (tractus palaeospinothalamicus), mainly nerve tracts from the formatio reticularis, but also from tractus spinothalamicus and tractus trigeminothalamicus, go to the medial nuclei of the thalamus (nuclei centralis lateralis, centralis medialis, and parafascicularis). These nuclei are assumed to be connected with limbic areas of the brain and with the hypothalamus. In the evolutionarily younger lateral system (tractus neo-spinothalamicus) the trajectories of the tractus spinothalamicus and tractus trigeminothalamicus join in the lateral somatosensory nuclei of the thalamus (ventro-basal-nucleus) and then connect with the somatosensory cortex in the postcentral gyrus (e.g., Apkarian, 1995).

#### *12.2.2.2 Descending inhibitory pathways*

An important mechanism of regulating the nociceptive input to the brain is mediated by a system of brain stem nuclei, exerting inhibition by neuronal fibers descending to the segments of the spinal cord. This "descending inhibition" is regulated by the nociceptive influx and is normally exerted by opiate-mediated inhibition of the transmission neurons in the spinal cord. The axons of these nociceptive dorsal horn cells connect via the anterolateral tract of the spinal cord (tractus anterolateralis) with the formatio reticularis in the brain stem (tractus spinoreticularis) and with the thalamus (tractus spinothalamicus). Collateral fibers from the anterolateral tract go to the periaquaeductal gray (PAG, substantia grisea) to initiate the inhibition. There are connections from the PAG to the locus coeruleus, another brain stem nucleus. It operates synergistically with the PAG in the opiodergic modulation of pain (Bodnar, Paul, & Pasternak, 1991). Nucleus raphe magnus (NRM) is the third brain stem area involved in pain inhibition (Basbaum, Marley, O'Keefe, & Clanton, 1977; Abbott, Melzack, & Leber, 1982). From this area, inhibitory fibers descend within the dorsolateral funiculus (DLF) to the nociceptive neurons in the dorsal horn of the spinal cord where they inhibit the afferent influx (Watkins & Mayer, 1982).

### ***12.2.3 Brain areas involved in nociception and pain***

In Craig's view of the homeostatic small fiber system, there is a specific area in the brain representing body perception—the insula cortex in the depth of the sylvian fissure—however, this is not an exclusive center of pain representation. Modern imaging methods such as magnetic resonance imaging or positron-emission-tomography have shown that there is no "pain center" in the brain, but a "neuromatrix" of functional brain areas subserving the various components of the pain experience (Derbyshire, 2000; Treede, Kenshalo, Gracely, & Jones, 1999).

The *primary somatosensory cortex* (area SI) is the part of the brain in the central area where most of the afferent information from the ventral posterior-lateral nuclei of the thalamus (VPL) reaches the cortex (Millan, 1999; Apkarian, 1995, 1996). This brain area is assumed to mediate the sensory-discriminative aspects of pain such as localization of a stimulus or estimating its magnitude. The *secondary somatosensory cortex* (area SII) receives parallel nociceptive input mainly from the medial nuclei of the thalamus (ventral posterior inferior, VPI; ventral medial posterior, VMPo) a smaller part from VPL. The SII area is supposed to be involved in pain-related attention and learning (Treede et al., 1999). The *insula cortex* is reciprocally connected with SII (therefore sometimes called area SIII), but receives also afferents from the posterior thalamic nuclei and projects to the amygdala and to the perirhinal cortex. Therefore the insula is supposed to be a higher-order integration area for somatosensation, which also modulates affective and motor pain responses (Derbyshire, Jones, Gyulai, Clark, Townsend, and Firestone, 1997).

The *anterior cingulate cortex (ACC)* influences vegetative functions and also psychomotoric und locomotoric drive (Treede et al., 1999; Treede, Apkarian, Bromm, Greenspan, & Lenz, 2000). The ACC includes an activation system which is located in the more posterior parts of the ACC and is supposed to be specific for pain. The anterior parts of the ACC mediate general activation and attention.

The *amygdala* is well known to be involved in affective-motivational processing of information in general and especially in mediating fear and aversive conditioning. The extended connectivity between the amygdala, ACC, insula, and prefrontal cortex provides the neurophysiological foundation for the integration of pain with fear, context information, and higher cognitive and motivational functions mediated by the prefrontal areas.

### *12.2.4 Nociception and perceptual qualities*

Some qualities of pain perception are dependent on specific properties of the nociceptive structures involved, such as the type of active nociceptor, the type of afferent fiber, and the organ system affected (Willis, 1988). The different nerve conduction velocities in nociceptive Aδ and C-fibers are assumed to determine two specific qualities of pain: *First pain* is a well-localized pricking pain quality which is due to activation of myelinated fast conducting (15–31 m/s) and fast adapting Aδ-fibers. *Second pain* is mediated by slow C-fibers (0.8 m/s), experienced as a slowly waxing and waning pain quality that has a pronounced burning component in skin areas, and a dull, throbbing quality in musculature, skeleton, or intestines (Table 12.1).

The physiological processes underlying the perception of pain have been further specified by comparative studies of humans and animals. In these studies, the subjective pain judgments in humans have been compared with the discharge frequencies of CMH-fibers, measured directly by small needle electrodes applied to the nerve fiber in animals. This technique is termed "microneurography." In this way, the subjective pain intensity has been shown to be connected with the CMH-fiber activity at comparable physical intensities. This finding is corroborated by selective blockade of AMH-fibers and CMH-fibers during thermal stimulation in humans: heat pain perception mainly depends on the activation of CMH-fibers, at least at stimulus intensities near the pain threshold (Raja et al., 1990). Furthermore, the perceived pain intensity and the discharge frequency in CMHs show a concurrent increase with stimulus intensity, showing that a coding of intensity is also performed in these fibers (Zimmermann & Handwerker, 1984; LaMotte & Campbell, 1978a, 1978b; Raja et al., 1990). These findings demonstrate that pain perception is functionally connected with response thresholds and response characteristics of C-fiber nociceptors (LaMotte & Campbell, 1978a, 1978b; van Hees & Gybels, 1981; Raja et al., 1990).

However, receptor excitation and subjective pain perception cannot be simply equated, and the deviations in this relationship are not yet fully clarified. For instance, a low-level excitation of CMH-fibers is not yet perceived as painful (van Hees & Gybels, 1981; Raja et al., 1990). Therefore, the nociceptive receptor threshold is not the same as the subjective pain threshold. Furthermore, the time course of CMH-fiber activation does not correspond to the perceived time course of pain in repetitive or tonic stimulation models. The discharge frequency of the CMHs decreases slowly during tonic contact heat; however, pain perception during the same time interval increases (LaMotte, Thalhammer, & Robinson, 1983) or remains constant (Meyer & Campbell, 1981). The same is valid for tonic mechanical stimulation (Raja et al., 1990). These inconsistencies between perceived pain and nociceptive activity require the assumption of neuronal mechanisms as temporal and spatial summation of afferent signals to explain the constituents of the pain experience (Raja et al., 1990; LaMotte et al., 1982).

## 12.3 Dynamic processes in nociceptive sensory networks

During the last two decades, important insight into the physiological and pathological processes of the nociceptive system has been gained. This has been achieved by diverse methods, ranging from single cell and nerve fiber recordings to functional neuroimaging. However, a complete picture of all the interwoven processes is still not in sight. Particularly, the connections between the microscopic processes on a cellular level and the macroscopic processes in medium and large-scale assemblies of neurons are widely unexamined, not to speak of an integration of psycho(physio) logical aspects. In the following, mechanisms mediating dynamic change in the nociceptive sensory networks are discussed under the heading of neuronal plasticity, and dynamic change in perception is discussed under the aspect of learning. These mechanisms demonstrate the far-reaching capabilities of the nociceptive system to reorganize itself, or in other words, to adapt continuously to altered general conditions. Normally, these processes of dynamic change are adaptive and have some benefit for the organism, for example, when a functional deficit caused by the impairment of one specific brain area is being compensated by cortical reorganization (Flor, 2003). But the various mechanisms of dynamic change may also lead to maladjustment and a dysfunctional state, as in chronic pain syndromes.

### *12.3.1 Neuronal mechanisms of dynamic change*

In peripheral and spinal nociception, certain stimulus configurations or activation patterns in the afferent nerve may cause short-lived and reversible changes and modulations, but also long-term and irreversible modifications of the neuronal transmission pathways (see figure inset in Table 12.2, representing the peripheral, spinal, and cerebral levels of the nociceptive pathways). The underlying neurobiological

*Table 12.2* Taxonomy of mechanisms mediating dynamic change in nociception and pain perception[a]

| | | *Activation* | *Modulation* | *Modification* |
|---|---|---|---|---|
| | Pain perception | Perceptual sensitization | Hyperalgesia[b] | Hyperalgesia[b] |
| | | | Allodynia[b] | Allodynia[b] |
| | | Habituation | | |
| 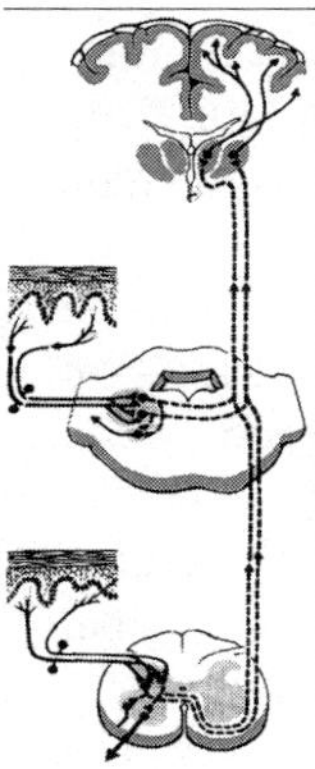 | Brain neuromatrix[c] | Automatic processes | Associative learning | Associative learning |
| | | | Cortical reorganization | Cortical reorganization |
| | | Descending inhibition | Descending inhibition | Descending inhibition |
| | Spinal nociception[c] | Wind-up in dorsal horn neurons | Central sensitization | Structural changes in spinal transmission |
| | | Facilitation | Long-term potentiation | |
| | | | Long-term depression | |
| | Peripheral nociception[c] | Autosensitization of nociceptors | Heterosensitization of nociceptors | Structural changes in nociceptors |
| | | Fatigue of nociceptors | Fatigue of nociceptors | |

[a] Extended version of a table based on Woolf & Salter (2000). Facilitative and inhibiting mechanisms, the latter given in shaded layout.

[b] A hypersensitivity to painful stimulation is called *hyperalgesia*, whereas a hypersensitvity to normally nonpainful stimuli is called *allodynia*.

[c] Three main levels of nociceptive pathways: peripheral cutaneous nociceptor fibers entering the dorsal horn of the spinal cord and ascending via the anterolateral tract to the thalamus in the brain. From there on, a neuromatrix of various brain areas receive nociceptive influx.

processes have been termed "neuronal plasticity," which can be classified into three categories, according to their time course and potential reversibility (Woolf & Salter, 2000; see columns in Table 12.2).

1. *Activation-dependent plasticity* refers to transient dynamic changes in nociceptive processing, being fully reversible within seconds or minutes. Such mechanisms include both facilitatory and inhibitory processes on all levels of nociception. In the periphery, the nociceptor excitability may increase (autosensitization) or decrease (fatigue) during repetitive stimulation of the same skin area. Skin damage by repetitive noxious stimuli or by burning may trigger inflammatory processes, increasing the sensitivity of the nociceptor (heterosensitization) by contact with the algetic substances

mediating inflammation (e.g., bradykinine, prostaglandine, and others). An ongoing afferent input from a peripheral nociceptor might also trigger sensitization in dorsal horn transmission neurons, which is well known from animal experiments as the so-called "wind-up" phenomenon (Mendell, 1966). Comparative studies in humans and animals have shown that wind-up is the neuronal correlate of the subjective short-term sensitization experienced under repetitive or tonic stimulation conditions (Price, Mao, Frenk, & Mayer, 1994; see also Section 12.2.2).

2. *Modulations* are termed dynamic changes in nociception lasting for minutes, hours, or even days, which may still be fully reversible. Again, there are facilitating and inhibiting processes at work. Long-term potentiation (LTP) is the strengthening of the synaptic connectivity between two neurons by applying a high-frequency stimulus pattern to one spinal neuron in animal experiments or by corresponding electrical stimulation of the skin in human experiments (Klein, Magerl, Hopf, Sandkühler, & Treede, 2004). By changing the stimulus properties to low-frequency stimulation, the conditions can be reversed: a long-term depression (LTD) inhibits synaptic connectivity, which might be of therapeutic value by modulating spinal transmission by transcutaneous electric nerve stimulation (TENS).
3. *Modification,* finally, includes non- or only slowly reversible changes in nociception, caused by altered gene regulation in the cell, which have a long-lasting influence on the excitability and connectivity of a neuron. These mechanisms are assumed to be central in establishing persistent pathological pain.

The neurophysiological processes underlying neuronal plasticity in nociception are well examined in animal models, usually comprising the same molecular processes as known from the neurobiology of memory formation in the brain. The *N*-methyl-D-aspartate (NMDA) receptor mechanism underlying the wind-up phenomenon, or the LTP, is a prominent example of these processes (e.g., Kandel, 2001). This origin of the plasticity-in-pain research has also led to the term "pain memories" for these mechanisms (Sandkühler, 2000; Kleinböhl, Baus, Hornberger, & Hölzl, 2005).

### *12.3.2 Psychological mechanisms of dynamic change*

In the taxonomy of learning mechanisms and related memory systems, the simplest mechanisms are the so-called *automatic processes*, represented in perception by habituation and perceptual sensitization (Milner, Squire, & Kandel, 1998).

#### *12.3.2.1 Automatic processes: Perceptual sensitization*

Sensitization in perception is defined as an increase of the subjective stimulus intensity during constant repetitive or continuous stimulation. In body perception, sensitization is a characteristic feature of the pain sensation (Greene & Hardy, 1962; LaMotte, 1979). In fact, sensitization seems so closely linked with the pain experience that attempts were made to use the occurrence of sensitization during tonic stimulation as an objective criterion for the pain threshold (Severin, Lehmann, & Strian, 1985). Perceptual sensitization is usually examined with repetitive phasic or continuous tonic stimulation with thermal, mechanical, or chemical stimulation of the skin or the musculature. In such stimulus models, a reversible short time sensitization in the time interval below one minute is prominent, which can be measured again after a short break (Kleinböhl, Hölzl, Möltner, Rommel, Weber, & Osswald, 1999; Kleinböhl, Baus, Hornberger, & Hölzl, R., 2005).

In accordance with its assumed neural cause this effect has also been termed *temporal summation*. The underlying neural mechanism has been identified in the above-mentioned wind-up phenomenon already known from animal experiments. There is an activation-dependent increase of sensitivity of class 2 or wide dynamic range neurons in the dorsal horn of the spinal cord, which is found with repetitive nociceptive stimulation at frequencies faster than 0. 3 Hz (Mendell, 1966). Continuous excitation of these neurons by nociceptive C-fiber afferents removes the block of an ion channel with a receptor sensitive for NMDA. This allows for an influx of calcium ions into the cell, thus further depolarizing the cell membrane and leading to an accelerated release of action potentials, the so-called wind-up. This neural process and its modulation or blockade by NMDA receptor antagonists (e.g., MK 801, ketamine, memantine, amantadine) are well examined in animal experiments (e.g., Woolf & Thompson, 1991; Ren, 1994). Psychophysical experiments in humans have shown that subjective sensitization might be at least in part a perceptual correlate of this spinal mechanism (Price et al., 1994).

### *12.3.2.2 Automatic processes: Habituation*

Habituation is defined as a decrease of the subjective intensity experience during repetitive or continuous stimulation at constant intensities. Thus habituation can be regarded as a perceptual process complementary to sensitization, although the underlying neuronal processes are supposed to be very different. In the classical interpretation of habituation, a sequential comparison process between a stored image of a stimulus and its repetitive presentation is assumed. The result of this comparison process determines the response to the actual stimulus: an agreement of stored and actual stimulus image leads to a decrease in response intensity (Sokolov, 1960). The response to new stimulation (orienting response) and habituation are well examined for nearly all sense modalities (e.g., Lang, Davis, & Öhman, 2000). For pain perception, there are only a limited number of studies available, probably because sensitization normally dominates in pain perception.

### *12.3.2.3 Associative learning: Operant conditioning*

In the taxonomy of higher-order learning mechanisms and related memory systems, operant and classical conditioning are termed associative learning mechanisms (Milner et al., 1998). Since the work of Fordyce and others, operant conditioning is considered an important psychological mechanism for the development and also for the treatment of chronic pain (Fordyce, 1984; Philips, 1987; Philips & Grant, 1991). Although this is common knowledge in pain research, studies on operant conditioning of pain are scarce and mostly limited to modifying the observable pain behavior.

Operant reinforcement of pain has been examined so far particularly with external social reinforcement, where reward and punishment were performed by means of verbal comments on pain behavior (extrinsic reinforcement). An example is the verbal comment on the participant's rating of pain intensity on a rating scale, such as "very well done" (reinforcement) or "badly performed" (punishment). The resulting dynamic change has been operationalized by explicit judgments of perceived pain intensities, which implies the possibility of various distortions in quantifying the judgment. Usually, with this type of study, it cannot be decided whether pain perception or only the linguistic judgment criterion has been modified by operant learning. This issue has been resolved by the operant procedure presented in Section 12.4.3.

Several other mechanisms of dynamic change in nociception and pain exist, but we limit the presentation to those for which appropriate validated procedures of assessment are available, which are presented in the next section.

## 12.4 Measurement of dynamic processes in pain

A thorough examination of the functions of the nociceptive system in humans requires a versatile toolbox of psychophysical and psychophysiological measuring procedures. Specific stimulus patterns have to be defined as probes, to tap selected mechanisms of nociception and pain on various levels of processing. This experimental pain stimulation provides a powerful framework to shed light on the multidimensional functionality and interaction of these mechanisms. Far from providing a complete compendium of psychophysical pain assessment, this section rather focuses on a selection of three psychophysical procedures, which capture dynamic properties of one or more of the previously described neuronal mechanisms and learning.

### *12.4.1 Assessment of pain dynamics during repetitive phasic stimulation*

Measuring sensitization has a long tradition in animal research on pain, with Mendell's discovery of the neuronal wind-up phenomenon being a major milestone (Mendell, 1966). However, psychometric evaluations of time course–intensity interactions in humans have only been addressed occasionally in the last two decades (e.g., Arendt-Nielsen, Andersen, & Jensen, 1996; Nielsen & Arendt-Nielsen, 1998). The classical approach in measuring perceptual sensitization in humans makes use of short stimulus pulses that are repetitively presented. Infrared lasers emitting thermal radiation are highly useful for this kind of stimulus model because they provide stimulus durations in the millisecond range and selectively activate nociceptive fibers (AMH-II in hairy skin; Bromm & Treede, 1983; 1984). The related experimental models based on this technique have been termed *temporal-summation models*, representing a promising approach to assess dynamic processes in the nociceptive system. Assessment of temporal summation focuses on the perceptual sensitization experienced during repetitive stimulation with constant intensity. This strategy leaves aside various other mechanisms of dynamic change, which are assumed to overlay the perceptual measures of habituation and sensitization to varying degrees. Therefore, a modified temporal summation procedure has been conceived which could capture this overlay of several dynamic nociceptive processes working concurrently to produce altered pain perception (Kleinböhl, Trojan, Konrad, & Hölzl, 2006).

In the new psychophysical procedure, repetitive heat pulses of 100 ms duration were applied to the skin by a PC-controlled $CO_2$-laser system. The laser beam was projected to the radial nerve area of the left hand by a scanning device that allowed automatic change of stimulation areas on the skin. This changing of stimulus site is usually performed to avoid local sensitization (auto- and heterosensitization; c.f. Section 12.3.1 and Table 12.2). A repetitive series of heat pulses is called a trial (Figure 12.2). Participants estimated the perceived magnitude of a first single pulse on a scale. This judgment served as a reference point for the perceived change during the subsequent repetitive series of ten pulses. The series was applied at the same intensity as the initial reference pulse and at one of three frequencies of repetition (Figure 12.2). Participants were instructed to focus their judgment on a gradual temperature change experienced between the first stimulus and the last of the repetitive stimulation trial.

Psychophysical scaling was performed with visual analog scales (VAS) presented on a computer screen. Participants were asked for four perceptual judgments: an intensity rating of the first and the last single laser pulse of the series, an estimate of the perceived intensity change during the repetitive pulse series, and finally, a rating of the aversiveness of the pulse series. Two measures of perceptual change were derived from these judgments: first, the difference between the ratings of the first and the last laser pulse, reflecting dynamic change in first pain perception, and second, the subjective rating of the dynamic change experienced during repetitive stimulation, rather connected to slow second pain.

The results in healthy participants showed that short-term sensitization occurred at stimulus frequencies above 0.3 Hz, the typical edge frequency for spinal wind-up to occur (Figure 12.3). Moreover, stimulus frequency had an overall influence on both measures of perceived dynamic change: The change of sensory magnitude (VAS) and the perceived temperature change $\Delta S$ both increased with stimulus frequency at all intensities used. In contrast, stimulus intensity effects were different for the measures of perceptual change: the change of sensory magnitude (VAS) depended on intensity only at the highest frequency (1.8 Hz). For the direct rating of perceived change (the $\Delta S$ response, "S" stands for "sensation"), stimulus intensity had a significant effect, showing an increase of perceptual sensitization with increasing intensity at all repetition rates (Figure 12.3).

The controlled stimulation protocol further allowed assessing the effects of multiple stimulations of the same skin area during medium-term time spans, showing habituation for these specific stimuli. Over the blocks of trials, each one related with a change in stimulated skin area, no long-term perceptual changes occurred.

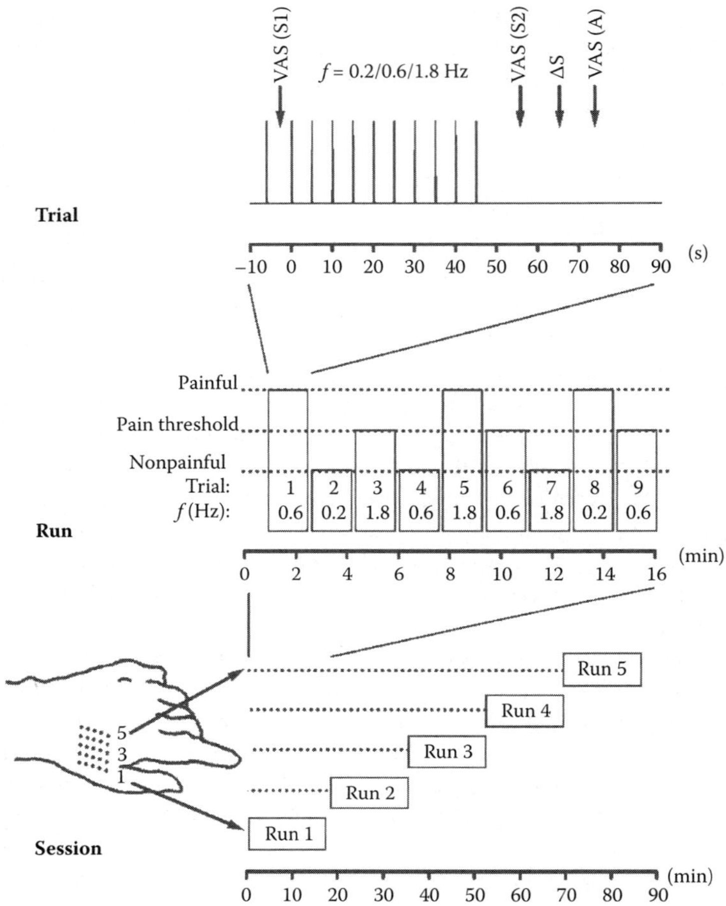


*Figure 12.2* Psychophysical phasic pain procedure with radiant heat stimulus protocol and psychophysical scaling. One session consists of 5 runs, including 9 trials per run and 11 single laser pulses per trial. *Trial:* A series of 10 laser pulses at one of three frequencies *f* (0.2, 0.6, or 1.8 Hz) was applied after an initial reference pulse. Within each trial, a set of psychophysical ratings was obtained: absolute magnitude estimation of the initial reference pulse (VAS(S1)) and the last pulse (VAS(S2)) of the repetitive series; direct estimation of perceived temperature change during repetitive stimulation (ΔS), and a magnitude estimate of the overall "aversiveness" of the entire trial (VAS(A)). Perceptual change during repetitive stimulation was assessed first, by the difference of stimulus magnitude ΔVAS = VAS(S2) – VAS(S1), and second, by the measure of perceived temperature change ΔS. *Run:* Within a fixed pseudorandom sequence of 9 trials, each of the 3 frequency × 3 intensity conditions of the design was applied once. *Session:* Five runs were applied during one experimental session. The stimulation patch in the left-hand radial nerve area consisted of 5 successively stimulated spots, which were additionally moved laterally with the start of each run (start positions 1–3–5 in the inset). All locations were positioned on a regular grid (1 cm). Perceptual measures were analyzed per trial (short-term effects; <1 min), per run (medium-term effects; 1–15 min), and per session (long-term effects; 15-90 min). (Figure from Kleinböhl et al., 2006: *Clinical Neurophysiology 117,* p. 122, fig.1; Elsevier Ireland Ltd.)

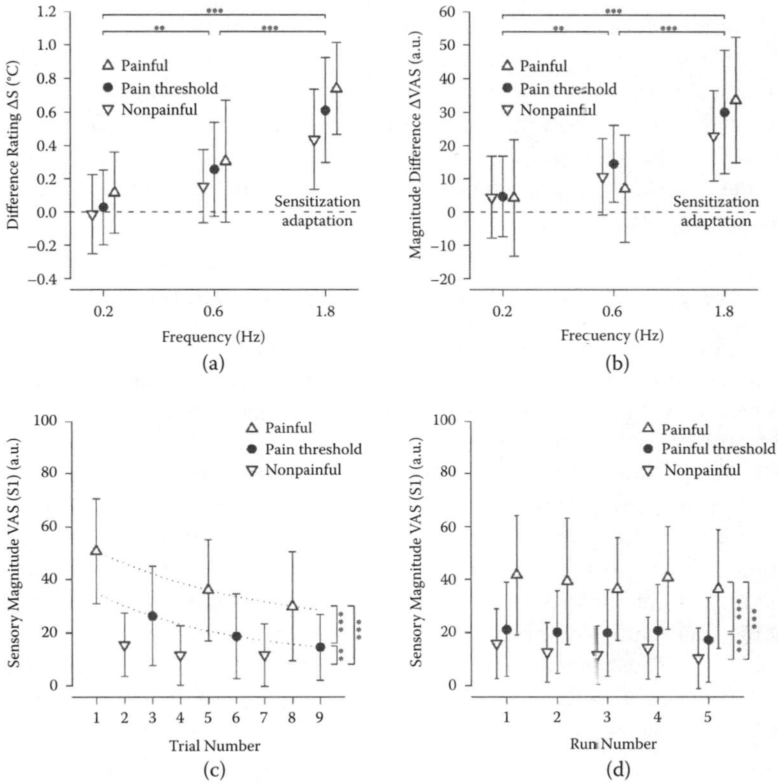


*Figure 12.3* Repetitive phasic pain stimulation and the overlay of dynamic mechanisms of perceptual change. Sensitization and habituation occur concurrently in this procedure, depending on the time interval observed, the frequency applied, the intensity, skin area, and the repetitive stimulation of the same skin patch. (a) Difference of magnitude estimates ΔVAS (mean ± SD), related to first pain sensations of laser pulses, over stimulus frequency for non-painful intensity (▽), pain threshold intensity (●), and painful intensity (△). Perceptual sensitization increases with repetition rate above 0.2 Hz. (b) Perceived difference rating of temperature change ΔS (mean ± SD) related to second pain sensations during repetitive stimulation, over stimulus frequency. Second pain-related perceptual sensitization increases with frequency in the same dose-dependent manner as the index of first pain-related sensitization, but an additional intensity effect is seen ($p < .05$). Data collapsed over 2 sessions, $N = 10$ participants, 90 trials each. (c) Medium-term habituation of sensory magnitude estimates of the reference pulse at a constant stimulus location over the 9 pseudorandomized trials within a run (trial within run main effect: $F = 17.8$; $p < .05$ adjusted). Dotted lines: exponential fit of the habituation curve for the two upper intensity classes. (d) Long-term effects of sensory magnitude estimates of the reference pulse over 5 runs during a session (run within session main effect: $F = 1.41$; $p > .10$ n.s.). The brackets in (c) and (d) indicate the adjusted significance of contrasts over trials (nonpain versus pain threshold: $F = 31.0$; $p < .01$; pain threshold vs. pain: $F = 55.9$; $p < .001$; nonpain vs. pain: $F = 59.6$; $p < .001$). (Figures from Kleinböhl et al., 2006: *Clinical Neurophysiology 117,* p. 124, figs.1, 2; Elsevier Ireland Ltd.)

The procedure permits the concurrent assessment of short-, medium-, and long-term dynamic processes of sensitization and habituation in pain processing by dissecting these mechanisms with a sophisticated stimulus protocol of repetitive stimulation (Figure 12.3). The main underlying neuronal mechanisms are assumed to be related to spinal wind-up and cutaneous nociceptive fiber fatigue, respectively. The method is therefore suitable for quantitative sensory testing of dynamic pain processing over different time spans, which is relevant in clinical testing of pain and in drug assessment.

### *12.4.2 Assessment of pain dynamics during tonic stimulation*

Tonic stimulation is a constant stimulus in the minutes or subminute range, during which dynamic changes in pain processing can be observed. Several experimental pain measurement procedures with tonic stimulation have been developed, but most of them are limited in their applications, because the control of the stimulus characteristics is rather crude. Examples for those tonic pain procedures are the "submaximal effort tourniquet test" and the "cold pressor test" (Handwerker & Kobal, 1993). The tourniquet test makes the musculature of a cuffed arm work under ischemic conditions, leading to a deep aching pain. The cold pressor achieves similar pain by placing the arm in cold water near the freezing point (approx. 4°C). Both methods assess the time until participants cannot bear the pain anymore, as a threshold of pain tolerance. These methods cannot easily be repeated and by capturing only one threshold parameter in the intensity continuum of pain, no dynamic processes can be assessed. Variants using continuous ratings during these tonic stimulation modes produce highly variable estimates and are difficult to interpret (e.g., Davis, Pope, Crawley, & Mikulis, 2004).

Based on an earlier method for the measurement of subjective sensitization (Severin et al., 1985), a new tonic heat pain test, the "dual sensitization procedure" (Kleinböhl et al., 1999) was developed (Figure 12.4). The procedure incorporates an assessment of pain threshold, and an assessment of a stimulus-response function for tonic stimuli as well as a twofold measure of pain sensitization or habituation.

Tonic heat stimuli are applied with a contact heat thermode to the skin, for instance, to the thenar of the hand. The stimulator is a small metal plate with a precisely adjustable temperature, controlled by a PC system. Each heat stimulus starts from baseline (40°C) to a preset temperature, typically one of several values above and below the previously assessed pain threshold. During a "reference interval" of 5 s participants are instructed to memorize the sensation on their hand. During the next 25 s of constant tonic stimulation, participants will typically perceive changes in temperature, an increase indicating sensitization and a decrease indicating habituation. At the end of the tonic stimulation the perceived dynamic change is assessed in a twofold way.

First, a direct and overt scaling of the perceived temperature change is performed; participants are asked to rate the amount of change (in 1/10°C) after 30 s of constant stimulation by comparing the present sensation with the sensation in the reference interval. A negative perceived temperature change indicates habituation, whereas

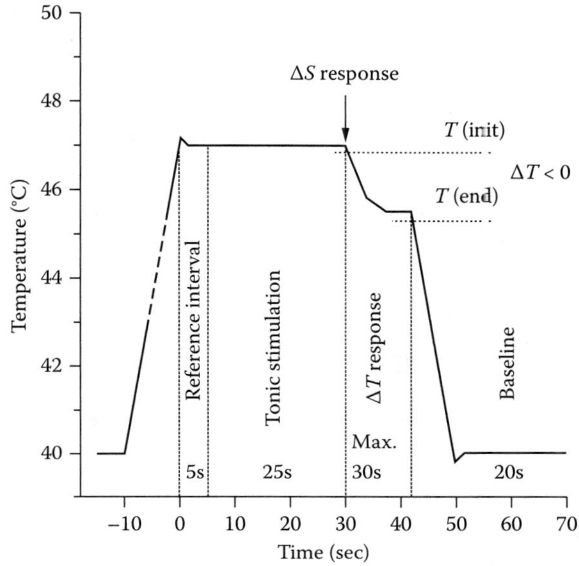


*Figure 12.4* Psychophysical "dual sensitization" procedure for the assessment of perceptual changes in humans (Kleinböhl et al., 1999). In this procedure, the change in perceived intensity is assessed during constant contact heat stimuli of 30 s duration. A subjective measure of perceived change ΔS is assessed on a magnitude scale (explicit judgment). The second measure of perceived change (ΔT) is acquired by method of production, where participants reproduce the same temperature sensation as perceived during the reference interval. The difference between the two temperatures is the second measure of perceived change (implicit measure).

positive ratings indicate sensitization (ΔS response, "S" again stands for "sensation"). Second, an indirect and covert scaling of the perceived temperature change is acquired. The task of the participants is to actively readjust the thermode temperature to reproduce their initial sensation during the reference interval. The measure of perceived change is then computed as the difference of end-temperature T(end) minus initial temperature T(init), negative values indicating sensitization and positive values habituation (ΔT response, where T stands for "temperature"). The latter technique, termed "behavioral discrimination," avoids the common response bias of subjective ratings by inferring the perception of participants covertly by their behavior (Kleinböhl et al., 1999).

Repeating this procedure at several intensities below and above subjective pain threshold allows the assessment of individual response profiles for sensitization and habituation in the domain of overt subjective evaluation of perceived change (ΔS), as well as for its counterpart of behavioral discrimination (ΔT). This measurement of dynamic change in pain perception is able to capture profound differences between healthy participants and chronic pain patients with musculoskeletal pain (Figure 12.5). Healthy participants are characterized by habituation in the first place, whereas patients display a strong sensitization (Figure 12.5). Both subjective and

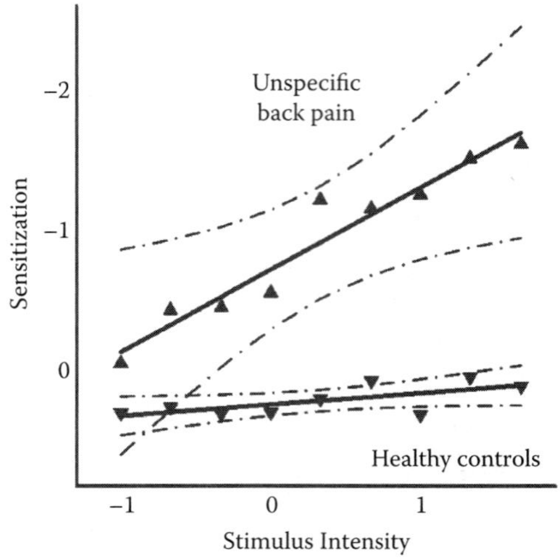


*Figure 12.5* Sensitization to tonic heat as a function of relative temperature in chronic back pain patients and controls. Mean temperature gradients of the behavioral sensitization measure with linear regressions (thick lines) and 95% confidence intervals (thin lines). Symbols indicate mean values over relative stimulus temperature for the groups (–1°C << pain threshold = 0 << + 1°C). Behavioral sensitization differentiates back pain patients from healthy controls, with patients showing enhanced sensitization already at nonpainful temperatures.

behavioral measures differentiate patients with normal phasic pain thresholds from healthy persons. In particular, in patients with spine-related musculoskeletal pain, enhanced sensitization appeared already well below pain threshold and increased further with stimulus intensity (Figure 12.5).

These results show that chronic musculoskeletal pain is not only characterized by an increased sensitivity toward painful and nonpainful stimuli, but also by altered characteristics of information processing in the nociceptive system. The temperature where sensitization is elicited is generally shifted to lower values, and the increase of sensitization with higher temperatures is more pronounced. This enhanced sensitization in chronic pain must reflect an overlay of different mechanisms of dynamic change in pain and nociception. At the least, the short time dynamics mediated by spinal wind-up seems to be present in the data, obviously amplified in patients by other mechanisms on the spinal or even cerebral level.

### *12.4.3 Assessment of pain dynamics mediated by operant learning*

Assessing operant learning mechanisms, the third class of dynamic change mechanisms in nociception and pain, requires a complex psychophysical procedure, combined with operant reinforcement. In the development of such an operant conditioning procedure, a starting point has been the pathogenetic marker of enhanced sensitization, which has been found mainly in patients with musculoskeletal pain (Kleinböhl et al., 1999). From previous pharmacological studies it had become clear that spinal wind-up cannot be the exclusive cause of enhanced pain sensitization (see Section 12.3.1 on neuronal mechanisms of pain). A modification of perceptual sensitization during tonic heat pain by an operant learning procedure would be strong proof for the relevance of such learning mechanisms for the emergence of pain hyperalgesia and for a modulation of pain perception leading to chronic pain. To show this experimentally, the "dual sensitization" procedure described previously has been modified in several ways (Figure 12.6).

1. The pathogenetic marker, enhanced sensitization measured by behavioral discrimination, has been chosen as the behavior to be modified by its consequences, determined by an operant schedule of reinforcement.
2. Sensitization has been measured in a twofold way, as in the dual sensitization procedure, by an overt subjective and by a covert procedure. Participants were instructed to keep the sensation constant during tonic heat stimulation by continuous adjustment of the temperature. Dynamic change during this adjustment phase is therefore measured indirectly as the difference between start and end temperature.
3. Reinforcement has been operationalized as intrinsic reinforcement, that is, within the sensory modality under examination. A reduction in stimulus intensity or pain served as negative reinforcement, and an increase of stimulus intensity as punishment. This was combined with standard methods of operant response shaping of increased sensitization and habituation (see Hölzl, Kleinböhl, & Huse, 2005, for details).

Healthy participants (24) were randomly assigned to two groups taking part in either operant sensitization or habituation learning. Painful and not painful initial stimulus temperatures were compared in participants in two separate sessions, each including 80 trials of thermal stimulation applied with a thermode system to the thenar eminence (see Figure 12.7).

The experimental study demonstrated for the first time an "implicit" operant modulation of pain perception; both habituation and sensitization learning have been successful. The sensitization response ($\Delta T$) was varied thereby in only 1–2 hours of operant conditioning in an order of magnitude resembling the enhanced sensitization found as a pathogenetic marker in chronic back pain patients. Pain perception has been changed by operant learning in two specific ways: first, the specific learning conditions increased the occurrence of behavior indicating sensitization or habituation. Second, subjective magnitude estimation and actual stimulus temperature fell apart with progressive training during sensitization learning: with stimulus temperature decreasing, the perceived intensity remained constant (Figure 12.7). Participants were not aware of the causality between their temperature regulation and the following reinforcement; the learning therefore occurred without their awareness, or implicitly. All test persons had adhered to provide exact sensory judgments, motivated by the cover instruction to perform a quantitative sensory testing.

The study demonstrated that it is possible to shape short-term sensitization and habituation to tonic thermo-nociceptive stimuli in healthy participants by implicit

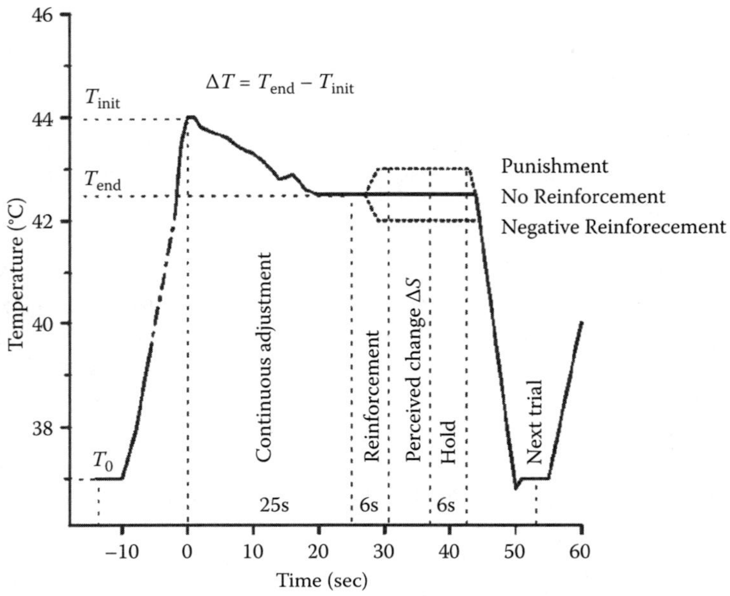


*Figure 12.6* Trial structure of operant conditioning procedure. Stimuli start from baseline temperature $T_0$ = 37°C up to a preset initial stimulus temperature $T_{init}$ (0.7°C/s). Participants continuously adjust the thermode temperature under the instruction to keep temperature constant. The adjusted change $\Delta T$ is the difference of end temperature $T_{end}$ and start temperature $T_{init}$. Reinforcement as a specified temperature decrease or increase is made contingent on criterion responses to be enhanced or weakened (downregulation in sensitization learning, upregulation in habituation learning). The perceived change $\Delta S$ is a visual analog rating of perceived temperature change during reinforcement (Hölzl et al., 2005). (Figure from Hölzl et al., 2005, *Pain 115,* p. 14, fig.1; Elsevier Ireland Ltd.).

operant reinforcement of discriminative behavior with contingent acute pain reduction and without participants' knowledge of contingencies. Consequently, implicit learning of enhanced pain sensitization may be a suitable model to assess operant plasticity of pain perception, in addition to basic sensory and neuronal mechanisms mediating dynamic change in nociception and pain.

## 12.5 Summary and final considerations

The assessment of dynamic mechanisms in nociception and pain has been presented in three sections. First, the complex neuronal structures subserving nociception and pain have been described on the level of peripheral nociception, the level of spinal nociception, and, finally, the level of the brain. This first section has been complemented by an overview of the few neurophysiological properties that translate directly into perceptual qualities. Second, the prominent mechanisms of dynamic change in nociception and pain were presented on a neurophysiological level, namely the mechanisms of neuronal plasticity, which are triggered under certain stimulus

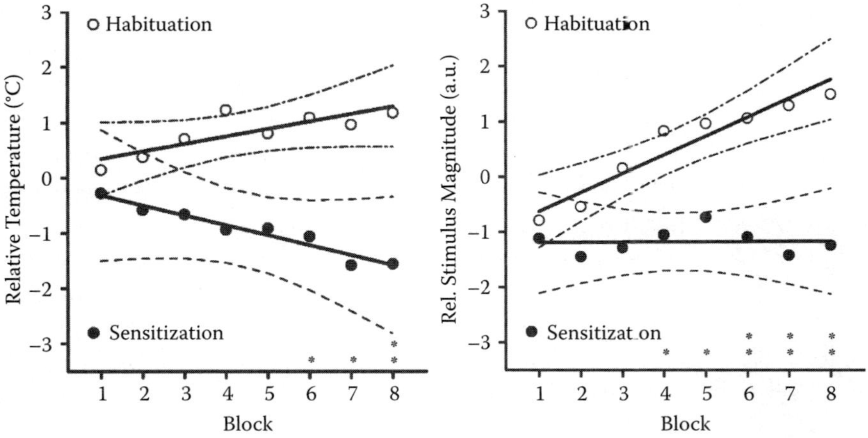


*Figure 12.7* Time course of stimulus temperatures in operant learning of short-term sensitization and habituation. (A) Learning curves as block to block means (linear regression trend with 95% confidence intervals). Stimulus temperatures differ significantly after 50 trials or five blocks (*$p < .05$, **$p < .01$; linear trend contrast: $p = .0007$**). Implicit (w/o awareness of contingencies) operant shaping of short-term sensitization or habituation by contingent decrease or increase of stimulus intensity is effective (Hölzl et al., 2005). (Figure from Hölzl et al., 2005, *Pain 115,* p. 16, fig.2b; p. 17, fig. 3b; Elsevier Ireland Ltd.).

conditions and affect nociception and pain within different time spans. Basic mechanisms of learning were selected as higher-order psychological mechanisms of dynamic change in pain: nonassociative learning or automatic processes represented by habituation and sensitization, and associative learning, represented by operant conditioning. Third, the assessment of some of the typical dynamic properties of nociceptive processing has been exemplified by three psychophysical measurement procedures and their implementation. Although there are many more psychophysical methods for assessing various aspects of pain processing, the focus has been put on three procedures that were specifically developed for measuring dynamic change in pain perception (Table 12.3).

The procedures introduced here capture several mechanisms mediating dynamic change in pain to various degrees. The selectivity for circumscribed mechanisms depends on factors such as the physical stimulation model (phasic, tonic), the specific procedural properties and the operationalization of target effect variables (e.g., rating scales for sensitization or habituation). The resulting measurement parameters hardly represent "pure" properties of a certain mechanism. It must be assumed that these parameters will always be constituted by an overlay of several mechanisms working in parallel and affecting the perception of dynamic change (Table 12.3). Therefore, exact proportions of the influence of specific neuronal mechanisms on pain cannot easily be given. However, the dissection of the specific neuronal and psychological contributions to perceptual phenomena can be improved by validating the psychophysical procedures under specific

*Table 12.3* Assessment of dynamic change mechanisms in pain perception[a]

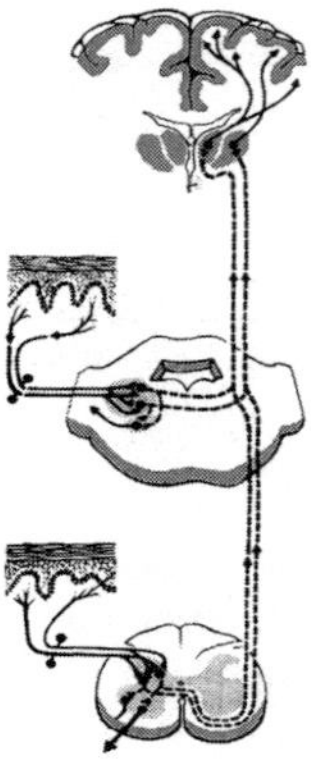

| | *Repetitive stim. (phasic pain)* | *Dual sensitization (tonic pain)* | *Operant conditioning (tonic pain)* |
|---|---|---|---|
| Pain perception | **Sensitization** | **Sensitization** | **Sensitization** |
| | **Habituation** | **Habituation** | **Habituation** |
| Brain neuromatrix | **Automatic processes** | **Automatic processes** | **Automatic processes** |
| | | | **Associative learning** |
| | Descending inhibition | Descending inhibition | Descending inhibition |
| Spinal nociception | **Wind-up** | **Wind-up** Central sensitization? | **Wind-up** Central sensitization? |
| | (Descending) inhibition | (Descending) inhibition | (Descending) inhibition |
| Peripheral nociception | Autosensitization of nociceptors | Autosensitization of nociceptors | Autosensitization of nociceptors |
| | **Fatigue of nociceptors** | | |

[a] Psychophysical procedures and mechanisms of dynamic change they are assumed to assess in the first place (indicated in boldface). Facilitative and inhibiting mechanisms are given (inhibition in shaded layout).

experimental conditions or in specific samples. This strategy might be pursued by pharmacological interventions such as blocking the spinal wind-up with NMDA-antagonists, and also by investigating patient groups with chronic pain syndromes. The methodological principles of measuring pain dynamics in human are summarized as follows:

1. *Stimulus model:* The spatiotemporal characteristics of experimental pain stimulation provide a first selection of the specific nociceptive pathways to be addressed. This is achieved by defining intensity, time course, and stimulation site on the body appropriately. Mechanisms of dynamic change in pain can be measured with phasic pain repetitive stimulation at different frequencies or with constant tonic stimulation over different time spans.
2. *Psychophysical scaling:* Two types of subjective judgments of perceived change are used. Direct scaling techniques, measuring the magnitude of perceived change by asking participants to make a subjective judgment on a scale are usually prone to various kinds of bias (Poulton, 1989). In contrast, indirect behavioral measurement of perceived change can be operationalized as unbiased no-knowledge procedures, where subjects operate on a task such as keeping apparent temperature constant, giving information

about perceived change by their temperature regulation behavior during the task.

3. *Experimental modulation* of dynamic change in pain perception can be used to dissect underlying subprocesses mediating the change, for instance, by applying pharmacological probes, including the topical application of capsaicin in peripheral nociception, or the application of NMDA-antagonists (ketamine, amantadine) affecting mainly spinal nociception. More complicated interventions are made on higher-order processes, such as the modulation of pain perception achieved by operant learning. These specific interventions or probes allow a certain degree of differentiating circumscribed components of pain processing and the underlying nociceptive mechanisms (Table 12.3).
4. The experimental pain psychophysical procedures and the most relevant mechanisms they capture are validated by comparing the measures of dynamic change for healthy participants and chronic pain patients. Thus, the relevant measurement parameters having differential validity can be isolated, which may point to the pathogenetic relevant mechanisms of altered dynamic change in chronic pain syndromes.

## References


Abbott, F. V., Melzack, R., & Leber, B. F. (1982). Morphine analgesia and tolerance in the tail-flick and formalin tests: Dose-response relationships. *Pharmacology Biochemistry Behavior, 17,* 1213–1219.

Apkarian, A. Vania. (1995). Functional imaging of pain: New insights regarding the role of the cerebral cortex in human pain perception. *Seminars in Neurosciences, 7*(4), 297 ff.

Apkarian, A. Vania. (1996). Primary somatosensory cortex and pain. *Pain Forum, 5*(3), 188–191.

Arendt-Nielsen, L., Andersen, O. K., & Jensen, T. S. (1996). Brief, prolonged and repeated stimuli applied to hyperalgesic skin areas: A psychophysical study. *Brain Research, 712*(1), 165–167.

Basbaum, A. I., Marley, N. J., O'Keefe, J., & Clanton, C. H. (1977). Reversal of morphine and stimulation produced analgesia by subtotal spinal cord lesions. *Pain, 3,* 43–56.

Bodnar, R., Paul, D., & Pasternak, G. W. (1991). Synergistic analgesic interactions between the periaquaeductal gray and the locus coeruleus. *Brain Research, 558,* 224–230.

Bromm, B., & Treede, R. D. (1983). $CO_2$ laser radiant heat pulses activate C nociceptors in man. *Pflugers Archiv: European Journal of Physiology, 399*(2), 155–156.

Bromm, B., & Treede, R. D. (1984). Nerve fibre discharges, cerebral potentials and sensations induced by $CO_2$ laser stimulation. *Human Neurobiology, 3*(1), 33–40.

Cervero, F. (1986). Dorsal horn neurons and their sensory inputs. In T L. Yaksh (Ed.), *Spinal afferent processing* (pp. 197–216). New York: Plenum Press.

Craig, A. D. (2002). How do you feel? Interoception: The sense of the physiological condition of the body. *National Review of Neuroscience, 3*(8), 655–666.

Craig, A. D. (2003a). Interoception: The sense of the physiological condition of the body. *Current Opinions in Neurobiology, 13*(4), 500–505.

Craig, A. D. (2003b). A new view of pain as a homeostatic emotion. *Trends in Neuroscience, 26*(6), 303–307.

Darian-Smith, I. (1984). Thermal sensibility. In I. Darian-Smith (Ed.), *Sensory processes II. Handbook of physiology, Sect. 1, Vol. 3* (pp. 879–913). Bethesda, MD: American Physiological Society.

Davis, K. D., Pope, G. E., Crawley, A. P., & Mikulis, D. J. (2004). Perceptual illusion of "paradoxical heat" engages the insular cortex. *Journal of Neurophysiology, 92*(2), 1248–1251.

Derbyshire, S. W. (2000). Exploring the pain "neuromatrix." *Current Review of Pain, 4*(6), 467–477.

Derbyshire, S. W. G., Jones, A. K. P., Gyulai, F., Clark, S., Townsend, D., & Firestone, L. L. (1997). Pain processing during three levels of noxious stimulation produces differential patterns of central activity. *Pain, 73,* 431–445.

Droste, C. (1988). Schmerzperception und periphere Schmerzlokalisation bei Angina pectoris. *Zeitschrift für Kardiologie, 5,* 15–33.

Flor, H. (2003). Cortical reorganisation and chronic pain: Implications for rehabilitation. *Journal of Rehabilitation Medicine, 41* (Suppl), 66–72.

Fordyce, W. E. (1984). Behavioural science and chronic pain. *Postgraduate Medical Journal, 60*(710), 865–868.

Greene, L. C., & Hardy, J. D. (1962). Adaptation of thermal pain in the skin. *Journal of Applied Physiology, 17,* 693–696.

Handwerker, H. O., & Kobal, G. (1993). Psychophysiology of experimentally induced pain. *Physiological Reviews, 73*(3), 639–671.

Heppelmann, B., Messlinger, K., Schaible, H. G., & Schmidt, R. F. (1991). Nociception and pain. *Current Opinion in Neurobiology, 1*(2), 192–197.

Hölzl, R., Erasmus, L., & Möltner, A. (1996). Detection, discrimination and sensation of visceral stimuli. *Biological Psychology, 42*(1–2), 199–214.

Hölzl, R., Kleinböhl, D., & Huse, E. (2005). Implicit operant learning of pain sensitization. *Pain, 115*(1–2), 12–20.

Hylden, J. L. K., Hayashi, H., Bennett, G. J., & Dubner, R. (1985). Spinal lamina I neurons projecting to the parabrachial area of the cat midbrain. *Brain Research, 336,* 195–198.

Kandel, E. R. (2001). The molecular biology of memory storage: A dialogue between genes and synapses. *Science, 294*(5544), 1030–1038.

Kenshalo, D. R., Leonard, R. B., Chung, J. M., & Willis, W. D. (1979). Responses of primate spinothalamic neurons to graded and to repeated noxious heat stimuli. *Journal of Neurophysiology, 42,* 1370–1389.

Klein, T., Magerl, W., Hopf, H. C., Sandkühler, J., & Treede, R. D. (2004). Perceptual correlates of nociceptive long-term potentiation and long-term depression in humans. *Journal of Neuroscience, 24*(4), 964–971.

Kleinböhl, D. (1996). *Psychophysikalische Korrelate von Anpassungsprozessen bei lang andauernden Schmerzreizen bei Gesunden und chronischen Schmerzpatienten.* Aachen: Shaker.

Kleinböhl, D., Baus, D., Hornberger, U., & Hölzl, R. (2005). Schmerzgedächtnis und Sensibilisierung. *PsychoNeuro, 31*(2), 84–91.

Kleinböhl, D., Hölzl, R., Möltner, A., Rommel, C., Weber, C., & Osswald, P. M. (1999). Psychophysical measures of sensitization to tonic heat discriminate chronic pain patients. *Pain, 81,* 35–43.

Kleinböhl, D., Trojan, J., Konrad, C., & Hölzl, R. (2006). Sensitization and habituation of AMH and C-fiber related percepts of repetitive radiant heat stimulation. *Clinical Neurophysiology: Official Journal of the International Federation of Clinical Neurophysiology, 117*(1), 118–130.

LaMotte, R. H. (1979). Intensive and temporal determinants of thermal pain. In D. Kenshalo (Ed.), *Sensory functions of the skin in primates*. Oxford: Pergamon Press.

LaMotte, R. H., & Campbell, J. N. (1978a). C-fiber afferents in monkey with human judgments of thermal pain. *Journal of Neurophysiology, 41,* 509–528.

LaMotte, R. H., & Campbell, J. N. (1978b). Comparison of responses of warm and nociceptive c-fiber afferents in monkey with human judgements of thermal pain. *Journal of Neurophysiology, 41,* 509–528.

LaMotte, R. H., Thalhammer, J. G., Torebjörk, H. E., & Robinson, C. J. (1982). Peripheral neural mechanisms of cutaneous hyperalgesia following mild injury by heat. *The Journal of Neuroscience, 2*, 765–781.

LaMotte, R. H., Thalhammer, J. G., & Robinson, C. J. (1983). Peripheral neural correlates of magnitude of cutaneous pain and hyperalgesia: A comparison of neural events in monkey with sensory judgments in human. *Journal of Neurophysiology, 50,* 1–26.

Lang, P. J., Davis, M., & Öhman, A. (2000). Fear and anxiety: Animal models and human cognitive psychophysiology. *Journal of Affective Disorders, 61*(3), 137–159.

Loeser, J. D., & Treede, R. D. (2008). The Kyoto protocol of IASP basic pain terminology. *Pain, 137*(3), 473–477.

Mendell, L. M. (1966). Physiological properties of unmyelinated fiber projections to the spinal cord. *Experimental Neurology, 16,* 316–332.

Mense, S., Hoheisel, U., Kaske, A., & Reinert, A. (1997). Muscle pain: Basic mechanisms and clinical correlates. In T. S. Jensen, J. A. Turner, & Z. Wiesenfeld-Hallin (Eds.), *Proceedings of the 8th World Congress on pain. Progress in Pain Research and Managment* (pp. 479–496).

Meyer, R. A., & Campbell, J. N. (1981). Myelinated nociceptive afferents account for the hyperalgesia that follows a burn to the hand. *Science, 213*, 1527–1529.

Millan, M. J. (1999). The induction of pain: An integrative review. *Progress in Neurobiology, 57*(1), 1–164.

Milner, B., Squire, L. R., & Kandel, E. R. (1998). Cognitive neuroscience and the study of memory. *Neuron, 20*(3), 445–468.

Nielsen, J., & Arendt-Nielsen, L. (1998). The importance of stimulus configuration for temporal summation of first and second pain to repeated heat stimuli. *European Journal of Pain, 2*(4), 329–341.

Philips, H. C. (1987). Avoidance behaviour and its role in sustaining chronic pain. *Behaviour Research and Therapy, 25*(4), 273–279.

Philips, H. C., & Grant, L. (1991). The evolution of chronic back pain problems: A longitudinal study. *Behaviour Research and Therapy, 29,* 435–441.

Poulton, E. C. (1989). *Bias in quantifying judgments*. Hove: Erlbaum.

Price, D. D., Mao, J., Frenk, H., & Mayer, D. J. (1994). The *N*-methyl-D-aspartate receptor antagonist dextromethorphan selectively reduces temporal summation of second pain in man. *Pain, 59,* 165–174.

Raja, S. N., Meyer, R. A., & Campbell, J. N. (1990). Hyperalgesia and sensitization of primary afferent fibres. In H. L. Fields (Ed.), *Pain syndromes in neurology* London: Butterworths.

Ren, K. (1994). Wind-up and the NMDA receptor: From animal studies to humans. *Pain, 59,* 157–158.

Rexed, B. (1952). The cytoarchitectonic organization of the spinal cord in the cat. *Brain Research, 51*, 415–495.

Sandkühler, J. (2000). Learning and memory in pain pathways. *Pain, 88*(2), 113–118.

Severin, F., Lehmann, W. P., & Strian, F. (1985). Subjective sensitization to tonic heat as an indicator of thermal pain. *Pain, 21,* 369–378.

Sherrington, C. S. (1906). *The integrative action of the nervous system.* New Haven, CT: Yale University Press.

Sokolov, E. N. (1960). Neuronal models and the orienting reflex. In M. A. Brazier (Ed.), *The central nervous system and behavior* (pp. 187–276). New York: Joshua Macy Foundation.

Torebjörk, E. (1994): Nociceptor dynamics in humans. In G. Gebhart, D. L. Hammond, & T. S. Jensen (Eds.), *Progress in pain research and management, Vol. 2: Proceedings of the 7th World Congress on Pain* (pp. 277–284). Seattle: IASP Press.

Treede, R. D., Apkarian, A. V., Bromm, B., Greenspan, J. D., & Lenz, F. A. (2000). Cortical representation of pain: Functional characterization of nociceptive areas near the lateral sulcus. *Pain, 87*(2), 113–119.

Treede, R. D., Kenshalo, D., Gracely, R., & Jones, A. (1999). The cortical representation of pain. *Pain, 79,* 105–111.

Treede, R. D., Meyer, R. A., & Campbell, J. N. (1998). Myelinated mechanically insensitive afferents from monkey hairy skin: Heat-response properties. *Journal of Neurophysiology, 80*(3), 1082–1093.

van Hees, J., & Gybels, J. (1981). C nociceptor activity in human nerves during painful and nonpainful skin stimulation. *Journal of Neurology, 44,* 600–607.

Watkins, L. R., & Mayer, D. J. (1982). Organization of endogenous opiate and nonopiate pain control systems. *Science, 216,* 1185–1192.

Willis, W. D. (1988). Dorsal horn neurophysiology of pain. *Annals of the New York Academy of Sciences, 531,* 76–89.

Woolf, C. J., & Salter, M. W. (2000). Neuronal plasticity: Increasing the gain in pain. *Science, 288*(5472), 1765–1769.

Woolf, C. J., & Thompson, S. W. (1991). The induction and maintenance of central sensitization is dependent on *N*-methyl-D-aspartic acid receptor activation: Implications for the treatment of post-injury pain hypersensitivity states. *Pain, 44*(3), 293–299.

Zimmermann, M. (1993). Physiologie von Nozizeption und Schmerz. In H.-D. Basler, C. Franz, B. Kröner-Herwig, H.P. Rehfisch & H. Seemann (Eds.), *Psychologische Schmerztherapie*. (pp.46–88). Berlin: Springer.

Zimmermann, M., & Handwerker, H. O. (1984). *Schmerz—Konzepte und ärztliches Handeln.* Berlin: Springer.

# 13 Measurement-related issues in the investigation of active vision

*Boris M. Velichkovsky,*[1,2] *Frans Cornelissen,*[3]
*Jan-Mark Geusebroek,*[4] *Sven-Thomas Graupner,*[1]
*Riitta Hari,*[5] *Jan Bernard Marsman,*[3]
*Sergey A. Shevchik,*[2] *and Sebastian Pannasch*[1]

[1]Applied Cognitive Research Unit
Department of Psychology
Dresden University of Technology
Dresden, Germany

[2]Institute of Cognitive Studies
Kurchatov Research Center "Kurchatov Institute"
Moscow, Russia

[3]University Medical Centre Groningen
Groningen, The Netherlands

[4]Institute of Informatics
University of Amsterdam
Amsterdam, The Netherlands

[5]Brain Research Unit, LTL
Helsinki University of Technology
Espoo, Finland

## 13.1 Introduction

In humans, as in all higher primates, vision is the dominant sensory modality. The essential role of eye movements in visual perception has been well known for a long time and has been repeatedly demonstrated (e.g., Findlay, 1998; Hayhoe & Ballard, 2005). This natural sampling of information from the environment requires that visual perception is investigated within the framework of "active vision" (Findlay, 1998). Due to the uneven distribution of light-sensitive receptors across the retina, the highest visual acuity is limited to the small foveal area (about two degrees of arc or double the thumbnail size of an extended arm). With increasing eccentricity—in parafoveal and peripheral regions—vision becomes blurred and the perception of color is reduced. These constraints make eye movements mandatory for perceiving the environment. Therefore, saccades—fast ballistic movements—are executed to bring the gaze from one point to another. The relatively stable periods in between are called fixations. The intake of visual information occurs within fixations but is largely suppressed during saccades. In many everyday situations, such as reading a text or inspecting an image, oculomotor activity can be described as interplay between fixations and saccades.

Sometimes, additional mechanisms are necessary to achieve clear and stable perception. For instance, if the object of interest is moving relative to a stationary background, smooth-pursuit movements (*dynamic fixations*) are observed (Lencer & Trillenberg, 2008), whereas movements of the head or body are compensated by the vestibulo-ocular reflex (Goldberg & Hudspeth, 2000). Within fixations, the eyes are not completely stationary, but they undergo several types of micromovements (for a recent review see Collewijn & Kowler, 2008). However, for the purpose of this chapter, the focus is on fixations and saccades, both of which can be characterized by several measurement parameters.

In relation to saccades, frequently measured parameters are the amplitude, maximum (or peak) velocity and direction, as well as the latency until a saccade is triggered. With respect to fixations, the prominent parameters are their duration and spatial distribution. Visual tasks are normally accompanied by the execution of saccadic eye movements about 3–4 times per second. In an everyday task, such as tea-making, the amplitudes of saccades vary in size from only a few degrees up to 130 degrees (Land, 2004), although in the latter cases the viewing is also supported by coordinated motion of the head and shoulders. The amplitude of saccades is directly related to variation of the size and overall shape of the image (von Wartburg, Wurtz, Pflugshaupt, Nyffeler, Lüthi, & Müri, 2007). A positive correlation between the amplitude of saccades and the saccadic velocity has been repeatedly demonstrated and is also known as *main sequence*, a term that has been adopted from astrophysics (Bahill, Clark, & Stark, 1975). In most situations, allocation of visual attention seems to be in a good correspondence with the direction of the eyes (e.g., Fischer, 1999).

The time that the eyes are stationary in relation to a particular region or object is denominated *fixation duration*. This time varies from less than 100 ms to several seconds, resulting in a positively skewed distribution with a pronounced peak between 200 and 300 ms. Because the intake of visual information is mostly limited to the time of fixations, the understanding of factors that influence the duration of fixation is essential in research on visual perception and gaze control. The duration of fixations is related to the difficulty of the ongoing task (Just & Carpenter, 1976; Velichkovsky, 1999). Investigations of different tasks, such as reading (Rayner, 1978), visual search (Vaughan, 1982), driving (Velichkovsky, Joos, Helmert, & Pannasch, 2005; Velichkovsky, Rothert, Kopf, Dornhoefer, & Joos, 2002) and static scene perception (Henderson, Weeks, & Hollingworth, 1999) have produced different models to explain the control of fixation duration. It has been suggested that fixations are controlled by the extraction of sensory information (Just & Carpenter, 1980), cognitive processes such as memory storage (Shebilske, 1975), and by the processes of eye movement programming (Zingale & Kowler, 1987).

In this chapter, we provide an overview of three classes of measurement issues that are central to investigation of eye movements and active vision: (1) physical measurements related to potential optical hazards to eyes and the related safety concerns, as well as statistical evaluation of natural-image parameters; (2) approaches to the analysis and interpretation of behavioral data on distribution of visual fixations across the image; and (3) the need for additional neurophysiological recordings. These latter problems currently are the focus of interest of the scientific community as their solution is a prerequisite for enhancing our understanding of brain mechanisms of visual cognition and control of eye movements.

## 13.2 Issues in eyetracking, optical measurement, and image statistics

Interest in active vision has a long history (for a review see Wade & Tatler, 2005). The first devices to make eye movement recordings were developed over 100 years ago (e.g., Dodge, 1900; Stratton, 1906). The early use of eyetracking in psychological research was often accompanied by severe inconveniences (e.g., vacuum devices were directly attached to the eyeball). Thus recording time was limited up to a few minutes. Nowadays registering eye movements is more comfortable and often does not require any contact of the system to the head or body. These advantages make it possible to measure eye movements for longer periods; in fact there are no longer any time limits. This technological progress makes eyetracking more and more appropriate for practical applications in industrial settings, as well as in studies of infants and of various patient groups. For instance, patients suffering from a lack of possibilities to communicate with the environment can benefit from eye typing systems to recover a part of their communicative abilities (Bates, Donegan, Istance, Hansen, & Räihä, 2007; Pannasch, Helmert, Velichkovsky, Malischke, & Storch, 2008). With the everyday application of eyetracking, questions concerning the safety of this technique arise, especially when it is used frequently for longer time periods of days, months, and years.

As a rule, today's contactless eyetracking systems use an infrared (IR) illumination produced via IR light-emitting diodes (LEDs). There are two reasons for this type of lighting in eyetracking systems. First of all, the use of a light source in the scene enhances the quality of the image in terms of contrast and intensity levels, and it facilitates detailed image analysis and gaze estimation. On the other hand, IR optical radiation is invisible to the human eye, so that the lighting is comfortable and does not distract the user's attention. In addition, IR radiation is reflected by the corneal surface, creating bright reflection points, termed *glints* (see Figure 13.1). It is frequently assumed that the glint positions in the image do not change with eye rotations but only with eyeball translations, thus giving an easily measured reference for head position. Recently, the initial assumption has been revisited (Guestrin & Eizenman, 2006; Shih & Liu, 2004). In these alternative models for gaze estimation, the movement of the glint due to eyeball rotations is introduced and measured accordingly.

One particular measurement problem is related to biophysical aspects of video-based eyetracking. As illustrated by Figure 13.2, current guidelines identify a number of potential hazards to the eye from optical sources; these hazards have to be evaluated to assure safety (see Mulvey, Villanueva, Sliney, Lange, Cotmore, & Donegan, 2008). Human vision is biologically adapted to protect itself against intense broadband optical radiation (ultraviolet, visible, and infrared radiant energy) from the natural environment. In addition, humans use protection, such as hats and sunglasses, to shield against the harmful effects upon the eye from intense ultraviolet (UV)

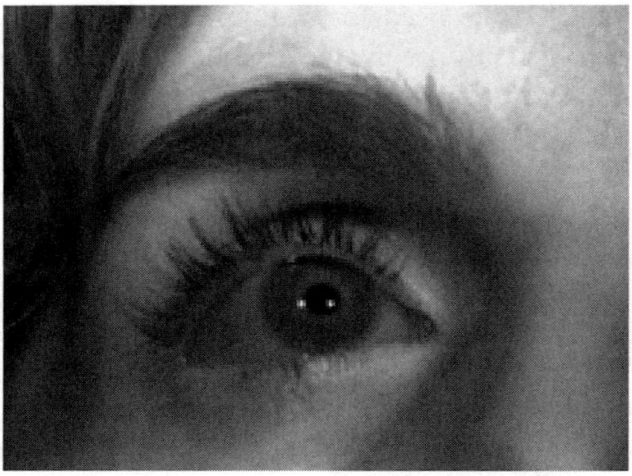

*Figure 13.1* An image of the human eye in video-based measurement of the ocular motility and the pupil diameter (two IR light sources are used).

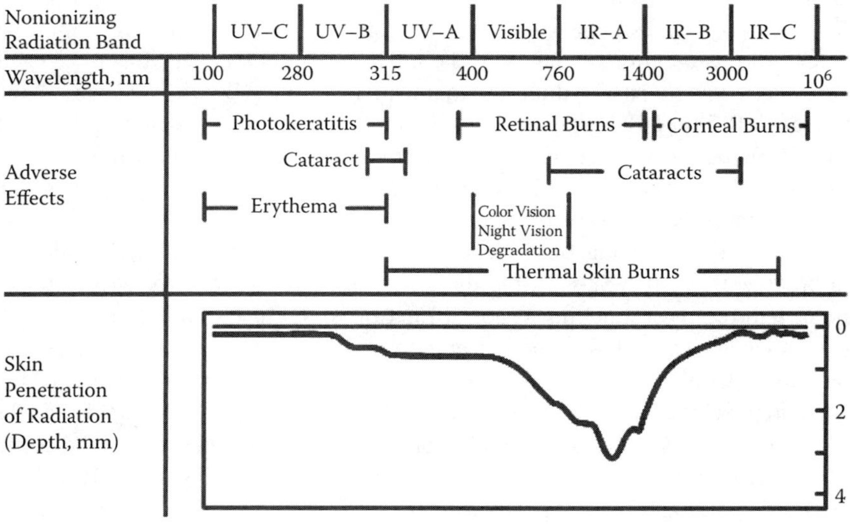


*Figure 13.2* The photobiological bands of the Commission Internationale de l'Éclairage (CIE) with spectral regions of optical hazards to human eyes and skin tissues (after Mulvey et al., 2008).

radiation and blue light present in sunlight over snow or sand. The aversion reflex effectively limits the light exposure of retina to a fraction of a second (about 200 ms or less) and thus protects the eye against injury from viewing bright light sources, such as the sun, lamps, and welding arcs. The infrared LEDs of modern eyetrackers do not, however, produce an aversion response, as they are barely visible, and their emission is limited to the near-infrared (IR-A, from 760 to 1400 nm) spectral band. If incandescent or discharge lamps that have been filtered to block most visible light and transmit IR-A are employed, some noticeable emissions are possible outside the IR-A. These emissions must be measured and evaluated separately.

Because the saccades are the movements that bring our eyes to a new location, the spatial position of landing is of particular interest. The early work on eye movements already showed that our eyes are guided to specific locations that are not randomly distributed over the whole scene (Buswell, 1935). Two possible sources that might influence saccadic target selection can be assumed: the task of the observer and the "saliency" of objects. The study by Alfred Yarbus (1967) revealed that presenting the same image with various instructions significantly affects the landing points of the saccades. For instance, when the age of the people in the image had to be rated, the faces were more often targeted by the gaze than if the material circumstances of the depicted family had to be estimated. In the latter case, saccades were guided mostly to furniture and other background objects (for a recent replication, see DeAngelus & Pelz, 2009). The other influencing factor is related to saliency, that is, the physical properties of the stimulus: the distinctiveness and prominence of physical features (e.g., contrast, shape, color, etc.) make an object more likely to become a saccade target than another object with other features (Itti & Koch, 2000).

Throughout evolution, environmental regularities have shaped sensory systems, and thereby have had a tremendous influence on visual perception and cognition (Geisler, 2008; Gibson, 1979). Hence, studying the statistical regularities present in natural scenes has great potential in the investigation of active vision. Accurate models of image statistics at the level appropriate for machine implementation may also reveal new mechanisms of visual processing in the brain (Karklin & Lewicki, 2009). In the current approaches, saliency maps of images are computed on a pixel-by-pixel basis. However, many perceptual tasks are concerned with a rougher impression of visual content rather than the exact image details. For example, scene categorization, such as knowing that a forest is a forest, generalizes over the various visual qualities of trees. Natural-image statistics are able to capture the appearance of many scene categories, although we only have a vague sort of understanding why. Another example, the perception of textures and materials, such as grass and trees, does not sort out every tiny leaf and twig, but captures some sort of impression of the visual image. As demonstrated by the work of impressionists and Gestalt psychologists, much of what we perceive is captured by a rough impression (Greene & Oliva, 2009; Koffka, 1935; Pelli & Tillman, 2008), rather than by precise depiction or exact pictorial assessment. However, what are the statistics gathering an impression of the scene? And how are these statistics used when we determine where to look next?

Natural images are highly structured in their spatial configuration. Where one would expect a different spatial layout, image statistics often follow a general Weibull-type spatial distribution (Geusebroek & Smeulders, 2005). Scholte, Ghebreab, Waldorp, Smeulders, and Lamme (2009) found a high correlation between the Weibull parameters and a simple model of the parvocellular and magnocellular pathways in the visual system. Thus one would expect image contrasts around fixation locations to reflect the Weibull statistics. Four types of natural-image statistics are expected according to the behavior of the integrated Weibull distribution: the power law, the exponential, the Gaussian, and the possibility that the Weibull distribution does not describe the data well (Yanulevskaya & Geusebroek, 2009).

To illustrate the different regimes of the integrated Weibull distribution, a set of several hundred natural images was recently analyzed on global statistics, local statistics, and statistics around eye fixations, that is, visually attended regions (Yanulevskaya & Geusebroek, 2009). For the global analysis, all images fit the Weibull statistic well, and could be further subdivided into 20% power-law and less than 5% Gaussian, the remainder fitting best to the exponential distribution. The power-law is one extreme, indicating strong overall contrast caused by a few edges. The Gaussian is the other extreme of the same distribution shape, indicating highly textured images. Figure 13.3 conveys an impression of the correlation between visual content and Weibull parameters. In a further local analysis, based on smaller image parts, 13% of the patches were rejected in the test for Weibull distribution. A visual inspection showed that these images contained only compression artifacts, or regions with regular patterns. The remaining 87% of the patches followed the Weibull distribution, whereby 26% were power-law distributed and 14% Gaussian.

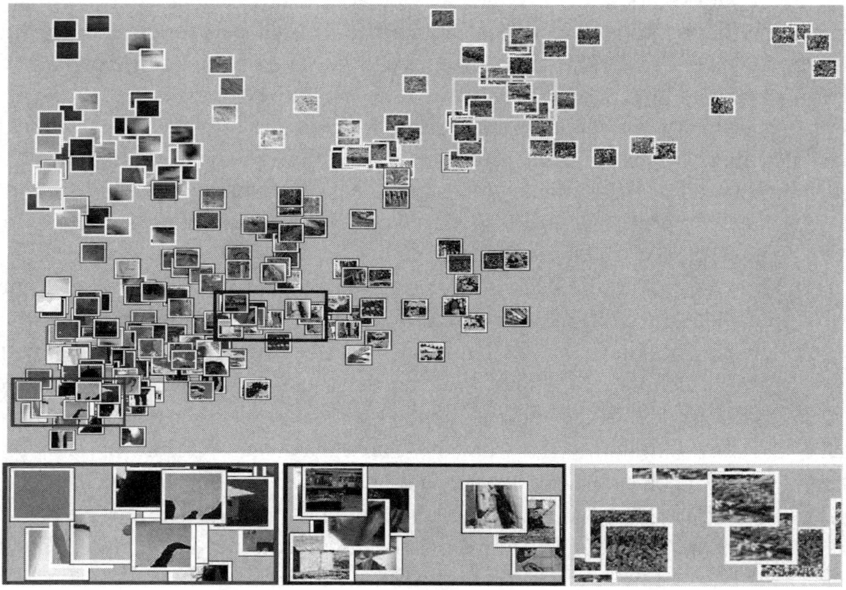

*Figure 13.3* Scatterplot of the Weibull parameters with contrast on horizontal and shape on vertical axes and each patch positioned at its respective value (after Yanulevskaya & Geusebroek, 2009). Images on the bottom left correspond to the power-law submodel. They contain uniform regions separated by strong edges. Patches in the middle part follow the exponential distribution showing smaller details. Two types of visual content demonstrate the Gaussian distribution: smooth patches with Gaussian-like noise (on the top left of the scatterplot) and patches with high frequency and contrast (on the top right and, as enlarged versions, in the bottom right inset).

This result can be expected, as local regions are likely to contain fewer edges and to have higher-frequency textures than the whole images. We compared eye fixation with the a priori baseline, as given by local analysis, using Weibull analysis of similarly sized local patches around eye fixation locations. Eye fixations were then 50% more likely to appear at power-law distributed patches than could be expected from local analysis. Furthermore, eye fixations were unlikely to appear at Gaussian distributed patches as they mainly exhibited low-contrast compression artifacts.

These findings were further exploited in eye fixation prediction, or equivalently salient region detection, by combining both the shape and contrast parameters of the Weibull distribution in a machine-learning approach. Eye fixation prediction has been related to simple statistics of several types of low-level image features, mainly related to contrast and local edge frequency. Due to the regularities in the statistics of natural images, many of these features are correlated. Given the abundantly present Weibull distribution in the statistics of such features for natural images, we study the local deviations of these statistics compared with "overall" image statistics over larger collections. These deviations become apparent when fitting the Weibull distribution to the local image (feature) data, and consecutively studying the distribution of the Weibull parameters over a single image in comparison to the parameter values found in a large set of natural images. The rough idea is that outliers in the parameters indicate a statistically salient image region with respect to "commonly" occurring image patches. In other words, regions are salient if their spatial statistics break with the generally observed statistics of natural scenes.

In detail, we consider the correlation between eye fixations and local image statistics, the latter being captured by the parameters of the Weibull distribution. Using eyetracking over a large collection of natural images and for many subjects, the probability distribution over Weibull parameters of fixated image regions can be measured. Knowing which locations have attracted attention, a complementary set of regions indicate the "nonfixated" regions, yielding a negative set of patches resulting in the Weibull parameter probability densities for "not-so-interesting" regions for human vision. Then, machine-learning techniques, such as logistic regression, can be devised to learn the distinction between fixated and nonfixated patches. Combined with purely bottom-up approaches, such as the method proposed by Itti and Koch (2000), a more adequate model for saliency prediction can be achieved.

This study illustrates an approach to active vision, which is a version of ecological optics long ago promulgated by James Jerome Gibson (1979). It is exclusively based on the measurement and statistical analysis of physical parameters of natural images. Indeed, it has often been suggested that eye guidance is mainly controlled by stimulus properties (Godijn & Theeuwes, 2002). Other authors consider saccadic target selection as being predominantly controlled by the task of the observer (Williams & Reingold, 2001). Recent observations revealed that task demands are of higher priority than low-level saliency features with respect to gaze behavior (Einhäuser, Rutishauser, & Koch, 2008). It was also suggested that a flexible combination of both approaches can properly account for the guidance of saccades (van Zoest & Donk, 2004; Ballard and Hayhoe, 2009).

## 13.3 Behavioral data analysis and interpretation

Since the earliest attempts, the interpretation of eye movement behavior has been mainly based on the analysis of fixations and saccades. In particular, analysis has been focused on parameters such as the duration and distribution of fixations, as well as the amplitude, velocity, and direction of saccades. However, as was already demonstrated by pioneers in this domain of research (e.g., Buswell, 1935; Yarbus, 1967), for the understanding of eye-movement behavior and the resulting perception, it is essential to consider also the inspected content, that is, text or image.

A promising approach to combine spatial and temporal characteristics of eye movements with the inspected material is the attentional landscape method introduced by Velichkovsky, Pomplun, and Rieser (1996). Instead of simply projecting the gaze tracking data on the original visual material, these authors proposed to elucidate the perception of ambiguous paintings (by Archimboldo, Dürer, and Escher) by rendering these pictures in terms of the distribution of visual fixations (see Figure 13.4). With this method it was possible to take into account both the saccadic suppression (i.e., a partial suppression of visual input between two fixations) and the fact that each fixation resolves only a narrow area of the visual scene. The limitations of visual spatial resolution were approximated by a Gaussian distribution with the standard deviation of 1 degree at each fixation point. In this way, it was possible to visualize when an observer perceived one or another version of ambiguous pictures (such as angels or devils in *Circle Limit IV* by Escher). The described attentional landscape approach is a step toward explicating the idiosyncratic perceptual experience of a person. It is nowadays a widely accepted instrument in usability research (e.g., Henderson, 2007; Wooding, 2002; Wooding, Mugglestone, Purdy, & Gale, 2002) and has also been used for an explication of the grounds for nonverbal decisions in clinical radiology (Burgert et al., 2007). Although the results of this approach look impressive, their interpretation is rather difficult and a statistical analysis of this type of information is complicated. An open question is whether the resulting visualization really says something about attention or just about fixation distributions.

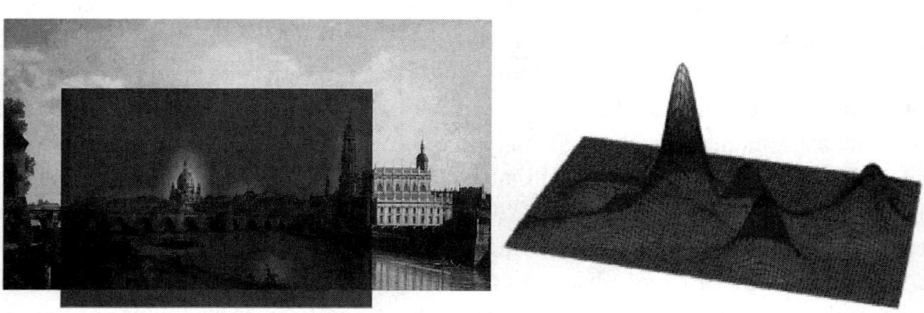

*Figure 13.4* An illustration of the attentional landscape approach with Canaletto's *View of Dresden* (copyright Gallery Alte Meister, Dresden, Germany) where the original painting is in the background, an empirically measured and computed *Fixation Map* is on the right, and the visualization is superimposed on the painting (image courtesy of Claudia Schmidt).

One critical issue is the equal treatment of all fixations for the creation of the attentional landscape visualizations. Beside task complexity and the intention of the observer, the quality and amount of visual information affect the duration of fixations. Mannan, Ruddock, and Wooding (1995) presented high- and lowpass-filtered and unfiltered photos and reported longest fixations for the lowpass-filtered scenes and shortest for the unfiltered material. With the development of the gaze contingent paradigm it became possible to manipulate regions of the presented text or scene according to the respective position of the eyes. For instance, van Diepen and d'Ydewalle (2003) used a gaze-contingent mask during visual search, preventing either foveal or peripheral processing of information. Prolonged fixations were reported for both manipulations, suggesting that both foveal and peripheral information modulate the lengths of fixations. During single fixations Loschky, McConkie, Yang, and Miller (2005) presented a multiresolutional display with high resolution at the fovea that decreased with eccentricity from the gaze center. Longer fixations were reported if the manipulation on the size of elements was perceivable.

Recently, evidence on qualitative differences in information processing during single fixations has been collected. It is known that the duration of fixations can be related to the level of cognitive processing (e.g., Velichkovsky, 2001) and therefore it seems to be implausible that all fixations would play the same role in active visual processing. In studies of eye movement behavior in static and dynamic environments, we found that a particular combination of fixation duration and amplitude of related saccades strongly correlates with the probability of correct recognition of objects and events (Velichkovsky, Rothert, Kopf, Dornhoefer, & Joos, 2002; Velichkovsky, Joos, Helmert, & Pannasch, 2005). According to these findings, a distinction is necessary between fixations serving the detailed processing of object features and those that are related to a dynamic spatial localization of the objects as undifferentiated blobs (*proto-objects*). Without consideration of this important difference in the modes of active vision, the representation produced in the attentional landscapes approach can only incorrectly reflect the perceptual process and perceived information.

Another critical issue in investigation of active vision is the influence of semantic and, in particular, social factors on human oculomotor activity. Even if the low-level saliency features are carefully controlled, one finds that facial area with eyes is the dominant attractor for human eye fixations (for an example, see Hari & Kujala, 2009). This tendency seems to persist also in nonhuman primates (Tomonaga & Imura, 2009). With a notable exception of autistic observers (Neumann, Spezio, Piven, & Adolphs, 2006), the eyes are always a very special target of attraction in our environment. The positions where eyes normally are in the scheme of face will be also fixated when there is no optical information on them in the physical image. These data illustrate one of the main functionalities of higher-order forms of visual attention, namely paying attention to the attention of another person (Velichkovsky, 1995). Overall, the results testify to the existence of a higher-order social saliency factor. The idea of joint attention states as the prerequisite for communicative and practical interaction of two persons is also manifested in an attentional emphasis on the objects of common interest. This Vygotskian idea is illustrated by some recent eyetracking studies, with one example shown in Figure 13.5.

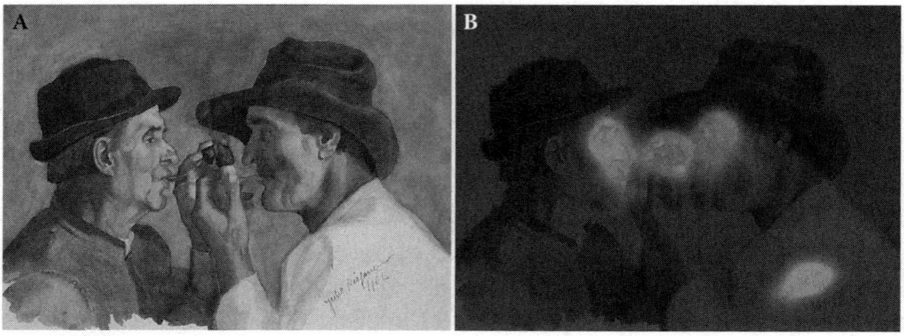


*Figure 13.5* A and B: typical distribution of gaze locations on a painting (*Lighting Pipes* by Juho Rissanen, 1902; copyright Ateneum Art Museum, Hannu Aaltonen, Finland). The fixation map is based on the data of 10 females and 10 males, who were allowed to view freely the image for 10 s (from Hari & Kujala, 2009; with permission of the publisher, *Physiological Reviews*).

Most of the current attempts aimed at understanding gaze control and mechanisms of visual processing in free viewing conditions come from the fields of experimental psychology and cognitive science. These studies often constrain themselves by the measurement and analyses on the behavioral level. To overcome these limitations and to reveal the underlying brain mechanisms, a broader interdisciplinary perspective is needed. For example, classical neuropsychological data demonstrate disturbances of active visual perception after frontal-lobe lesions (Luria, Karpov, & Yarbus, 1966). In nonhuman primates and other animals, invasive measuring procedures (e.g., single-cell recordings using implanted electrodes) are common and they are used also with complex natural images and realistic tasks (Cavanaugh & Wurtz, 2004; Maldonado, Babul, Singer, Rodriguez, Berger, & Grun, 2008). In human subjects, it would be beneficial to combine eyetracking with noninvasive neurophysiological measurements.

## 13.4 Active vision in human electrophysiology and neuroimaging

The idea to combine eyetracking with noninvasive methods of measuring human brain activity is not new. Several attempts have been made to analyze eye movements together with physiological techniques, such as EEG (electroencephalography) and MEG (magnetoencephalography). Two different strategies can be applied when using such a combination. Because eye movements produce strong electromagnetic signals, eyetracking is used to control for those movements to remove their influences on the brain signals of interest. The other possible approach follows the idea that eye movements are genuine components of visual cognition. The research question then would be to identify brain processes that are involved during different stages in the inspection of a scene, including single visual fixations. In this case the aim is to describe how visual perception works during natural vision and what are the underlying brain processes. However, each of the neurophysiological measuring techniques has its advantages and disadvantages, as discussed in the remainder of this chapter.

Measuring EEG is the oldest and most broadly used method for studying ongoing brain activity, not only during visual perception but also during rest and in a variety of other tasks. Current EEG technology allows the measurement of brain activity with high temporal resolution and relatively good spatial accuracy. Thus EEG could be a suitable method to study brain activations during natural viewing of scenes. However, the integration and simultaneous recordings of eye movements and EEG has been only rarely accomplished in the past. As a matter of fact, motility of the eyeballs is one of the critical sources of artifacts in EEG. Because the cornea is positively charged compared with the retina, the eye behaves as an electric dipole: each movement of the eyeball generates an electromagnetic field that is detected on the scalp (EEG) and outside the head (MEG; Hari, 2004). Because the eyes move about three times a second, this activity strongly influences the raw EEG signal, with amplitudes often being larger than the actual EEG signal of interest. Many mathematical approaches have been proposed in the past to eliminate the contaminating influences of the eye movements (e.g., Delorme, Sejnowski, & Makeig, 2007; Gratton, Coles, & Donchin, 1983; Vigário, Jousmäki, Hämäläinen, Hari, & Oja, 1997). Although these methods significantly contribute to the improvement of the signal, there are considerable limitations in their application as they either do not remove the artifacts completely or may filter out some signals of interest.

Yagi (1995) was one of the first to mention the possible benefits of combining eyetracking with EEG for the analysis of brain dynamics in more natural settings. He introduced the term "eye fixation related potential" (EFRP), which describes the method of analyzing the EEG signal as time locked to the occurrence of fixations. The main idea of this method is to structure the electrophysiological data according to the events of information uptake during active vision. Even if this approach does not completely solve the problem of eye-movement-related artifacts in the EEG data, it allows researchers to investigate brain activity and vision during more complex and natural tasks. Subsequently, the EEG data can be analyzed in a more controlled way, on a fixation-by-fixation basis. New approaches use eyetracking not only for offline experimental control and segmenting of the data, but also for online manipulation of independent variables, such as in gaze-contingent experiments, with simultaneous measurement of electrophysiological responses either to the fixated site as such or on a specially selected test stimulus (Baccino & Manunta, 2005; Graupner, Velichkovsky, Pannasch, & Marx, 2007). The latter paradigm may be the method of choice as it allows testing the visual system with a specified delay after the saccade and, in this way, to avoid much of the interference with electromagnetic contamination from the moving eyeballs.

Apart from electromagnetic artifacts caused by the eyes, other effects can be observed in the brain when the eyes move. The signals prior to, during, and after a saccade are related to the processes of saccade preparation and generation, signal transduction along the optic nerve, and information processing within the visual and other cortical areas. All these activities are of crucial interest for understanding the active vision. A number of interesting signals have been identified in the EFRPs.

Presumably the most prominent signal is the so-called *lambda response*, which is a scalp-positive EEG deflection peaking 80–100 ms after the offset of a saccade (Rémond, Lesèvre, & Torres, 1965; Yagi, 1979). The largest amplitude of this peak is usually observed at occipital electrode sites (Graupner et al., 2007). Some authors have argued that the lambda response is equivalent to the P100 deflection of conventional visual evoked potentials (VEPs), elicited by abrupt visual stimuli (Billings, 1989; Kazai & Yagi, 2003). This interpretation was supported by dipole tracing for the lambda and P100 response, showing similar source locations, presumably in the calcarine fissure (Kazai & Yagi, 2003). However, other results exist, reporting a very lambda-like response generated in the parieto-occipital sulcus after eye blinks and saccades (Hari, Salmelin, Tissari, Kajola, & Virsu, 1994; Jousmäki, Hämäläinen, & Hari, 1996; Kazai & Yagi, 2003). The peak amplitude of the lambda response was found to be correlated with the amplitude of the preceding saccade (Yagi, 1979). Similar to the P100 deflection, the lambda response depends on the physical aspects of stimulation, such as luminance, contrast, spatial frequency, and color. Another component of an EFRP is the spike potential (Becker, Hoehne, Iwase, & Kornhuber, 1972), a scalp-negative deflection peaking 8–20 ms prior to the onset of a saccade. It likely results from synchronous firing of the motoneurons of ocular muscles (Riemslag, Van der Heijde, Van Dongen, & Ottenhoff, 1988; Thickbroom & Mastaglia, 1985). Additionally, characteristic EEG patterns have been reported in relation to the programming and execution of saccades (Evdokimidis, Smyrnis, Constantinidis, Gourtzelidis, & Papageorgiou, 2001; Skrandies & Laschke, 1997).

For a comparison of two sets of fixations, all these contributing factors need to be considered. For example, disregarding the matching of the saccadic amplitudes prior to the fixation will result in a systematic bias with respect to the lamda/P100 amplitudes (Yagi, 1979) which also might affect later EFRP components (N100, P200, etc.). Similar effects must be expected also for the subsequent saccade if not matched accordingly. However, due to a high variability of fixation durations during natural visual exploration, such influences of the subsequent saccades might be less pronounced because of temporal smearing. Differences in fixation duration between the two datasets can introduce additional bias because the onset of the following saccade will systematically vary.

Still another influencing factor in paradigms studying active vision has to be mentioned. It concerns the lack of control on the temporal and spatial distribution of fixations, that is, when in the course of scene inspection a particular object or region is fixated. When two subjects freely observe the same natural scene, two rather different sets of fixation may arise with respect to the *when* and *what* of the gaze pattern. Thus, image statistics of the fixated spots, such as local contrast, spatial frequency, luminance, and color might be different for the two sets of fixations which will also influence the obtained EFRP. Even if the eyetracking data enable researchers to gain this information during an experiment either online or offline, it is still an open question of how these details of the efficient sensory stimulation can be integrated in the data analysis. In any case, considering the mentioned points is mandatory for a proper interpretation of results.

The problem of eye-movement-related artifacts in EEG recordings does not only apply to the investigation of natural viewing of scenes. The relevance of such influences has been recently reported in a study with parallel recording of EEG and eye movements where subjects had to perform a simple object identification task. It was shown that some gamma-band activity in the EEG signal is highly correlated with the onset of saccades (Yuval-Greenberg, Tomer, Keren, Nelken, & Deouell, 2008). The authors explained this finding by the spike potentials that accompany the saccade onsets. That means that even in simple visual tasks eye movement behavior may vary systematically with the investigated conditions and its outcome on the EEG signal may translate into apparent but not always meaningful differences in the results.

A complementary approach to the eletrophysiological EFRP (EEG) and EFRF (MEG; the last F to refer to magnetic field) measurements is fixation-based event-related fMRI (FIBER fMRI; see Cornelissen, Marsman, Renken, & Velichkovsky, 2008). This is a perspective of deriving brain activation patterns related to rapid human visual behavior from a slow blood-oxygenation-level-dependent (BOLD) fMRI response. Until the present, fixations have not been considered as events of primary interest in neuroimaging studies. Nevertheless, we have been able to identify differences in brain activity, following different types of fixations in either viewing task or object inspected. Specifically, we investigated the processing of visual information following fixations made during natural viewing behavior. In the following, we briefly present results from a recent fMRI experiment, where subjects' gaze was recorded to control actual visual fixations to build a marker event for the FIBER fMRI analysis in three conditions: free viewing and two versions of instructed viewing, one of which emphasized looking at faces and another at houses. Figure 13.6 shows the stimulus display and other relevant aspects of the study.

First of all, two well-documented brain regions in correspondence with our stimuli—fusiform face area (FFA) and parahippocampal place area (PPA) bilaterally (Epstein, Harris, Stanley, & Kanwisher, 1999; Kanwisher, McDermott, & Chun, 1997)—were identified in every subject by standard localizer experiments. Furthermore, in the main series of experiments, distinguishable features between the BOLD responses following fixations were elicited. The result was achieved by reconstructing the hemodynamic response functions for each type of fixation in three task conditions.

In all cases, the BOLD response peaked around 3 seconds, which is a shorter latency than is commonly reported in conventional fMRI studies (Buckner, 1998). It is apparent that fixations during which houses were inspected (either in a specific house-viewing task or during free exploration of the stimuli) result in larger activation of PPA. FFA becomes active when faces were inspected under comparable conditions. At the same time, it seems that FFA is also active during house viewing in the face-viewing task. During free viewing the difference in activations of house and face fixations becomes more distinct in PPA in comparison with FFA activation. FFA does not differentiate between houses and faces on the basis of the amplitude of the response, even though the responses are still differently shaped. A distinction between the conditions is the existence of a double peak effect, specifically

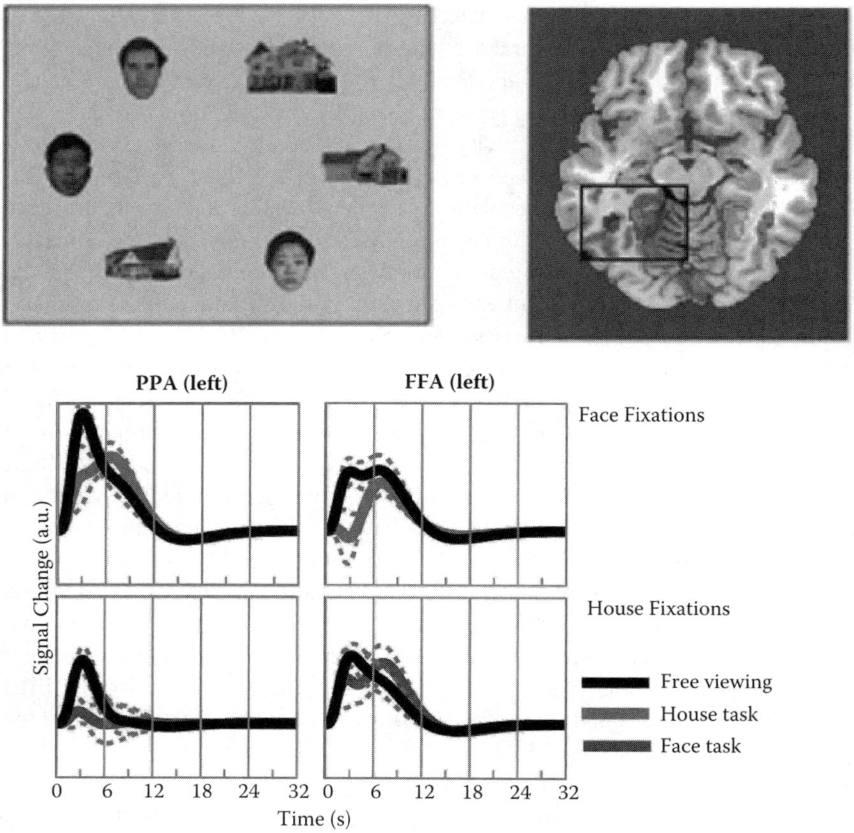


*Figure 13.6 (See color insert.)* Top left: Example stimulus. Top right: Investigated brain regions, FFA (blue) and PPA (red), left hemisphere activations are within the rectangle. Bottom: Estimated hemodynamic responses for fixations toward houses (upper row) and faces (underside row) in left FFA (left column) and left PPA (right column). Colors indicate task; dashed lines denote standard error of the mean. Vertical axes show percentages of the mean whole-brain signal.

visible during instructed (i.e., explicitly task-related) viewing compared with free viewing. Hence, we argue that this can be a task-related effect that is driven by repeated stimulation. The conclusion was corroborated by multivoxel pattern analyses (MVPA; Norman, Polyn, Detre, & Haxby, 2006) where we were able to classify the signals significantly above chance level according to the inspected object and the task. Interestingly, we found that classification of both house and face tasks is more efficient than classification of free viewing items.

These results demonstrate that brain-activity analyses can in an important respect enhance the behavioral analysis of eye movement data, namely to reveal the nature of the task at hand beyond simply showing—as eyetracking studies often do—which object or region of the image is currently fixated. We have shown that fMRI analysis based on fixations reveals meaningful spatiotemporal patterns of brain activation despite the suboptimal temporal characteristics of visual fixations and saccades with respect to hemodynamics in the brain. These findings open new paths to explore natural viewing behavior in the fMRI analysis of human brain activity. However, they also demonstrate the importance and benefits of combining neurocognitive methods and eyetracking for the control of experiments as well as for a better interpretation of the data.

## 13.5 Conclusion and outlook

As an interdisciplinary endeavor, further insights into brain mechanisms of human active vision will demand continuous efforts of experts from different domains of research. In this chapter, we illustrated the scope of relevant measurement problems by three groups of studies ranging from classical physical to psychological and neurobiological investigation. None of these approaches is nowadays completely satisfying and free of potential critical comments. However, in such a thorny field of measurement as active vision the old methodological principle of converging operations (Garner, Hake, & Eriksen, 1956) might be the best strategy. By using complementary, albeit imperfect instruments it is still possible to reach some reasonable conclusions. Several recent examples demonstrate the successful *transmethodical* convergence in studies of active vision, such as elucidation of mechanisms of global versus local processing (Cant, Arnott, & Goodale, 2009), investigation of visual attention as expressed in the patterns of eye movements (Velichkovsky et al., 2005), and "social salience" in cognitive-affective neuroscience (Hari & Kujala, 2009).

In the years to come, innovative research on visual perception and eye movements will be supported by new technological solutions and include new interdisciplinary directions. Beside the further improvement of existing measurement techniques (based on hard- or software achievements) there will be the development of new methods. For instance, the emerging method of magnetic induction tomography (MIT; Korjenevsky, Cherepenin, & Sapetsky, 2000; Vauhkonen, Hamsch, & Igney, 2008) aims at mapping the local distribution of the electrical conductivity inside the brain. Eddy currents are induced in the body by relatively weak magnetic stimulation and the resulting fields are measured by an array of receiver coils.

Moreover, the basic biochemical nature of the brain's wetware and neurotransmitters is assumed to become more influential in the future. The paradigmatic changes are motivated by the design of new applications and services under the influence of increasingly fast convergence of nano-, bio-, and information technologies with cognitive science (for a review, see Bainbridge & Roco, 2006). Such a *trans-technological* convergence could explode in the number of studies devoted to genetic and epigenetic mechanisms of human visual processing and cognition. In a middle-term perspective, new molecular methods of measurement will emerge based on the use of nano-sized sensors and dyes, such as in quantum-dots technology. Of course, before this quantum leap in investigation with human subjects will become a reality, much tighter safety problems have to be solved than in the case of the video-based eyetracking devices.

## Acknowledgment

Thanks are due to Birgitta Berglund, Jens R. Helmert, Alexander Kaplan, Fiona Mulvey, Joel Norman, Remco Renken, and Claudia Schmidt for their help in preparation of the manuscript. Our research was supported by grants from the European Commission (NEST-Pathfinder projects PERCEPT 043261 and MINET 043297, Network of Excellence COGAIN 511598), the Russian Foundation for Basic Research (Ofi-m 09-02-12222 and 09-06-12003), the Russian Ministry of Education and Science (P1265), and ERC Advanced Grant #232946.

## References

Baccino, T., & Manunta, Y. (2005). Eye-fixation-related potentials: Insight into parafoveal processing. *Journal of Psychophysiology, 19*(3), 204–215.

Bahill, A. T., Clark, M. R., & Stark, L. (1975). The main sequence, a tool for studying human eye movements. *Mathematical Biosciences, 24*(3–4), 191–204.

Bainbridge, W. S., & Roco, M. C. (2006). *Managing nano-bio-info-cogno innovations: Converging technologies for improving human performance*. Dordrecht: Springer.

Ballard, D. H., & Hayhoe, M. M. (2009). Modelling the role of task in the control of gaze. *Visual Cognition, 17*(6/7), 1185–1204.

Bates, R., Donegan, M., Istance, H. O., Hansen, J. P., & Räihä, K.-J. (2007). Introducing COGAIN: Communication by gaze interaction. *Universal Access in the Information Society, 6*(2), 159–166.

Becker, W., Hoehne, O., Iwase, K., & Kornhuber, H. H. (1972). Readiness potential, pre-motor positivity and other changes of cortical potential in saccadic eye movements. *Vision Research, 12*(3), 421–436.

Billings, R. J. (1989). The origin of the occipital lambda wave in man. *Electroencephalography and Clinical Neurophysiology, 72*(2), 95–113.

Buckner, R. L. (1998). Event-related fMRI and the hemodynamic response. *Human Brain Mapping, 6*, 373–377.

Burgert, O., Örn, V., Velichkovsky, B. M., Gessat, M., Joos, M., Straub, G., Tietjen, C., Preim, B., & Hertel, I. (2007). Evaluation of perception performance in neck dissection planning using eye tracking and attention landscapes. In Jiorg, Y. & Sahiner, B. (Eds.). *Medical imaging 2007: Image perception, observer performance, and technology assessment*. Proceedings Vol. 6515, Article No. 65150B.

Buswell, G. T. (1935). *How people look at pictures*. Chicago: University of Chicago Press.

Cant, J., Arnott, S., & Goodale, M. (2009). FMRI-adaptation reveals separate processing regions for the perception of form and texture in the human ventral stream. *Experimental Brain Research, 192*, 391–405.

Cavanaugh, J., & Wurtz, R. H. (2004). Subcortical modulation of attention counters change blindness. *Journal of Neuroscience, 24*(50), 11236–11243.

Collewijn, H., & Kowler, E. (2008). The significance of microsaccades for vision and oculomotor control. *Journal of Vision, 8*(14), 1–21.

Cornelissen, F. W., Marsman, J. B. C., Renken, R., & Velichkovsky, B. M. (2008). Predicting gaze behavior and cognitive task from cortical activity: A fixation based event related (FIBER) fMRI study. *Proceeding of the Third Biennial Conference on Cognitive Science* (pp. 553–557), Moscow: Science.

DeAngelus, M., & Pelz, J. B. (2009). Top-down control of eye movements: Yarbus revisited. *Visual Cognition, 17*(6/7), 790–811.

Delorme, A., Sejnowski, T., & Makeig, S. (2007). Enhanced detection of artifacts in EEG data using higher-order statistics and independent component analysis. *Neuroimage, 34*(4), 1443–1449.

Dodge, R. (1900). Visual perception during eye movement. *Psychological Review, 7*, 454–465.

Einhäuser, W., Rutishauser, U., & Koch, C. (2008). Task-demands can immediately reverse the effects of sensory-driven saliency in complex visual stimuli. *Journal of Vision, 8*(2), 1–19.

Epstein, R., Harris, A., Stanley, D., & Kanwisher, N. (1999). The parahippocampal place area: Recognition, navigation, or encoding? *Neuron, 23*, 115–125.

Evdokimidis, I., Smyrnis, N., Constantinidis, T. S., Gourtzelidis, P., & Papageorgiou, C. (2001). Frontal-parietal activation differences observed before the execution of remembered saccades: An event-related potentials study. *Cognitive Brain Research, 12*(1), 89–99.

Findlay, J. M. (1998). Active vision: Visual activity in everyday life. *Current Biology, 8*(18), R640–R642.

Fischer, M. H. (1999). An investigation of attention allocation during sequential eye movement tasks. *The Quarterly Journal of Experimental Psychology: Human Experimental Psychology, 3*, 649–677.

Garner, W. R., Hake, H. W., & Eriksen, C. W. (1956). Operationalism and the concept of perception. *Psychological Review, 63*, 149–159.

Geisler, W. S. (2008). Visual perception and the statistical properties of natural scenes. *Annual Review of Psychology, 59*, 167–192.

Geusebroek, J. M., & Smeulders, A. W. M. (2005). A six-stimulus theory for stochastic texture. *International Journal of Computer Vision, 62*(1–2), 7–16.

Gibson, J. J. (1979). *An ecological approach to visual perception*. Boston: Houghton Mifflin.

Godijn, R., & Theeuwes, J. (2002). Programming of endogenous and exogenous saccades: Evidence for a competitive integration model. *Journal of Experimental Psychology: Human Perception & Performance, 28*(5), 1039–1054.

Goldberg, M. E., & Hudspeth, A. J. (2000). The vestibular system In E. R. Kandel, J. H. Schwartz, & T. M. Jessell (Eds.), *Principles of neural science* (4th ed., pp. 801–815). New York: McGraw-Hill.

Gratton, G., Coles, M. G., & Donchin, E. (1983). A new method for off-line removal of ocular artifact. *Electroencephalography and Clinical Neurophysiology, 55*(4), 468–484.

Graupner, S.-T., Velichkovsky, B. M., Pannasch, S., & Marx, J. (2007). Surprise, surprise: Two distinct components in the visually evoked distractor effect. *Psychophysiology, 44*(2), 251–261.

Greene, M. R., & Oliva, A. (2009). Recognition of natural scenes from global properties: Seeing the forest without representing the trees. *Cognitive Psychology, 58*(2), 137–176.

Guestrin, E. D., & Eizenman, M. (2006). General theory of remote gaze estimation using the pupil center and corneal reflections. *IEEE Transactions on Biomedical Engineering, 53*(6), 1124–1133.

Hari, R. (2004). Magnetoencephalography in clinical neurophysiological assessment of human cortical functions. In E. Niedermeyer & F. Lopes da Silva (Eds.), *Electroencephalography: Basic principles, clinical applications, and related fields* (5th ed., pp. 1165–1197). New York: Lippincott; Williams & Wilkins.

Hari, R., & Kujala, M. V. (2009). Brain basis of human social interaction: From concepts to brain imaging. *Physiological Reviews, 89*(2), 453–479.

Hari, R., Salmelin, R., Tissari, S., Kajola, M., & Virsu, V. (1994). Visual stability during eye-blinks. *Nature, 367*, 121–122.

Hayhoe, M., & Ballard, D. (2005). Eye movements in natural behavior. *Trends in Cognitive Sciences, 9*(4), 188–194.

Henderson, J. M. (2007). Regarding scenes. *Current Directions in Psychological Science, 16*(4), 219–222.

Henderson, J. M., Weeks, P. A., & Hollingworth, A. (1999). The effects of semantic consistency on eye movements during complex scene viewing. *Journal of Experimental Psychology: Human Perception & Performance, 25*(1), 210–228.

Itti, L., & Koch, C. (2000). A saliency-based search mechanism for overt and covert shifts of visual attention. *Vision Research, 40*(10–12), 1489–1506.

Jousmäki, V., Hämäläinen, M., & Hari, R. (1996). Magnetic source imaging during a visually guided saccade task. *NeuroReport 1996, 7*, 2961–2964.

Just, M. A., & Carpenter, P. A. (1976). Eye fixations and cognitive processes. *Cognitive Psychology, 8*(4), 441–480.

Just, M. A., & Carpenter, P. A. (1980). A theory of reading: From eye fixations to comprehension. *Psychological Review, 87*(4), 329–354.

Kanwisher, N., McDermott, J., & Chun, M. M. (1997). The fusiform face area: A module in human extrastriate cortex specialized for face perception. *Journal of Neuroscience, 17*(11), 4302–4311.

Karklin, Y., & Lewicki, M. S. (2009). Emergence of complex cell properties by learning to generalize in natural scenes. *Nature, 457*, 83–86.

Kazai, K., & Yagi, A. (2003). Comparison between the lambda response of eye-fixation-related potentials and the P100 component of pattern-reversal visual evoked potentials. *Cognitive, Affective, & Behavioral Neuroscience, 3*(1), 46–56.

Koffka, K. (1935). *Principles of gestalt psychology*. New York: Harcourt.

Korjenevsky, A., Cherepenin, V., & Sapetsky, S. (2000). Magnetic induction tomography: Experimental realization. *Physiological Measurement, 21*(1), 89–94.

Land, M. F. (2004). The coordination of rotations of the eyes, head and trunk in saccadic turns produced in natural situations. *Experimental Brain Research, 159*(2), 151–160.

Lencer, R., & Trillenberg, P. (2008). Neurophysiology and neuroanatomy of smooth pursuit in humans. *Brain and Cognition, 68*(3), 219–228.

Loschky, L. C., McConkie, G. W., Yang, J., & Miller, M. E. (2005). The limits of visual resolution in natural scene viewing. *Visual Cognition, 12*(6), 1057–1092.

Luria, A. R., Karpov, B. A., & Yarbus, A. L. (1966). Disturbances of active visual perception with lesions of the frontal lobe. *Cortex, 2*, 202–212.

Maldonado, P. E., Babul, C. M., Singer, W., Rodriguez, E., Berger, D., & Grun, S. (2008). Synchronization of neuronal responses in primary visual cortex of monkeys viewing natural images. *Journal of Neurophysiology, 100*, 1523–1532.

Mannan, S., Ruddock, K. H., & Wooding, D. S. (1995). Automatic control of saccadic eye movements made in visual inspection of briefly presented 2-D images. *Spatial Vision, 9,* 363–386.

Mulvey, F., Villanueva, A., Sliney, D., Lange, R., Cotmore, S., & Donegan, M. (2008). Exploration of safety issues in eyetracking. In Communication by Gaze Interaction, IST-2003-511598: Retrieved from http://www.cogain.org/results/reports/COGAIN-D5.4.pdf

Neumann, D., Spezio, M. L., Piven, J., & Adolphs, R. (2006). Looking you in the mouth: Abnormal gaze in autism resulting from impaired top-down modulation of visual attention. *Social Cognitive and Affective Neuroscience, 1*, 194–202.

Norman, K. A., Polyn, S. M., Detre, G. J., & Haxby, J. V. (2006). Beyond mind-reading: Multi-voxel pattern analysis of fMRI data. *Trends in Cognitive Sciences, 10*(9), 424–430.

Pannasch, S., Helmert, J. R., Velichkovsky, B. M., Malischke, S., & Storch, A. (2008). Eye typing in application: A comparison of two systems with ALS patients. *Journal of Eye Movement Research, 2*(4), 1–8.

Pelli, D. G., & Tillman, K. A. (2008). The uncrowded window of object recognition. *Nature Neuroscience, 11*(10), 1129–1135.

Rayner, K. (1978). Eye movements in reading and information processing. *Psychological Bulletin, 85*(3), 618–660.

Rémond, A., Lesèvre, N., & Torres, F. (1965). Etude chrono-topographique de l'activité occipitale moyenne recueillie sur le scalp chez l'homme en relation avec les déplacements du regard (complexe lambda) [Chrono-topographic study of middle occipital activity recorded on the scalp in humans in relation to eye movements (lambda complex)]. *Revue Neurologique, 113*(3), 193–226.

Riemslag, F. C., Van der Heijde, G. L., Van Dongen, M. M., & Ottenhoff, F. (1988). On the origin of the presaccadic spike potential. *Electroencephalography and Clinical Neurophysiology, 70*(4), 281–287.

Scholte, H. S., Ghebreab, S., Waldorp, L., Smeulders, A. W. M., & Lamme, V. A. F. (2009). Brain responses strongly correlate with Weibull image statistics when processing natural images. *Journal of Vision, 9*(4), 29.

Shebilske, W. (1975). Reading eye movements from an information processing point of view. In D. Massaro (Ed.), *Understanding language* (pp. 291–311). New York: Academic Press.

Shih, S. W., & Liu, J. (2004). A novel approach to 3-D gaze tracking using stereo cameras. *IEEE Transactions on Systems Man and Cybernetics Part B-Cybernetics, 34*(1), 234–245.

Skrandies, W., & Laschke, K. (1997). Topography of visually evoked brain activity during eye movements: Lambda waves, saccadic suppression, and discrimination performance. *International Journal of Psychophysiology, 27*(1), 15–27.

Stratton, G. M. (1906). Symmetry, linear illusions, and the movements of the eye. *Psychological Review, 13*(2), 82–96.

Thickbroom, G. W., & Mastaglia, F. L. (1985). Presaccadic 'spike' potential: Investigation of topography and source. *Brain Research, 339*(2), 271–280.

Tomonaga, M., & Imura, T. (2009). Faces capture the visuospatial attention of chimpanzees (*Pan troglodytes*): Evidence from a cueing experiment. *Frontiers in Zoology, 6*, 14–27.

van Diepen, P. M. J., & d'Ydewalle, G. (2003). Early peripheral and foveal processing in fixations during scene perception. *Visual Cognition, 10*(1), 79–100.

van Zoest, W., & Donk, M. (2004). Bottom-up and top-down control in visual search. *Perception, 33*(8), 927–937.

Vaughan, J. (1982). Control of fixation duration in visual search and memory search: Another look. *Journal of Experimental Psychology: Human Perception & Performance, 8*(5), 709–723.

Vauhkonen, M., Hamsch, M., & Igney, C. H. (2008). A measurement system and image reconstruction in magnetic induction tomography. *Physiological Measurement, 29*(6), 445–454.

Velichkovsky, B. M. (1995). Communicating attention: Gaze position transfer in cooperative problem solving. *Pragmatics and Cognition, 3*(2), 199–222.

Velichkovsky, B. M. (1999). From levels of processing to stratification of cognition: Converging evidence from three domains of research. In B. H. Challis & B. M. Velichkovsky (Eds.), *Stratification in cognition and consciousness* (pp. 203–235). Amsterdam: John Benjamins.

Velichkovsky, B. M. (2001). Levels of processing: Validating the concept. In M. Naveh-Benjamin, M. Moscovitch, & H. L. Roediger III (Eds.), *Perspectives on human memory and cognitive aging: Essays in honour of Fergus I.M. Craik* (pp. 48–71). Philadelphia: Psychology Press.

Velichkovsky, B. M., Joos, M., Helmert, J. R., & Pannasch, S. (2005). Two visual systems and their eye movements: Evidence from static and dynamic scene perception. In B. G. Bara, L. Barsalou, & M. Bucciarelli (Eds.), *Proceedings of the XXVII Conference of the Cognitive Science Society* (pp. 2283–2288). Mahwah, NJ: Lawrence Erlbaum.

Velichkovsky, B. M., Pomplun, M., & Rieser, H. (1996). Attention and communication: Eye-movement-based research paradigms. In W. H. Zangemeister, H. S. Stiel, & C. Freksa (Eds.), *Attention and cognition* (pp. 125–154). Amsterdam: Elsevier.

Velichkovsky, B. M., Rothert, A., Kopf, M., Dornhoefer, S. M., & Joos, M. (2002). Towards an express diagnostics for level of processing and hazard perception. *Transportation Research, Part F, 5*(2), 145–156.

Vigário, R., Jousmäki, V., Hämäläinen, M., Hari, R., & Oja, E. (1997). Independent component analysis for identification of artifacts in magnetoencephalographic recordings. In M. I. Jordan, M. J. Kearns, & S. A. Solla (Eds.), *Advances on neural information processing systems* (Vol. 10, pp. 229–235). Cambridge, MA: MIT Press.

von Wartburg, R., Wurtz, P., Pflugshaupt, T., Nyffeler, T., Lüthi, M., & Müri, R. (2007). Size matters: Saccades during scene perception. *Perception, 36*(3), 355–365.

Wade, N. J., & Tatler, B. W. (2005). *The moving tablet of the eye: The origins of modern eye movement research.* Oxford: Oxford University Press.

Williams, D. E., & Reingold, E. M. (2001). Preattentive guidance of eye movements during triple conjunction search tasks: The effects of feature discriminability and saccadic amplitude. *Psychonomic Bulletin & Review, 8*(3), 476–488.

Wooding, D. S. (2002). Eye movements of large populations: II. Deriving regions of interest, coverage, and similarity using fixation maps. *Behavior Research Methods, Instruments, & Computers, 34*(4), 518–528.

Wooding, D. S., Mugglestone, M. D., Purdy, K. J., & Gale, A. G. (2002). Eye movements of large populations: I. Implementation and performance of an autonomous public eye tracker. *Behavior Research Methods Instruments & Computers, 34*(4), 509–517.

Yagi, A. (1979). Saccade size and lambda complex in man. *Physiological Psychology, 7*(4), 370–376.

Yagi, A. (1995). Eye fixation-related potential as an index of visual function. In T. Kikuch, H. Sakuma, I. Saito, & T. Tsuboi (Eds.), *Biobehavioral self-regulation* (Vol. 32, pp. 177–181). Tokyo: Springer-Verlag.

Yanulevskaya, V., & Geusebroek, J. M. (2009). Significance of the Weibull distribution and its sub-models in natural image statistics. *Visapp 2009: Proceedings of the Fourth International Conference on Computer Vision Theory and Applications, 1*, 355–362.

Yarbus, A. L. (1967). *Eye movements and vision.* New York: Plenum Press.

Yuval-Greenberg, S., Tomer, O., Keren, A. S., Nelken, I., & Deouell, L. Y. (2008). Transient induced gamma-band response in EEG as a manifestation of miniature saccades. *Neuron, 58*(3), 429–441.

Zingale, C. M., & Kowler, E. (1987). Planning sequences of saccades. *Vision Research, 27*(8), 1327–1341.

# 14 Electrical and functional brain imaging

*Pasquale Anthony Della Rosa and Daniela Perani*

Department of Neuroscience
Università Vita Salute San Raffaele
Milan, Italy

## 14.1 Introduction

In the fourth century BC, Hippocrates wrote

> Men ought to know that from nothing else but the brain comes joys, delights, laughter and sports, and sorrows, griefs, despondency and lamentations. And by this, in an especial manner, we acquire wisdom and knowledge .... And by the same organ we become mad and delirious, and fears and terrors assail us .... All these things we endure from the brain when it is not healthy .... In these ways, I am of the opinion that the brain exercises the greatest power in the man. (trans. 1972)

The history of our quest to understand the brain is certainly as long as human history itself. In the early 1900s, Walter Dandy introduced a process called pneumoencephalography that involved draining the cerebrospinal fluid from around the brain and replacing it with air, altering the relative density of the brain and its surroundings, to cause it to show up better on an X-ray. This technique carried significant risks to the patient under investigation; however, the surgical information given by this method was remarkably precise and greatly enlarged the capabilities and accuracy of neurosurgical treatment. At the beginning of the 1970s the advent of modern neuroimaging techniques brought about a radical change in the application of methods and instruments to assess and quantify brain–behavior relationships.

Magnetic resonance imaging (MRI) and computed tomography (CT) were developed in the 1970s and 1980s. For the first time, the brain anatomy appeared in vivo with a great power in structural details. Next came SPECT and PET scans, which allowed scientists to map brain function because, unlike MRI and CT, these scans could create more than just static images of the structures in the brain. These functional imaging in vivo techniques can provide physicians and scientists with several molecular parameters such as brain perfusion and metabolism, receptor density, neurotransmitters, and enzyme activity, measurements only partially available in post mortem specimens before the advent of these techniques.

MRI and PET scanning established a milestone from which scientists were able to develop functional MRI (fMRI) providing the possibility to "directly" observe cognitive activities and quantify them. In recent years, neurophysiological and functional neuroimaging techniques have provided measures of brain activity that have increased our ability to study the neural basis and the cerebral organization of sensorimotor and cognitive brain functions. These techniques fall roughly into two classes: the electromagnetic approach measuring brain activity directly by recording the electromagnetic fields generated by certain neuronal populations and the hemodynamic approach estimating brain activity by detecting blood-dependent changes indirectly coupled with modifications in neural activity. These methods differ in a number of aspects among which are the prerequisites for detecting a signal, the homogeneity with which neural activity is sampled from different parts of the brain, and more importantly the relative accuracy in determining *when* versus *where* neural activity takes place. These two approaches, therefore, provide complementary views of neural activity and the deep insight we gained about brain function in the last two decades largely derives from scientific studies employing these two techniques.

In this chapter, we illustrate the essentials of both types of approaches and how they may be employed to measure the relationship between the brain and cognitive activities which rule our behavior in everyday life.

## 14.2 When does brain activity occur?

### *14.2.1 Electroencephalogram (EEG) and brain rhythms*

Electroencephalography is a medical imaging technique that reads scalp electrical activity generated by brain structures. The electroencephalogram (EEG) is defined as electrical activity of an alternating type recorded from the scalp surface after being picked up by metal electrodes. Thus electroencephalographic measurement is a completely noninvasive procedure that can be applied repeatedly to patients, healthy adults, and children with virtually no risk or limitation. When neurons are activated, local current flows are produced. EEG measures mostly the currents that flow during synaptic excitations of the dendrites of many pyramidal neurons in the cerebral cortex.

Differences in electrical potentials are caused by summed postsynaptic graded potentials from pyramidal cells that create electrical dipoles between soma (body of neuron) and apical dendrites (neural branches) and weak electrical signals detected by the scalp electrodes are massively amplified, and stored in computer memory. Between the electrodes and neuronal layers current penetrates through skin, skull, and several other layers allowing only the electrical activity generated by large populations of active neurons to be detected and recorded on the head surface. Due to the capability of reflecting both normal and abnormal electrical activity of the brain, EEG has been found to be a very powerful tool in the field of neurology and clinical neurophysiology and indeed in the domain of cognitive neuroscience. With respect to the latter, the number of neurons that discharge synchronously is captured, in a physiological sense, by the EEG "power," which is assumed to be a

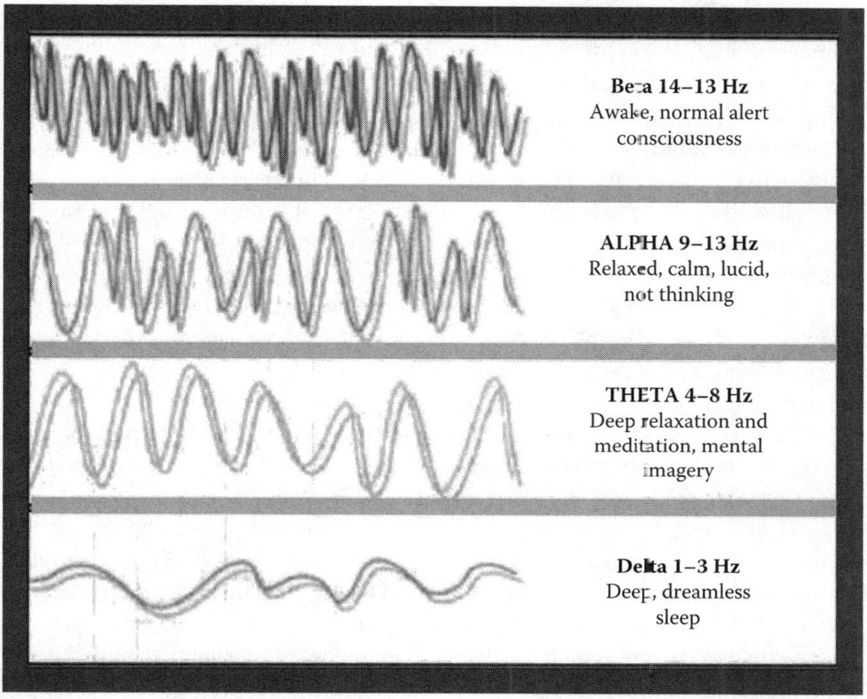


*Figure 14.1* Brainwave frequencies measured with EEG: beta waves (14-30 Hz) are seen during attention to task and focus; alpha waves (9-13 Hz), an idling rhythm, seen during relaxation and meditation; theta waves (4-8 Hz), seen in the dreamlike state between sleep & wakefulness; delta waves (1-3 Hz) occur primarily during sleep.

measure that reflects the capacity or performance of cortical information processing. EEG power can be measured in different frequency ranges (e.g., alpha, beta, gamma, or theta waves; see Figure 14.1), however, the best-known and most extensively studied frequency of activity in the human brain is the normal alpha rhythm.

Alpha activity is induced by closing the eyes and by relaxation, and reduced by eye opening or alerting by any mechanism (thinking, calculating). Since the work of Berger (1929) it was suggested that visual or other sensory task demands, specifically visual attention, are the primary factors that induce a suppression of the alpha rhythm (Mulholland, 1969; Ray & Cole, 1985). An individual brain operation relies upon the formation of functionally interconnected neurons in large neuronal assemblies in order to be carried out. The underlying mechanism is the synchronization of neurons characterized by a rhythmical pattern. When a neuronal assembly is set up a rhythmical increase in the total potential occurs, whereas a disruption of the neuronal assembly induces a decrease in total potential.

Alpha is the dominant frequency in the human scalp EEG of adults and due to its property of being an oscillatory component of the human EEG it has led to the development of techniques such as event-related desynchronization (ERD), capable of inducing changes in EEG alpha activity associated with sensory or task manipulations. The phasic structure of alpha activity refers to the alterations of synchronization and desynchronization periods and reflecting the formation and disruption of cortical neuronal assemblies, respectively. In this framework, periods of alpha synchronization and desynchronization do not indicate episodes of "rest state" and "active work," respectively, but are markers of two types of cortical processing equally active which differ only in the way the neighboring neurons are used.

In using ERD (Pfurtscheller & Aranibar, 1977), a typical example of an EEG epoch may come from a task in which subjects were asked to read a visually presented word and to make a semantic judgment by responding yes to a word denoting a living object and no to a word denoting a nonliving object (Klimesch, Doppelmayr, Pachinger, & Russegger, 1997). A warning signal was presented immediately preceding the word and subjects had to judge the words.

During the first second of the epoch, namely the "reference interval," the subjects showed pronounced rhythmic alpha activity. After subjects were presented with many trials, the anticipation of the warning signal already led alpha to desynchronize even before the actual signal appeared (see Figure 14.2).

The basic principle for measuring ERD is that a typical phasic change occurs in the alpha rhythm over the time course of a trial. After a response, the subject relaxes and waits for the next stimulus to come up. During this state of relaxed but alert wakefulness the brain idles, highlighting a pronounced alpha activity during the reference interval before each trial. Even before the warning signal actually appears, the alpha rhythm becomes suppressed, because the subject prepares and anticipates the beginning of the next trial. If alpha suppression is regarded as a marker of desynchronization, it would indicate that large populations of neurons no longer oscillate in synchrony while information is processed.

Thus, ERD can be calculated as the percentage of a band power change while performing a specific task with respect to a reference or resting interval (Pfurtscheller &

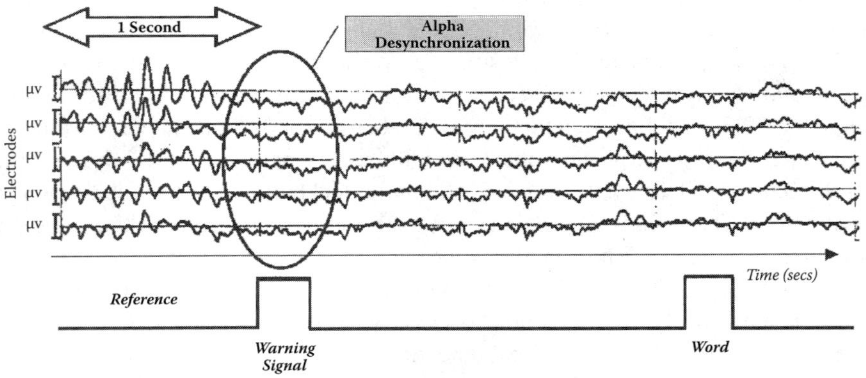


*Figure 14.2* Alpha desynchronization measured with EEG. A typical phasic change occurs in the alpha rhythm over the time course of a trial indicating that the alpha rhythm becomes suppressed.

Aranibar, 1977), and represents a measure reflecting the extent to which synchrony is lost. The standard measure of ERD quantifies a shift in signal band power in terms of the difference between a baseline period before the event occurs and a period following the event. Typically, the ERD is evaluated as the average response over a set of single trials. One method for estimating the ERD is the power method which allows the computation of the power spectral density (PSD) of the data. PSD is a measure of how power in a signal changes as a function of frequency. Spectral analysis detects periodic oscillations (amplitude and frequency) and has been employed in a great variety of signal processing applications. This method allows us not only to compute the PSD for specific time segments, but also to compare statistically the PSD between data segments. Hence differences in the PSD between reference periods versus active periods can be found easily.

By convention an ERD corresponds to a negative value (i.e., a decrease in power) whereas event-related synchronization (ERS) (Pfurtscheller, 1992; Klimesh, 1996) refers to an increased signal power. It is important to note that changes of signal power are quantified only with respect to the deviation from a fixed, constant baseline level. However, it is possible to generalize the conventional ERD framework with respect to the choice of reference by measuring the relative deviation of the event-related power from a dynamic baseline. The dynamic reference can be estimated from catch trials, that is, as averaged power across trials without processing the event under study. The main advantage of the generalized ERD (gERD) measure is due to its ability to reliably study ERD responses even in the presence of dynamical cortical states by using the natural relaxation dynamics of the unperturbed EEG rhythm as reference obtained from catch trials.

### *14.2.2 Evoked potentials (ERPs)*

Evoked potentials or event-related potentials (ERPs) are significant voltage fluctuations resulting from an external or internal stimulus. Mental operations, such as those involved in perception, selective attention, language processing, and memory, proceed over time ranges in the order of tens of milliseconds, for which reason ERPs are a suitable methodology for studying cognitive processes of both normal and abnormal nature (e.g., in neurological or psychiatric disorders). Amplitudes of ERP components are often much smaller than spontaneous EEG components, so they are extracted from a set of single recordings by digital averaging of epochs (recording periods) of EEG time-locked to repeated occurrences of sensory, cognitive, or motor events. The spontaneous background EEG fluctuations, which are random relative to the time the stimuli occurred, are averaged out, leaving the event-related brain potentials. These electrical signals reflect only that activity which is consistently associated with the stimulus processing in a time-locked way. The ERP thus reflects, with high temporal resolution, the patterns of neuronal activity evoked by a stimulus.

An ERP waveform consists of a series of peaks and troughs; however, these voltage deflections reflect the sum of several relatively independent underlying or *latent* components. It is extremely difficult to isolate the latent components so that they can be measured independently, and this is the biggest barrier to designing and interpreting ERP experiments. Consequently, one of the keys to successful ERP research is to distinguish between the observable peaks of the waveform and the unobservable latent components.

After extracting the signal, researchers generally focus on some specific feature of the resulting ERP waveform (e.g., a peak or trough), and this particular feature then becomes the component of interest. According to Donchin & Heffley (1978), a "component" is a part of the ERP waveform with a delimited scalp distribution (referring to the neurons underlying the ERP) and a defined relationship to experimental variables (linked to the cognitive function carried out by the activity of this population of neurons).

There are three measurable aspects of the ERP component: amplitude, latency, and scalp distribution (Johnson, 1992). The amplitude of a component provides an index of the extent of neural activation; namely it captures how the component responds functionally to experimental variables. The latency refers to the point in time at which the peak occurs and reveals the timing of activation, and the scalp distribution gives information on the overall pattern of activated brain areas and reflects the pattern of voltage gradient over the scalp at any point in time.

Therefore, components can be defined in terms of a combination of the specific operation being performed and a neuroanatomical generator site. By this definition, a component may occur at different times under different conditions, as long as it arises from the same module and represents the same cognitive function. Furthermore the same cognitive function may occur and peak in different parts of a cortical area leading to changes in its scalp distribution and polarity.

Different techniques have been developed which use different approaches in order to trace the specific markers of ERP components according to their temporal and spatial characteristics.

Techniques such as PCA (principal component analysis) and ICA (independent component analysis; for a review of both techniques see Donchin and Heffley, 1978) use the correlational structure of an ERP dataset to define a set of components, and these techniques therefore derive components that are based on functional relationships. Specifically, different time points are grouped together as part of a single component to the extent they tend to vary in a correlated manner, under the assumption that time points which reflect a common cognitive process should in theory show an overlapping pattern of variation. As we have noted above, variation in ERP voltage across the scalp is attributed to variation in the psychological processes that are engaged in a situation. The purpose of PCA and ICA in this context then is to identify aspects of the waveform that show temporal covariation over both experimental conditions and scalp locations.

Despite the complications arising when trying to identify the generator sites of specific ERP components, the scalp distribution of the ERP can add extremely useful information to component amplitudes and latencies. Comparison of the scalp distributions of ERPs elicited by different stimuli allow us to infer whether two types of stimuli engage different patterns of neural activity which in turn may underlie different functional processes (for a review see Johnson, 1993). Hence, given the combination of both temporal and spatial information embedded in the ERP waveform recorded at many different sites over the scalp, we are able to define the temporal characteristics (both onset and duration) of brain activity specifically related to a type of stimulus.

The clearest way of representing ERP data, especially when recording from a large number of electrodes, is with maps. Two types of maps can be created for any dataset: voltage and current source density (CSD) ones. Both types of maps are traced directly from the original amplitude data; however, each gives a different perspective of the brain's activity (for a complete tutorial, see Picton, Lins, & Scherg, 1995). Voltage maps are extracted from the ERP amplitudes collected at each electrode site, providing a picture of the summed activity from all active brain areas, as scalp-recorded ERP activity reflects the summation of all the neural activity, both cortical and subcortical, during any given temporal window. On the other hand, the amplitudes are spatially filtered with an algorithm that "cleans up" the amount of activity conveyed by subcortical and distant cortical areas before CSD maps are generated. The resulting maps depict a spatially sharpened, reference-free display of positive and negative current densities that highlights local (cortical) differences between generators (Nunez, 1981; Picton et al., 1995), and is particularly useful in forming hypotheses about neural sources in superficial cortex (Perrin, Pernier, Bertrand, & Echallier, 1989).

An essential difference between these mapping methods is that they assign a different weight to the contribution of subcortical activity. However, it is generally useful to calculate both types of maps in order to pinpoint and take into consideration the differences between the voltage and CSD maps. This is because, although CSD maps allow one to infer neocortical sources, the activity of deeper generators (e.g., subcortical nuclei), would only be revealed in the voltage maps. It is important to note that both types of maps are employed only for visual inspection of brain activity and do nothing to quantify the activity patterns they display unless they undergo statistical analysis which may allow us to infer quantitative differences between them.

More direct techniques that allow ERP sources to be directly inferred from scalp fields themselves have also been developed. Among the most advanced techniques is the Brain Electrical Source Analysis (BESA) procedure (Sherg, 1990). This procedure is grounded in the assumption that the ERP waveform represents the summation of the activity of a number of different sources of fixed location within the brain, and that these sources can be appropriately modeled as "equivalent dipoles" in a solution fitted to the observed data pattern. A BESA solution specifies these sources in terms of their number, location, orientation, and time courses and relative strengths of their activity. Such solutions can be verified by computing the scalp fields that they would generate and determining the goodness-of-fit between these predicted fields and those measured empirically. An important feature of the BESA procedure is that the location of the sources can be defined by the experimenter based on a priori anatomical knowledge or on the location of brain activity derived from a complementary technique such as fMRI scanning. A second important advantage of this procedure is that the contribution made by each source to the ERP can be regarded as an independent ERP component. Thus, in principle this technique allows us to reduce ERP data in terms of a small number of underlying components each associated with its own "defined" source in the brain.

However, the core limitation of analyzing ERP waveforms with the BESA approach is that the results are constrained by a priori assumptions made by the experimenter. Although there may be a long history and a robust grounding in the literature concerning the best or appropriate source of a component it will always remain a choice and therefore a seed of bias introduced by the experimenter.

The first step for adding more information and refining EEG/ERP analyses is to find a reference-independent measure (Dien, 1998) and this may be accomplished by comparing topographies (Lehmann, 1987; Michel, Murray, Lantz, Gonzalez, Spinelli, & Grave de Peralta, 2004.) That is, the configuration of the electric field at the scalp (i.e., the topographic map) remains constant and the extent of topographic similarity or dissimilarity can be quantified and statistically tested. Thus, topographic analyses (i.e., quantification of scalp distribution differences) can be performed on the ERP amplitudes in order to test the significance of the differences shown by the maps. The most important feature of this technique is that topographic differences can be translated in terms of neurophysiology. Only changes in the configuration of the underlying intracranial sources (given the exclusion of artifacts such as eye movements, muscle activity, etc.) can induce alterations in the topography of the electric field at the scalp, although the opposite will not verify itself (for a review see Fender, 1987 and Murray et al., 2008). Hence, qualitatively and quantitatively distinct ERP scalp topographies reflect different patterns of neural activity associated with the respective experimental conditions. Topographic dissociations could recall both the engagement of distinct neural populations or differences in the relative activity levels in the members of a common population. Such differences potentially stand for a neural double dissociation, which implies that two experimental manipulations lie upon functionally distinct cognitive processes.

However, all these procedures do not solve the "inverse problem": that is, they do not provide a unique solution to account for the distribution of scalp activity on the basis of the activity of a number of intracranial sources. This issue is common to both EEG and MEG and is discussed in the next section.

## 14.3 Event-related potential (ERP) studies

### *14.3.1 ERP components*

ERP components can be grouped in two main classes. The *early*, or *sensory*, components underlie sensory stimuli in all modalities and are associated with a series of deflections in the ERP that are related to the transmission of sensory information from the peripheral sensory system to the cortex. For example, after auditory stimuli, one can detect responses with a latency less than 50 ms and these deflections have been shown to correspond to the activation of various nuclei in the brainstem that are associated with the transmission of auditory information. These components are compulsory in the sense that they will be observed in every individual unless the sensory systems in question are impaired.

The second class is referred to as *late* or *cognitive* components. These are the components that occur later in the ERP (from about 100 ms) and are thought to represent activity at the level of the cortex. Examples of such components are the N100, N200, and P300 and the so-called N400, a large negative deflection in the ERP elicited by anomalous words. The number roughly indicates the time in milliseconds at which the component occurs. These cognitive components can vary as a function of attention, task relevance, and the nature of the processing required by the stimulus. On some occasions they may even occur when an expected stimulus does not occur.

However, a clear-cut boundary between early and late components is difficult to trace as many early sensory components have been shown to be modifiable by cognitive manipulations (e.g., attention) and many of the later cognitive components have been shown to be influenced by physical attributes of the eliciting conditions (e.g., modality of the stimulus).

Components serve at least three purposes. First, they represent a common denominator that allows communication across experiments and scientific fields. Second, they are a bridge between ERP data and other measures of brain activity. Third, components can be interpreted as physiological markers for specific cognitive processes. In order to enhance the sensitivity of ERP components to particular cognitive or sensorimotor processes we can adopt specific strategies to establish clear connections between specific ERP components and specific processes.

### 14.3.2 Some examples of ERP components

Specific to language processing several ERP components with different temporal and spatial characteristics have been identified indicating that distinct mechanisms may mediate at least semantic and syntactic processes (Hagoort & Brown, 2000a, 2000b).

The development of ERP language research began with the seminal study by Kutas and Hillyard (1980) on the semantic processing of written sentences. These authors examined the ERPs produced when their subjects read sentences that ended either with a semantically congruent or incongruent word. They observed a component that peaked about 400 ms after the onset of the incongruent word. This so-called N400 component is a broad negative wave distributed over posterior areas of the brain (see Figure 14.3a). Moreover this component has been observed under a wide range of conditions: in different languages, including English, Dutch, German, French, and Italian; in different modalities, including visual, auditory, and even sign language; and with different experimental procedures (Kutas & Van Petten, 1994). Thus, it seems that the amplitude of the N400 component provides a proper measure of the difficulty encountered by the reader in integrating the lexical element in the preceding context.

Interestingly, the presentation of syntactic violations such as verb subcategorization violations did not produce an N400 component, but rather an increase in the positivity

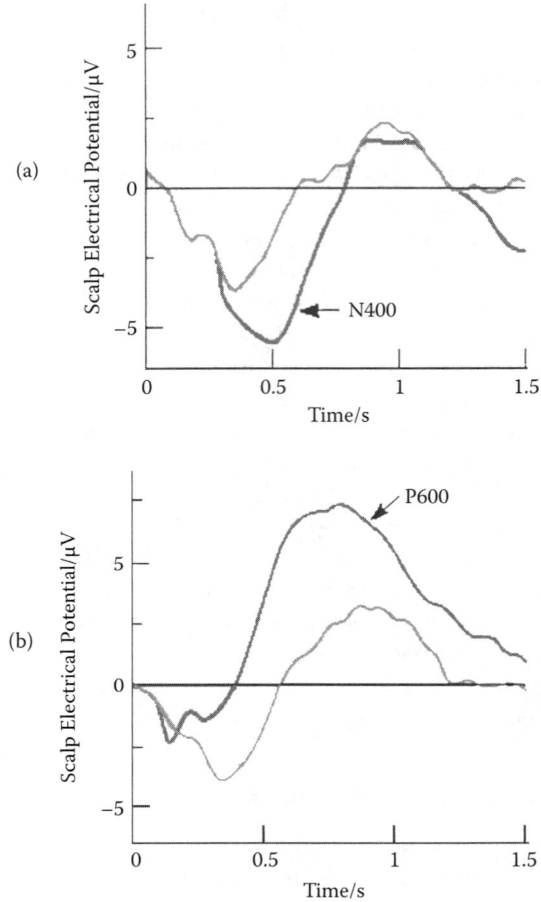


*Figure 14.3* *(See color insert.)* (a) N400 component. This component has the form of a negative wave peaking about 400 ms after the onset of a semantically incongruent word. Event-related potential trace for "The shirt was ironed" (blue line) versus "The thunderstorm was **ironed**" (red line). The key word is ironed, and the deviation is called the N400. (Reprinted from Friederici, 2002.) (b) P600 component. The presentation of syntactic violations produces an increase in the positivity at around 600 ms after stimulus presentation. Posterior event-related potential trace for "The shirt was ironed" (blue line) versus "The shirt was **on** ironed" (red line). The key word is ironed, and the deviation is called the P600. (Reprinted from Friederici, 2002.)

with a biparietal distribution (the centro-posterior areas of the brain), several hundred milliseconds later. This effect has been called P600 (Osterhout & Holcomb, 1992) or late positive syntactic shift (Hagoort, Brown, & Groothusen, 1993; see Figure 14.3b). Furthermore studies on memory have isolated two topographically distinct ERP correlates of recognition memory, the parietal and mid-frontal old/new effects that are dissociated by variables that selectively modulate recollection and familiarity, respectively.

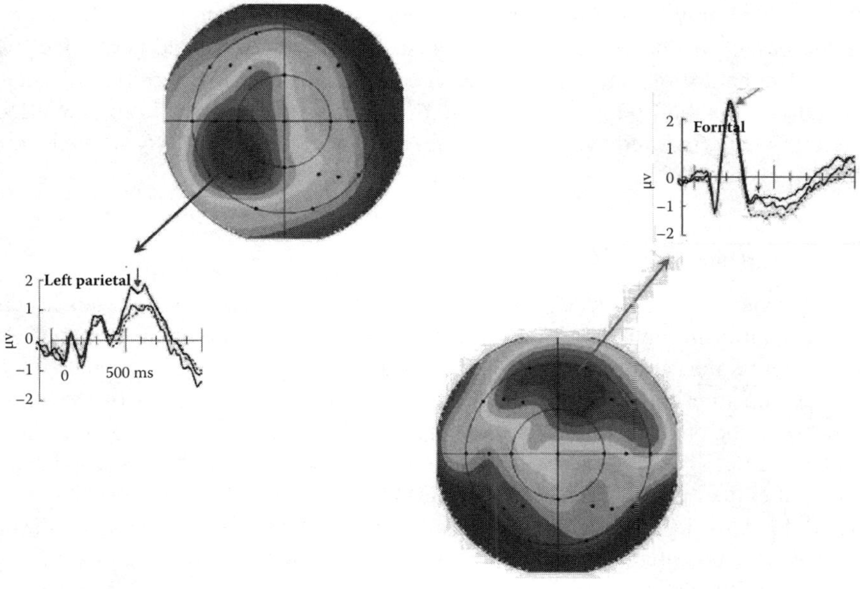


(a) (b)

*Figure 14.4* *(See color insert.)* ERP old/new effects. (a) Grand-average ERPs from left parietal with the parietal old/new effect indicated by the purple arrow. (b) Grand-average ERPs from frontal electrodes with the mid-frontal old/new effect indicated by the green arrow. Repeated measures analyses of variance (ANOVAs) focused on mean amplitudes from 300 to 500 msec. Data adapted from Curran (2000).

It has been more than 25 years since the first reports showed that ERPs elicited by correctly classified old (studied) items are more positive-going than those elicited by correctly classified new (unstudied) test items (Warren, 1980). Investigators have manipulated several variables in order to tease apart these ERP "old/new effects" (Yovel & Paller, 2004; Duarte et al. 2004). Findings from these studies suggested that recollection, which refers to the retrieval of episodic information in response to a recognition test item, has a distinct ERP signature, now often termed the "parietal" old/new effect (see Figure 14.4a.). The effect is shaped as a phasic, positive-going, parietally maximal ERP modulation that originates around 400–500 ms post-stimulus onset and commonly peaks on the left side of the scalp. It is important to note that this effect has been functionally and topographically dissociated from other posteriorly distributed ERP effects that occur in the same timeframe, but rather respond to factors such as stimulus probability and response confidence (Woodruff et al., 2006).

In a study by Rugg et al. (1998) subjects performed either a *deep* (sentence generation) or a *shallow* (alphabetic judgment) task on each word studied, followed by a recognition test. The authors found that this posterior effect was elicited exclusively by old items subjected to deep study. Unlike the posterior effect, a mid-frontal effect was observed only for items correctly judged as old (see Figure 14.4b). Rugg et al. (1998), based on this evidence, proposed that the mid-frontal old/new effect was an ERP signature of familiarity-driven recognition whereas recognition of deeply studied words relied on both recollection (indexed by the parietal old/new effect) and familiarity (indexed by the mid-frontal old/new effect); shallowly studied words were instead identified largely on the basis of their familiarity.

### *14.3.3 A glimpse of MEG*

As mentioned above, the electrical activity of active cells in the brain produces currents spreading through the head. Furthermore, these currents produce magnetic fields which can be measured above the scalp surface through magnetoencephalography (MEG). The amplitude of the magnetic fields produced spontaneously by the human brain are of the order picotesla (more than one million times smaller than the earth's magnetic field). These very low field strenghts can be recorded by so-called superconducting quantum interference devices (SQUIDS) through a special pick-up coil cooled down to superconductivity by liquid helium. The magnetic field, in contrast to the electric potential, has a direction, usually illustrated by magnetic field lines. A current flowing along a straight line produces circular magnetic field lines that are concentric with respect to the current line. The coil picks up only the strength of the magnetic field in the direction perpendicular to the coil area and exploiting a specific quantum effect the magnetic flux through the coil can be measured. This important feature makes MEG insensitive to current sources that are directed toward or away from the scalp (like the top of a cortical gyrus) referred to as "radial" sources. MEG measures instead tangential sources, which are parallel to the scalp.

MEG can be considered as the most direct correlate of online brain processing obtainable noninvasively because it combines both high temporal precision with a high spatial resolution. MEG can be employed to disclose both evoked and ongoing brain activity. Evoked responses to various sensory stimuli can be withdrawn from the background activity using time-locked averaging. Furthermore the responses can be used as tools to study functions of brain areas at a millisecond time scale once the neural generators of evoked responses are isolated.

One of the advantages of exploiting the properties of MEG can be summarized in the example that follows. Given the fact that attention was known to affect auditory evoked EEG potentials (Näätänen, 1992), it was only MEG that allowed us to gain deeper insight on the functioning of the supratemporal auditory cortex, enabling us to characterize the role of the sensory-specific cortex during auditory attention. Results from one MEG study showed that the maximum effect of attention occurred around 200 ms and the supratemporal auditory cortex processed in a different way low- or high-pitch tones when attention was oriented to either of them in a monaural context (Rif et al., 1991). However, another MEG study has found evidence for an early modulation of cortical activity as early as 20–40 ms after the sound onset due to attention, which may somehow recall an early selection of input for further processing. These results suggested that modulation starts even earlier and specifically when attention is directed to one ear during binaural stimulation than when

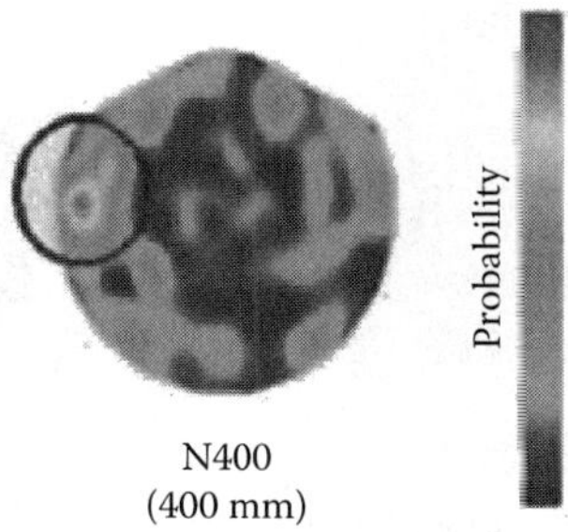


*Figure 14.5* The N400 component localized with MEG. The source of the N400 ERP in MEG appears a distinct cluster in the superior temporal lobe, near the auditory cortex.

one frequency channel is attended during stimulation exclusively directed to one ear (Woldorff et al., 1993). Moreover, MEG allows tracking of activation of the auditory cortices separately in both hemispheres (Mäkelä et al., 1993), whereas the corresponding EEG signals from the left and right auditory cortices summate at the scalp midline and source modeling is required in order to disentangle them.

Another example of the capability held by MEG to localize generators of ERP components is summarized below. In the section above we discussed the N400 ERP component elicited by semantically incongruent sentences. This component elicits a sustained field showing the same scalp topography for several hundred milliseconds. In the same time window, a slightly different waveform morphology appears to denote MEG responses to visual words between 200 and 500 ms after word-onset. The N400 time window has been explored with MEG using the classical N400 paradigm where expectations for the final word, in sentences are violated ("He spread the warm bread with socks"; Halgren et al., 2002; for a review see Pylkkanen and Marantz, 2003). For example, Helenius and colleagues (1998) manipulated the predictability of visual sentence final words to localize the source of the N400 ERP and pinpointed several areas responsive to semantic congruity, although a distinct cluster was localized in the superior temporal lobe, near the auditory cortex (see Figure 14.5).

### *14.3.4 The inverse problem in EEG and MEG*

"The deduction of neuronal currents from the measured external electric potential or magnetic field distribution" is referred to as "the inverse problem" and unfortunately does not have a unique solution (Hämäläinen et al,. 1993). However, some solutions are more likely than others as EEG and MEG signals are not due to spurious distributions of electric neuronal generators. They are ruled instead by electrophysiological and neuroanatomical constraints and obey the laws of electrodynamics as well. Hence, we can reach an approximate solution to the inverse problem by establishing constraints derived from anatomy, physiology, and other data, in order to limit the number of possible solutions to a smaller amount, and estimate the source topographies in a confident manner. Low-resolution brain electromagnetic tomography (LORETA; Pascual-Marqui,

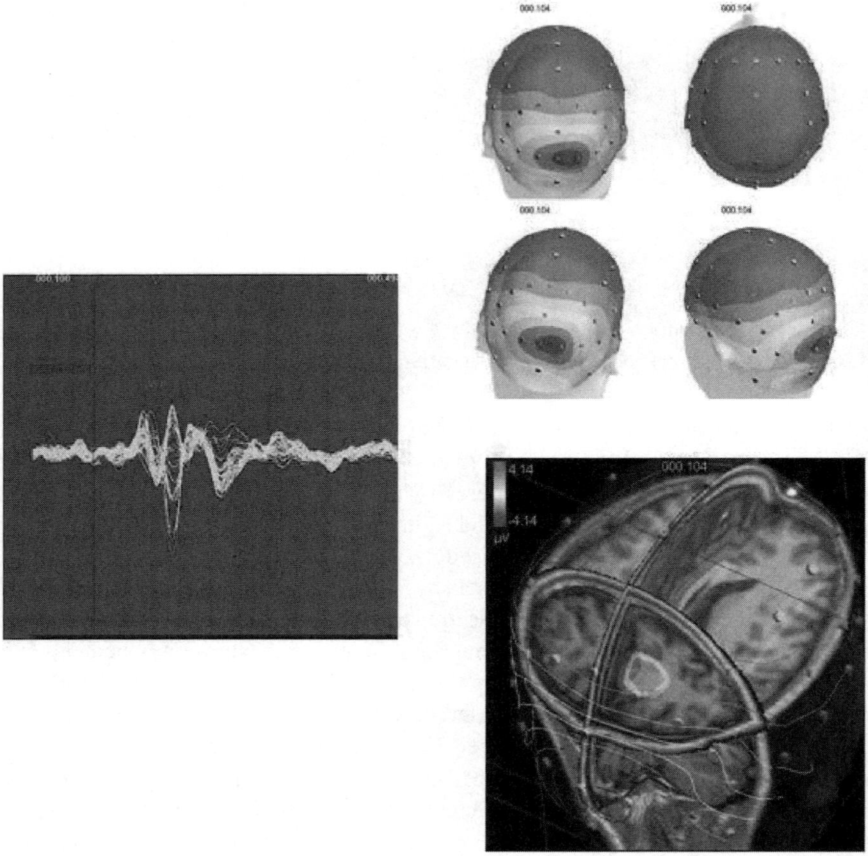

*Figure 14.6* Source modeling using LORETA. The LORETA inverse solution corresponds to the 3D distribution of electric neuronal activity modeled on the cortex.

Michel, & Lehmann,1994; Pascual-Marqui, 1999) is a functional imaging method based on the electrophysiological and neuroanatomical constraints in which the cortex can be modeled as a collection of volume elements (voxels) in the digitized atlas in order to trace sources (see Figure 14.6). The LORETA inverse solution (which is consistent with the EEG/MEG measurements) corresponds to the 3-D distribution of electric neuronal activity that has maximum similarity (i.e., maximum synchronization), in terms of orientation and strength, between neighboring neuronal populations (represented by adjacent voxels). The cortical surface can be modeled as a set of surface elements with a given a priori orientation and LORETA can look up to this neuroanatomical constraint, and derive the inverse solution that maximizes only the synchronization of strength between neighboring neuronal populations. According to calculations reviewed by Hämäläinen et al. (1993), a typical cluster of neurons must cover at least 40 to 200 mm² of the cortical surface.

The LORETA solution has been validated by confronting topographies with data obtained using other imaging techniques or from lesion studies and intracranial recordings where the source sites and signal waveforms have been largely confirmed (see, for review, Pascal-Marqui, Esslen, Kochi, and Lehmann, 2002).

To conclude, MEG and EEG trace the same neuronal activation patterns, just from a different perspective, and provide complementary information in order to reconstruct the brain's current distributions as accurately as possible.

## 14.4 Where do things happen in the brain?

### *14.4.1 PET and (f)MRI*

Event-related potentials and magnetic fields can help us learn "when" dfferent things happen in the brain to characterize the spatiotemporal pattern of brain activity in basically all areas of neuroscience, but how do we precisely find out about "where"? PET and fMRI can localize with high spatial resolution regions of activation while the brain is involved in a given mental task, whereas ERPs and MEG can help us in defining the time course of these activations. PET and fMRI both fall under the category of active recording techniques due to the ways in which they "interfere" with normal brain metabolism.

PET allows us to measure in detail the functioning of distinct areas of the human brain while a patient or a normal subject is comfortable, conscious, and alert. Before the advent of the PET scanner, we could only infer what went on within the brain from postmortems or animal studies. Now we are able to use radioactivity to measure cerebral metabolism, cerebral blood flow, or neuroreceptors and neurotransmitters to study the chemical process involved in the working of healthy or diseased human brains in a way previously impossible. PET can give us a detailed picture of the brain at work in vivo allowing scientists and doctors to depict how it functions.

Functional magnetic resonance imaging does not require radioactivity and can give very high spatial resolution images reflecting neuronal activation. A large part of the metabolic needs of the brain relies upon oxygen and glucose to maintain synaptic activity and the intake of these energy resources to sustain a constant neural activity occurs through the cerebral blood flow. This observation is important because it proves that changes in regional blood flow can provide more meaningful parameters than direct measurements of cerebral metabolism and fMRI allows us to pinpoint local changes in regional cerebral blood flow that may occur after physiological stimulation.

### *14.4.2 PET—positron emission tomography*

PET measures emissions from radioactively labeled chemicals that have been injected into the bloodstream and uses the data to produce two- or three-dimensional images of the distribution of radiochemicals throughout the brain. It also measures the distribution of particular organic molecules and compounds (e.g., water, glucose, neurotransmitters, enzymes) in the brain. However, organic molecules and compounds are not directly detectable because they do not emit electromagnetic signals. Therefore, a machine called a cyclotron is used to "label" these natural body compounds, such as glucose or water, with small amounts of radioactivity to constitute positron-emitting isotopes of these molecules. The labeled compound, which is called a radiotracer, is then injected into the bloodstream, which carries it to the brain passing through the blood-brain barrier and after a short time period the isotopes are dispersed throughout the brain.

The isotopes, along with the blood, flow to the areas of the brain with the highest metabolic needs that are assumed to be the most active at the given point in time. According to their chemical characteristics, they can also specifically bind to neuroreceptors or compete with enzymatic activity. At a specific time point the nuclei of the isotopes decay, giving off positrons. When a positron meets an electron, the collision (annihilation) produces two gamma rays having the same energy, but going in opposite directions. The gamma rays leave the patient's body and are detected by sensors in the PET scanner. The greater the activation of an area, the more gamma rays originate from that area.

A computer uses the data gathered by the sensors to construct multicolored two- or three-dimensional images that show where the compound acts in the brain, providing a complex picture of the subject's or patient's brain. The final PET images show areas of different color tones, each shade representing different molecular parameters of the underlying brain structures (see Figure 14.7). Using different compounds, PET can show blood flow, oxygen and glucose metabolism, neurotransmission, and drug concentrations in the tissues of the brain. Blood flow and oxygen and glucose metabolism reflect the amount of brain activity in different regions and enable scientists to learn more about the physiology and neurochemistry of the working brain.

For example in a recent study Garibotto et al. (2008) used fluorine-18-fluorodeoxyglucose positron (18FDG) to measure glucose consumption and assess the impact of education and occupation on brain glucose metabolism (rCMRglc) measured in aMCI (amnestic mild cognitive impairment) patients and in a very large sample of subjects with probable Alzheimer disease (pAD). The results showed a significant association between higher education/occupation and lower rCMRglc in posterior temporoparietal cortex and precuneus in pAD and aMCI patients which converted to AD, and no correlation in aMCI nonconverters and healthy controls. This means that pAD and aMCI converters with higher education/occupation had a more severe rCMRglc reduction than the ones with lower education/occupation, given the same cognitive impairment,. This study suggests that highly intelligent or educated individuals appear to be able to cope better with the onset of dementia.

In another study Tettamanti et al. (2005) used (11C) raclopride and positron emission tomography to measure modulations of the dopaminergic system induced by phonological or syntactic processing. They found that the level of accuracy in phonological processing significantly correlated with tracer binding potential in the left caudate nucleus and the speed in phonological processing significantly correlated with tracer binding potential in the left putamen. These findings show that the striatal dopaminergic system plays an essential role in grammatical processes that form the core of human language.

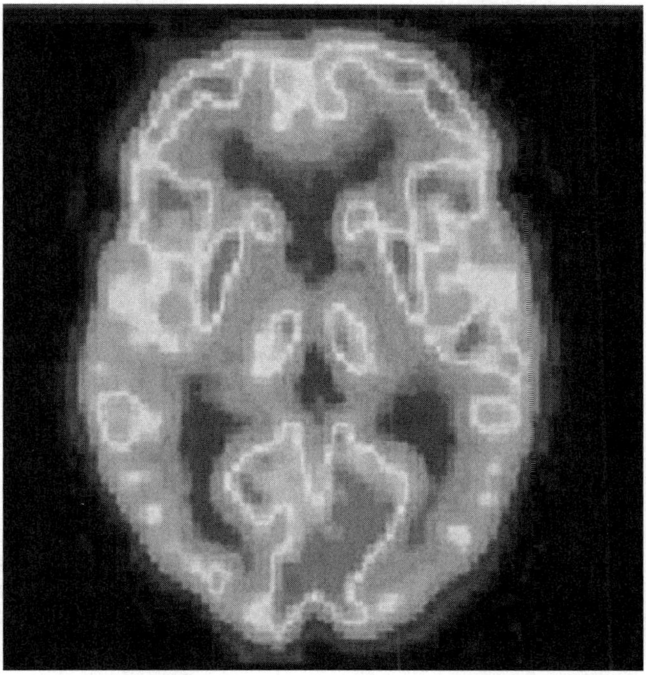

*Figure 14.7* *(See color insert.)* Example of a PET image showing areas of different color tones, each shade representing different molecular parameters of the underlying brain structures.

When the measurements refer to water molecules and regional cerebral blood flow (rCBF), labeled oxygen ($^{15}O_2$; oxygen from which an electron has been removed from its atom to create an unstable compound capable of emitting positrons) is used in so-called "triple oxygen" PET activation studies. In this case, areas of higher blood flow will have a larger amount of radioactive tracer, and thus emit a stronger signal. Blood flow is an indirect measure of local synaptic activity and cognitive functions have been studied mainly investigating increases in rCBF (cerebral activation) linked to the performance of cognitive tasks (e.g., language, memory, attention). These studies have used labeled oxygen ($^{15}O_2$) as the radiotracer in the form of water ($H_2{}^{15}O$) as the advantage of this tracer is that it decays in a short time (approximately 2 min). This means that it is possible to make several scans (up to 16 approximately) during a single session, thus enabling researchers to study different conditions while patients carry out different tasks. At the beginning of each PET scan, a small amount of labeled water is injected into a subject's vein, while her or his head is placed inside the PET scanner. After about 30 seconds, the tracer starts appearing in the brain and the next 30 seconds constitute the "critical window" when radiation reaches its peak in the brain. Images of rCBF are obtained during this critical window. Using data analysis methods, a 3-D representation of the brain is obtained in the form of a mapping of radioactivity distribution, which indicates cerebral activity linked to the cognitive task.

PET activation studies commonly employ blocked experimental paradigms because long intervals of time (30 seconds or more) are required to collect sufficient data to yield a good image. In a block design, different conditions in the experiment are presented as separate blocks of trials (i.e., reading a word in one block and naming a picture in a different block), with each block representing one scan during an experiment. Moreover, in order to observe the neural effect of some briefly occurring psychological process (e.g., the activation due to a flashing red light) in a PET experiment the stimulus needs to be presented repeatedly during a block of trials so that activations accumulate over the recording interval of a scan. One could then compare the activations in this scan to an appropriate control scan (baseline) in which the event did not occur. In this manner activations related to slowly changing factors such as a task-set can be captured.

For example, Perani, Schnur, Tettamanti, Gorno-Tempini, Cappa, and Fazio (1999) investigated the functional correlates of the semantic processing of pictures and words during picture and word matching tasks, in which they assessed cerebral activation with PET comparing the processing of stimuli belonging to different semantic categories (animate and inanimate). Regional cerebral blood flow was measured by recording the distribution of cerebral radioactivity following the injection of labeled oxygen. These results highlighted different brain networks subserving the identification of living and nonliving entities indicating a crucial role of the left fusiform gyrus in the processing of animate entities and of the left middle temporal gyrus for tools for both words and pictures.

### *14.4.3 Magnetic resonance imaging (MRI) and fMRI*

Unlike PET, MRI uses magnetic fields and radio waves to produce images of brain structures without injecting radioactive tracers. Patients or volunteers are placed in a large cylindrical magnet which creates a magnetic field around their head. Radio waves are sent through the magnetic field and sensors read the signals which are fed to a computer that uses the information to create high-dimensional images of the brain. MRI allows imaging of both surface and deep brain structures with a high degree of anatomical detail and detecting minute changes in these structures that occur over time. In the early 1990s Ogawa and Lee (1990), Ogawa, Lee, Kay, and Tank (1990) and Kwong et al. (1992) developed a technique called functional brain imaging that enables us to use MRI to image the brain as it functions. Functional MRI relies on the magnetic properties of blood to enable scientists to see images of blood flow in the brain as it is occurring. This technique takes advantage of the BOLD (blood oxygen level dependent) effect to trace changes in the local blood oxygenation of stimulated brain areas in humans (Bandettini, Wong, Hinks, Tikofsky, & Hyde, 1992; Kwong et al., 1992; Ogawa et al., 1992).

The generation of images that are related to blood flow exploits a property of hemoglobin that has different magnetic properties when it is not carrying oxygen (deoxyhemoglobin) than when it is carrying oxygen (oxyhemoglobin, or simply hemoglobin). The rationale is that more deoxygenated blood in an area causes a decrease in BOLD signal which is sensitive to changes in the concentration of deoxygenated

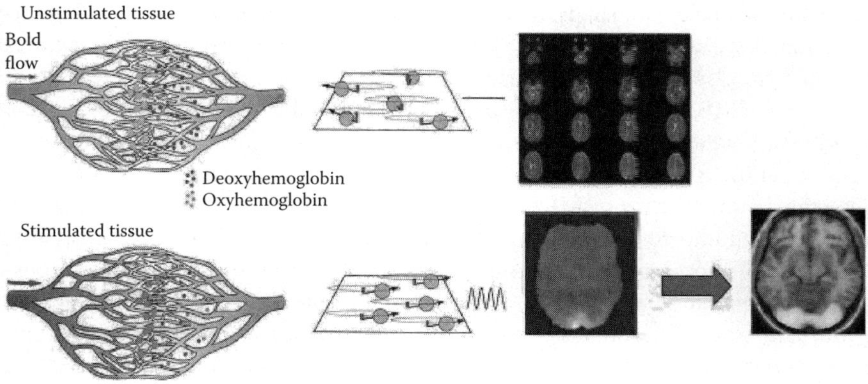


*Figure 14.8* The BOLD effect. More deoxygenated blood in an area causes a decrease in BOLD signal which is sensitive to changes in the concentration of deoxygenated hemoglobin across the vessels of the brain. Neural activity instead is accompanied by increased blood flow, which reduces the concentration of deoxygenated hemoglobin and produces a relative increase in signal (Ogawa & Lee, 1990; Logothetis, 2002). Therefore, fMRI measures changes in blood flow in an indirect manner, through the effects of changing percentages of deoxyhemoglobin (Howseman & Bowtell, 1999) producing images of brain activity.

hemoglobin across the vessels of the brain. Neural activity instead is accompanied by increased blood flow, which reduces the concentration of deoxygenated hemoglobin and produces a relative increase in signal (Ogawa & Lee, 1990; Logothetis, 2002). Therefore, fMRI measures changes in blood flow in an indirect manner, through the effects of changing percentages of deoxyhemoglobin (Howseman & Bowtell, 1999) producing images of brain activity as fast as every second (see Figure 14.8).

We are now able to characterize the nature of the BOLD contrast in a better way as it depends not only on blood oxygenation but also on cerebral blood flow and volume, representing a complex response controlled by several parameters (Boxerman et al., 1995; Buxton and Frank, 1997; Ogawa, Menon, Kim, & Ugurbil, 1998; see for a review Logothetis, 2003). However, evidence coming from simultaneous fMRI and electrophysiological recordings points to a direct relationship between the BOLD contrast mechanism and the neural responses elicited by a stimulus (Logothetis, Pauls, Augath, Trinath, & Oeltermann, 2001). This specific feature allows researchers to determine with great precision when brain regions become active and how long they remain active when patients or volunteers perform a task or are exposed to different types of stimuli.

### 14.4.4 *Neuroimaging experiments with fMRI*

Functional neuroimaging experiments are commonly built to investigate complex psychological processes. The underlying assumption is that these complex functions can be broken down and imagined as combinations of constituent elementary operations. The rationale behind neuroimaging is to highlight brain activations commonly associated with elementary psychological processes and analyze what combinations of elementary processes are involved in a cognitive task (for details see Frackowiak, Friston, Frith, Dolan, & Mazziotta, 1997).

PET and fMRI provide enough spatial and temporal resolution to measure neural activity simultaneously in the entire brain allowing us to make meaningful conclusions about the roles specific brain regions play during cognition. It needs to be outlined that before starting a fMRI neuroimaging experiment, several important issues must be taken into consideration (e.g., a specific experimental hypothesis, appropriate methods) and above all the nature of the task chosen to draw specific types of inference from the study. The task must be designed in order to clearly tease apart the neural and psychological processes under investigation from the influence of interfering variables. Nuisance variables may be neural processes unrelated to the question of interest or technological artefacts or physiological artefacts (e.g., heart rate, respiration, etc.). To the extent that nuisance variables influence the brain activations in a task, they will harm and blur the interpretability of the data. Once an adequate task is chosen, important decisions need to be made concerning the right frame to fit around the task, namely, the experimental paradigm. The predominant paradigms for analyzing task-related changes using fMRI are blocked paradigms, such as those used for PET activation studies (see above) and so-called event-related designs.

Many fMRI studies have used blocked paradigms, in which subjects alternate between performing an active (i.e., reading a word) and a control task (i.e., a rest condition where they are asked to look at a fixation cross) for short time periods (e.g., 30 s), and then the images acquired during the active task blocks are statistically compared to the images acquired during the control task block. One advantage of using a blocked design with fMRI is that it offers more statistical power to detect a change.

For example, Canessa et al. (2005) used a block-design paradigm to investigate the effects of the content of stimuli on brain activation underlying deductive reasoning while subjects were solving two reasoning tasks: one version of the task described an arbitrary relation between two actions (descriptive: "If someone does …, then he does …"), whereas the other described an exchange of goods between two persons (social-exchange: "If you give me …, then I give you …"). When compared to control, both tasks activated frontal medial cortex and left dorsolateral frontal and parietal regions, confirming the major role of the left hemisphere in deductive reasoning. Although the two reasoning conditions were identical in logical form, the task with stimuli referring to contexts and situations with a social content was also associated with right frontal and parietal activations, mirroring the left-sided activations common to both reasoning tasks. These results suggest that the recruitment of the right hemisphere is dependent on the content of the stimuli presented.

The event-related paradigm has been developed to take advantage of the rapid data-acquisition capabilities of fMRI. This technique allows us to create images of the neural activity related to specific stimuli or cognitive events within a trial by spacing events with a specific time interval (usually 14–16 s; Aguirre, Zarahn, & D'Esposito, 1998; Dale & Buckner, 1997) in which the hemodynamic response to a single stimulus returns to baseline before the onset of the next stimulus. Signals from individual trials of the same task (i.e., reading single words) can be averaged together, in order to identify the time course of the hemodynamic response within a trial. This paradigm makes it possible to randomize trials from different conditions (i.e., presenting words that refer to animals or tools intermixed), which is essential for certain tasks and avoids habituation effects. Furthermore, activity related to selected types of trials may be isolated in blocks where different types of trials occur enabling us to draw inferences on processes that occur only on some trials.

The recent advent of "rapid" event-related fMRI techniques has permitted researchers to perform experiments in which successive events can be presented with a time interval between them as short as 750 ms (Dale, 1999). Note that rapid event-related fMRI allows us to minimize the effects of fatigue or boredom that may occur when long intervals separate the stimuli. This type of design is limited by the speed of the underlying hemodynamic response to a neural event, which peaks 5–8 s after that neural activity has peaked. Thus, if the time interval is not varied from trial to trial the neural events would occur too rapidly to be sampled effectively.

According to this framework, Canessa et al. (2008) presented subjects with pictures showing pairs of manipulable objects and asked whether the objects within each pair were used with the same manipulation pattern (action knowledge condition) or in the same context (functional knowledge condition) using an event-related design. Direct comparisons showed action knowledge, relative to functional knowledge, to activate a left frontoparietal network, whereas the reverse comparison yielded activations in the retrosplenial and the lateral anterior inferotemporal cortex. The authors interpreted these results as supporting the hypothesis of the existence of different types of information processing in the internal organization of semantic memory.

## 14.5 Statistical analysis of neuroimaging measurements

### *14.5.1 Functional specialization*

Several statistical methods are available for the analysis of neuroimaging data. Many functional imaging studies use the subtraction method, which compares the pattern of brain activation in two different conditions. The main determinants of the contrast are the task and the materials. For example, in the case of the Canessa et al. (2008) study investigating semantic memory, the task is kept constant, whereas the contrasted materials reflect the dimension of interest (in the present case type of knowledge but typically it could be category membership or modality of stimulus presentation). (See Cappa, 2008, for a review on imaging studies of semantic memory.)

Data in neuroimaging experiments are in the form of a matrix of signal intensity values in each region of the brain expressed in voxels (the smallest distinguishable box-shaped part of a three-dimensional image). Standard univariate analyses of fMRI data are employed to perform statistical tests independently on each voxel to identify significant activations in the brain. This approach inherently emphasizes the functional localization of cognitive functions over a functional integration, which is discussed in the next section.

Once a task is designed and data are collected, the statistical analysis of the data consists of two important steps: pre-processing of the images and statistical analysis of the resulting activations (Friston, Holmes, Poline, Price, & Frith, 1995a; Frackowiak et al., 1997). Preprocessing refers to image processing in which the various images in a set of data are prepared to be fed into a statistical analysis of possible differences. Briefly, the images must be aligned to correct for head motion and following alignment they are often normalized to a standard brain template so that results from several subjects can be used for comparison with other studies and inferences can be extended to the population of interest. Finally images are smoothed with a kernel in order to give the noise in the images a more Gaussian distribution. Following these preprocessing stages, statistical tests are performed on the data. A number of statistical strategies are available to analyze the data obtained in functional activation studies. In principle, the mean signal intensity can be compared on a voxelwise basis between images acquired during "Condition A" versus "Rest" (or "Condition B"). The significance of any observed difference can then be tested using a simple Student's *t*-test. The magnitude (*r*) and significance level (*p*-value) can then be described on a voxelwise basis and used to build color overlay maps, in which "activated pixels" are identified in color overlaid on a grayscale source image, usually a normalized template image (see Figure 14.9).

Researchers prevalently employ univariate techniques to localize the regions of activation by extracting meaningful signals and reducing noise. In this approach, the question is whether there is activation in a specific voxel and most of the data is

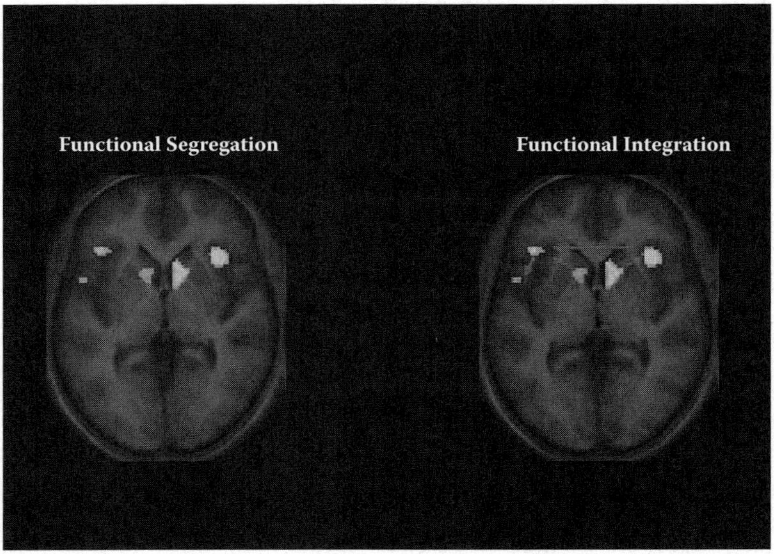


*Figure 14.9* Statistical approach to neuroimaging measurements. Functional specialization is the correspondence between a cognitive function and a specific area (or areas) in the brain. Functional integration refers to the interactions among specialized areas or neuronal populations.

regarded as noise. However, as in the case of ERPs, some researchers have implemented multivariate techniques such as ICA and PCA (see section on evoked potentials and Chapter 8 of this book for further details on these techniques), showing that meaningful information could be extracted not from each voxel but from activation patterns across the entire set of voxels (Haynes & Rees, 2005; Kamitani & Tong, 2005). In contrast to a univariate approach, the multivariate approach regards most of the data as meaningful signals.

Many fMRI experiments are commonly carried out to identify active voxels in a dataset, however, to determine meaningful activation thresholds in functional magnetic resonance imaging paradigms is complicated by several factors. These include the time-series nature of the data, the influence of physiological rhythms (e.g. respiration), and variations introduced by the experimental design.

A common way of determining significance of a statistical hypothesis test is to establish the significance level (usually denoted by *a)* or type I error rate of the test. The type I error rate can be used to establish a threshold as it stands for the probability that, if the voxel is truly not active, its statistic test would surpass the threshold, leading to the incorrect conclusion that it is instead active. This rule results in a large number of false positives or voxels declared active when they are truly not. The reason for this problem is that there are multiple individual voxel hypotheses being tested commonly referred to as "the multiplicity problem"; it occurs when multiple hypothesis tests are carried out at the same time and the possibility of errors occurring on each of these tests must be taken in consideration (Hochberg & Tamhane, 1987; Miller, 1981; Westfall and Young, 1993).

The interpretation of significance in this case is hampered by the enormous amount of multiple comparisons being made between voxels and clearly evokes some form of correction to the simple *t*-statistic. The simplest approach is the Bonferroni correction method, which approximates the actual probability of $N$ comparisons as $N$ times the $p$-value at any one voxel. The uncorrected (or voxelwise) $p$-values indicate the proportion of voxels in the image that will light up by chance, and the corrected (or familywise) $p$-values indicate the probability of false positive voxels occurring anywhere in the image (Friston, Holmes, Worsley, Poline, Frith, & Frackowiak, 1995b; for how to design a neuroimaging experiment, see Abutalebi & Della Rosa, 2008).

Regardless of which specific methods are used to analyze the data and to create a corrected statistical parametric map of the brain, one cannot entirely avoid this problem as the dichotomization of each individual voxel as active or not active does not provide an exhaustive explanation for the majority of scientific questions investigating the brain and its complex functions.

### *14.5.2 Functional integration*

In the past decade functional neuroimaging has highly succeeded in proving functional segregation as the underlying principle of organization in the human brain by revealing the link between a cognitive function and a specific area (or areas) in the brain. Functional segregation is commonly established by identifying the presence of activation foci in statistical parametric maps that are directly related to specific sensorimotor or cognitive processes manipulated experimentally. Newer approaches have instead focused on the integration of functionally specialized areas, defining neurophysiologcal activations in terms of distributed changes (Friston, Frith, Liddle, & Frackowiak, 1993b; see Figure 14.9).

Functional integration refers to the interactions among specialized areas or neuronal populations and to the degree to which these interactions are driven by the experimental context. Functional specialization and integration are complementary approaches, as the latter can be inferred only in the context of the former. Functional specialization implies the identification of regionally specific effects induced by a shift within stimuli or task conditions. Functional integration is inferred instead by accounting for the correlations among activity in different brain areas or by finding a causal link between the activity in one area in relation to activity in another area (Friston et al., 1993a, 1993b; McIntosh and Gonzalez-Lima, 1994; McIntosh, Grady, Ungerleider, Haxby, Rapoport, & Horwitz, 1994). Two aspects of functional interactivity can be characterized: functional and effective connectivity (Friston, 1994). Two brain regions are assumed to be functionally connected if activity within both is correlated; correlations can occur as the result of the association between activities from many sources which does not necessarily imply that the interaction between two areas is meaningful in terms of connectivity (e.g., stimulus-evoked transients in two neuronal populations that are not connected, or the modulation of two cortical areas by a common subcortical input). Functional connectivity simply reflects observed correlations without providing any direct insight concerning how these correlations are mediated. Once functional connectivity allows us to establish integration within a distributed system, effective connectivity is used to investigate the nature of this integration. Effective connectivity examines the direct influence of a neural source on a second. One key aspect of effective connectivity is that it is always grounded in an a priori model that defines the nature of the influence that one neuronal system exerts over another. This approach attempts to disentangle spurious correlations from those mediated by direct or indirect neuronal interactions. The parameters (usually the connection strengths) of the model are then extracted and are recognized as those allowing the model to emulate, as closely as possible, the observed regional activities (or interregional correlations).

Thus, functional connectivity does not necessarily imply a causal link, whereas effective connectivity does. There is a fundamental distinction between simply observing correlated activity and demonstrating effective connectivity in terms of the influence one neuronal system exerts over another in relation to some model of neuronal interactions. However, as pointed out by Friston (see Lee, Harrison, & Mechelli, 2003), effective connectivity is model dependent, whereas functional connectivity is not. The application of multivariate statistical analyses to fMRI data has allowed us to display clear pictures of the functional and effective connections within cortical networks.

Structural equation modeling (SEM). is a statistical approach enabling the characterization of the directionality of influence between regions of a network. With SEM, an a priori model composed of the regions (or "nodes") and the allowable connections of influence between them is defined and presumed to be driven by the task. The strengths of these connections (i.e., path coefficients) that best fit the model to the observed covariance structure between regions in the data are then estimated.

However, SEM is not able to take into consideration the temporal changes in the signals across regions and therefore ignores relative timing as a factor influencing signal directionality. Two recent techniques—dynamic causal modeling (DCM) and granger causality mapping (GCM)—overcome these weaknesses by limiting a priori assumptions about directionality and relying upon temporal measures across regions to establish effective connectivity.

DCM models respond at the neural level by accounting for the hemodynamic parameters of each region included in an a priori anatomical network. The dynamics of these neural responses are then fed to algorithms aimed at estimating how the coupling between regions in the system is modulated by different cognitive contexts or inputs. Mechelli, Price, Friston, & Ishai (2004) used DCM to analyze fMRI data specific to both a visual perception task and a visual imagery task. A DCM analysis on active regions sought to detect changes in coupling between regions induced by the task conditions. They concluded that during visual perception, bottom-up signals from early visual areas spread to category-specific visual regions (e.g., fusiform face area (FFA) for face perception).

GCM is another technique explicitly assessing directionality of signals in cortical networks. Specifically it identifies causal interactions between two regions by determining the extent to which the time series of area *X* predicts the future time series of area *Y*. This technique is grounded in the hypothesis that network dynamics evolve over time in a predictable manner therefore we can measure effective connectivity between two regions in a confident way. Roebroeck, Formisano, and Goebel (2005) applied GCM to a complex visuomotor task by using an area of the prefrontal cortex (PFC) as a "seed" region. They highlighted a significant connection from the PFC to the parietal cortex, indicating a direct influence of the PFC in guiding behavioral performance. The advantage of GCM over SEM and DCM is that it does not require an a priori anatomical network and can thus be used to pinpoint areas throughout the brain that show systematic links with a region of interest.

### *14.5.3 A glimpse of structural imaging (VBM and DTI)*

In recent years, a number of techniques have been developed to display neuroanatomical differences in vivo using MRI images. These techniques can be broadly classified into those that look for macroscopic differences in brain shape and those that aim at identifying dissimilarities in the local structure of brain tissue after accounting for macroscopic differences. The former, such as deformation-based morphometry (DBM), translate the anatomy of any individual brain in terms of deformation fields which allow the matching of each brain to a standard reference. The latter, which include voxel-based morphometry (VBM), compare different brains on a voxel-by-voxel basis after the deformation fields have been used to spatially normalize the images (Wright et al., 1995). The sensitivity of each technique for detecting major or minor differences within brain structures changes even though both enable us to examine the whole brain in an objective manner. Where there are global patterns of difference, multivariate approaches such as DBM are more powerful as the covariances between different structures can be taken into consideration. In contrast, mass univariate approaches such as VBM are more sensitive for isolating small-scale regional differences in gray or white matter.

For example, in one study, Brambati et al. (2004) performed an in vivo anatomic study of gray matter volume in a group of familial dyslexic individuals, using voxel-based morphometry. Focal abnormalities in gray matter volume were observed bilaterally in the planum temporale, inferior temporal cortex, and cerebellar nuclei, suggesting that the underlying anatomic abnormalities may be responsible for defective written language acquisition in these subjects. In a second study by Silani et al. (2005), voxel-based morphometry was used to assess the consistency among brain and morphometry data, and functional imaging addressed with a PET activation study (Paulesu et al., 2001) which revealed a common pattern of reduced activation during reading tasks in the left temporal and occipital lobes in subjects with developmental dyslexia. The authors provided evidence that altered activation observed within the reading system was associated with altered density of gray and white matter of specific brain regions such as the left middle and inferior temporal gyri and the left arcuate fasciculus supporting the view that dyslexia is associated with both local gray matter dysfunction and with altered connectivity among phonological areas within the language system.

Another recent structural imaging technique that is becoming increasingly popular in brain research and clinical practice is diffusion tensor imaging (DTI). DTI gives us the possibility to visualize and track white matter fascicli in two and three dimensions (see Figure 14.10). This MRI-based methodology (Basser et al., 1994) exploits the translational displacement of water molecules within white matter bundles which is made visible through diffusion MRI measurements (Le Bihan, 1995; Basser et al., 1994; Basser, 1995; Basser & Jones, 2002; Basser & Pierpaoli, 1996). Water molecules' motion (diffusion) is much faster along the white matter fibers than perpendicular to them (Basser et al., 1994; Basser, 1995; Basser & Pierpaoli, 1996, 1998). Therefore, "diffusion anisotropy," namely the difference between these two motions (parallel and perpendicular to the fibers) is the basis of DTI (see, for details, Basser & Jones, 2002).

This technique has been used to define the white matter architecture of normal brains as well as the preserved integrity of diseased brains (multiple sclerosis, stroke, aging, dementia, schizophrenia, etc.). For example VBM and DTI were successfully combined in a study by Borroni et al. (2008) to measure selective structural changes in early corticobasal degeneration syndrome (CBDS) and to evaluate the structural correlates of limb apraxia, a key feature of CBDS. This approach to in vivo structural anatomy combined VBM and DTI, the latter describing patterns of white matter connections between cortical areas, with neuropsychological data providing new evidence of gray matter and fiber tract abnormalities in early-phase disease and contributing to clarifying the neural basis of a neuropsychological deficit (apraxia) in CBDS.

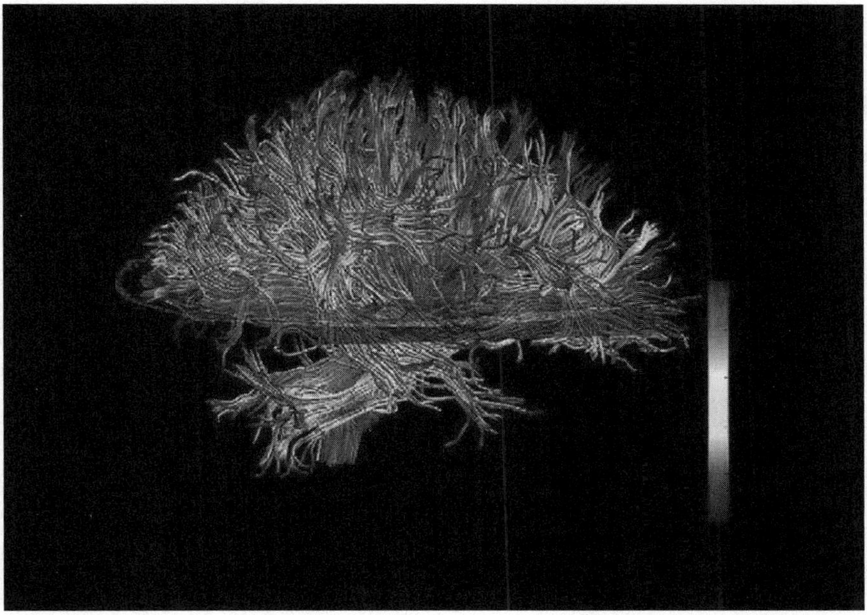

*Figure 14.10* Example of DTI image. DTI enables visualization and characterization of white matter fascicli in two and three dimensions.

## 14.6 Final remarks

In the past two decades a large body of functional neuroimaging studies has been devoted to the investigation of cognitive functions both in the intact human brain and in patients. The studies applying these techniques have not only confirmed the anatomical knowledge gained from early neuropsychological lesion studies, but have also found that cognitive functions appear to be subtended by more extended patterns of activity in the brain and are also less fixed to specific areas as previously hypothesized. All these techniques have opened a number of new perspectives in the understanding of the brain-function relationship and are widely used to characterize the spatiotemporal pattern of brain activity in basically all areas of neuroscience. New concepts and methods constantly arise and latest developments include the combination of EEG/MEG with functional magnetic resonance imaging (PET and fMRI), for combining the superior spatial resolution of the latter with the better temporal resolution of the former.

## References

Abutalebi, J., & Della Rosa, P. A. (2008). Imaging technologies. In Wei & Moyer (Eds.), *Blackwell guide to research methods in bilingualism*. Oxford: Blackwell.

Aguirre, G. K., Zarahn, E., & D'Esposito, M. D. (1998). The variability of human BOLD hemodynamic responses. *NeuroImage, 8*, 360–369.

Bandettini, P. A., Wong, E. C., Hinks, R. S., Tikofsky, R. S., & Hyde, J. S. (1992). Time course EPI of human brain function during task activation. *Magnetic Resonance Medicine*, *25*, 390–397.

Basser, P. J. (1995). Inferring microstructural features and the physiological state of tissues from diffusion-weighted images. *NMR in Biomedicine*, *7–8*, 333–344.

Basser, P. J., & Jones, D. K. (2002). Diffusion-tensor MRI: Theory, experimental design and data analysis—A technical review. *NMR in Biomedicine*, 15, 456–467.

Basser, P.J., Mattiello, J., & LeBihan, D. (1994). MR diffusion tensor spectroscopy and imaging. *Biophysical Journal*, *66*, 259–267.

Basser, P. J., & Pierpaoli, C. (1996). Microstructural and physiological features of tissues elucidated by quantitative-diffusion-tensor MRI. *Journal of Magnetic Resonance Series B*, *111*, 209–219.

Basser, P. J., & Pierpaoli, C. (1998). A simplified method to measure the diffusion tensor from seven MR images. *Magnetic Resonance in Medicine*, *39*, 928–934.

Berger, H. (1929). Uber das Elektroenkephalogramm des Menschen, *Archiv fur Psychiatrie und Nervenkronkheim*, *87*, 527–570.

Borroni, B., Garibotto, V., Agosti, C., Brambati, S. M., Bellelli, G., Gasparotti, R., Padovani, A., & Perani, D. (2008).White matter changes in corticobasal degeneration syndrome and correlation with limb apraxia. *Archives of Neurology*, *65*, 796–801.

Boxerman, J. L., Bandettini, P. A., Kwong, K. K., Baker, J. R., Davis, T. L., Rosen, B. R., & Weisskoff, R. M. (1995). The intravascular contribution to fMRI signal change: Monte Carlo modeling and diffusion-weighted studies in vivo. *Magnetic Resonance Medicine*, *34*, 4–10.

Brambati, S. M., Termine, C., Ruffino, M., Stella, G., Fazio, F., Cappa, S. F., & Perani, D. (2004). Regional reductions of gray matter volume in familial dyslexia. *Neurology*, *63*, 742–745.

Buxton, R. B., & Frank, L. R. (1997). A model for the coupling between cerebral blood flow and oxygen metabolism during neural stimulation. *Journal of Cerebral Blood Flow Metabolism*, *17*, 64–72.

Canessa, N., Borgo, F., Cappa, S. F., Perani, D., Falini, A., Buccino, G., Tettamani, M., & Shallice, T. (2008). The different neural correlates of action and functional knowledge in semantic memory: An FMRI study. *Cerebral Cortex*, *18*, 740–751.

Canessa, N., Gorini, A., Cappa, S. F., Piattelli-Palmarini, M., Danna, M., Facio, F., & Perani, D. (2005). The effect of social content on deductive reasoning: An fMRI study. *Human Brain Mapping*, *26*, 30–43.

Cappa, S. F., (2008). Imaging studies of semantic memory. *Current Opinion in Neurology*, *21*(6), 669–675.

Curran, T. (2000). Brain potentials of recollection and familiarity. *Memory and Cognition*, *28*, 923–938.

Dale, A. (1999). Optimal experimental design for event-related fMRI. *Human Brain Mapping*, *8*, 109–114.

Dale, A. M., & Buckner, R. L. (1997). Selective averaging of individual trials using fMRI. *Human Brain Mapping*, *5*, 329–340.

Dien, J. (1998). Issues in the application of the average reference: Review, critiques, and recommendations. *Behavioral Research Methods Instrumentation Computation*, *30*, 34–43.

Donchin, E., & Heffley, E. F. (1978). Multivariate analysis of event-related potential data: A tutorial review. In Otto, D. (Ed.), *Multidisciplinary perspectives in event-related brain potentials research* (pp. 555–572). Washington, DC: U.S. Environmental Protection Agency.

Duarte, A., Ranganath, C., Winward, L., Hayward, D., & Knight, R. T. (2004). Dissociable neural correlates for familiarity and recollection during the encoding and retrieval of pictures. *Brain Research & Cognitive Brain Research, 18*, 255–272.

Fender, D. H. (1987). Source localisation of brain electrical activity. In Gevins, A. S., & Remond, A. (Eds.). *Handbook of electroencephalography and clinical neurophysiology, Vol. 1: Methods of analysis of brain electrical and magnetic signals* (pp. 355–399). Amsterdam: Elsevier.

Frackowiak, R. S. J., Friston, K. J., Frith, C. D., Dolan, R. J., & Mazziotta, J. C. (1997). *Human brain function*. San Diego: Academic Press.

Friederici, A. D. (2002). Towards a neural basis of auditory sentence processing. *Trends in Cognitive Sciences*, *6* (2), 81.

Friston, K. J. (1994). Functional and effective connectivity in neuroimaging: A synthesis. *Human Brain Mapping*, *2*, 56–78.

Friston, K. J., Frith, C. D., & Frackowiak, R. S. J. (1993a). Time-dependent changes in effective connectivity measured with PET. *Human Brain Mapping*, *1*, 69–80.

Friston, K. J., Frith, C. D., Liddle, P. F., & Frackowiak, R. S. J. (1993b). Functional connectivity: The principal component analysis of large (PET) data sets. *Journal of Cerebral Blood Flow Metabolism, 13*, 5–14.

Friston, K. J., Harrison, L., & Penny,W. (2003). Dynamic causal modelling. *NeuroImage*, *19*, 1273–1302.

Friston, K. J., Holmes, A. P., Poline, J.-B., Price, C. J., & Frith, C. D. (1995a). Detecting activations in PET and fMRI: Levels of inference and power. *NeuroImage*, *4*, 223–235.

Friston, K. J., Holmes, A. P., Worsley, K. J., Poline, J.-B., Frith, C. D., & Frackowiak, R. S. J. (1995b). Statistical parametric maps in functional imaging: A general linear approach. *Human Brain Mapping*, *2*, 189–210.

Garibotto, V., Borroni, B., Kalbe, E., Herholz, K., Salmon, E., Holtoff, V., Sorbi, S., Cappa, S. F., Padovani, A., Fazib, F., & Peroni, D. (2008). Education and occupation as proxies for reserve in aMCI converters and AD: FDG-PET evidence. *Neurology*, *71*, 1342–1349.

Hagoort, P., & Brown, C. M. (2000a). ERP effects of listening to speech: Semantic ERP effects. *Neuropsychologia*, *38*, 1518–1530.

Hagoort, P., & Brown, C. M. (2000b). ERP effects of listening to speech compared to reading: The P600/SPS to syntactic violations in spoken sentences and rapid serial visual presentation effects, *Neuropsychologia*, *38*, 1531–1549.

Hagoort, P., Brown, C. M., & Groothusen, J. (1993). The syntactic positive shift (SPS) as an ERP-measure of syntactic processing, *Language and Cognitive Processing*, *8*, 439–483.

Halgren, E., Dhond, R. P., Christenson, N., Van Petten, C., Marinkovic, K., Levine, J. D., & Dale, A. M. (2002). N400-like magnetoencephalography responses modulated by semantic context, word frequency, and lexical class in sentences. *NeuroImage*, *17*, 1101–1116.

Hämäläinen, M., Hori, R., Ilmoniemi, R. J., Knuutila, J., & Lounasmaa, O. V. (1993). Magnetoencephalography—theory, instrumentation, and applications to non-invasive studies of the working human brain. *Review of Modern Physics*, *65*, 413–497.

Haynes, J. D., & Rees, G. (2005). Predicting the orientation of invisible stimuli from activity in human primary visual cortex. *Nature Neuroscience*, *8*, 686–691.

Helenius, P., Salmelin, R., Seivice, E., & Connolly, J. F. (1998). Distinct time courses of word and context comprehension in the left temporal cortex. *Brain*, *121*, 1133–1142.

Hippocrates. (n.d.) Functions of the brain. Adapted from Francis Adams (Trans.), *The Genuine Works of Hippocrates* (1972). Retrieved from http://www.humanistictexts.org/hippocrates.htm.

Hochberg, Y., & Tamhane, A. C. (1987). *Multiple comparison procedures*. New York: Wiley.

Howseman, A., & Bowtell, R. W. (1999). Functional magnetic resonance imaging: imaging techniques and contrast mechanisms. *Philosophical Transactions of the Royal Society of London B, 354*, 1179–1194.

Johnson, R., Jr. (1992). Event-related brain potentials. In Litvan, I., & Agid, Y. (Eds.), *Progressive supranuclear palsy: Clinical and research approaches* (pp. 122–154). New York: Oxford University Press.

Johnson, R., Jr. (1993). On the neural correlates of the P300 component of the event-related potential. *Psychophysiology, 30*, 90–97.

Kamitani, Y., & Tong, F. (2005). Decoding the visual and subjective contents of the human brain. *Nature Neuroscience, 8*, 679–685.

Klimesch, W. (1996). Memory processes, brain oscillations and EEG synchronization. *International Journal of Psychophysiology, 24*, 61–100.

Klimesch, W., Doppelmayr, M., Pachinger, T., & Russegger, H. (1997). Event-related desynchronization in the alpha band and the processing of semantic information. *Cognitive Brain Research, 6*, 83–94.

Kutas, M., & Hillyard, S. A. (1980). Reading senseless sentences: Brain potentials reflect semantic incongruity. *Science, 207*, 203–205.

Kutas, M., & Van Petten, C. (1994). Psycholinguistics electrified: event-related potential investigations. In Gernsbacher, M. A. (Ed.), *Handbook of psycholinguistics* (pp. 83–143). San Diego: Academic Press.

Kwong, K. K., Belliveau, J. W., Chesler, D. A., Goldberg, I. E., Weisskoff, R. M., Poncelet, B. P., Kennedy, D. N., Hoppel, B. E., Cohen, M. S., & Turner, R. (1992). Dynamic magnetic resonance imaging of human brain activity during primary sensory stimulation. *Proceedings of the National Academy of Sciences USA, 89*, 5675–5679.

Le Bihan, D. (Ed.). (1995). *Diffusion and perfusion MRI*. New York: Raven.

Lee, L., Harrison, L. M., & Mechelli, A. (2003). A report of the functional connectivity workshop, Dusseldorf 2002. *NeuroImage, 19*, 457–465.

Lehmann, D. (1987). Principles of spatial analysis. In Gevins, A. S., & Remond, A. (Eds.), *Handbook of electroencephalography and clinical neurophysiology, Vol. 1. Methods of analysis of brain electrical and magnetic signals* (pp. 309–354). Amsterdam: Elsevier.

Logothetis, N. K. (2002). On the neural basis of the BOLD fMRI signal. *Philosophical Transactions of the Royal Society of London B Biological Science, 357*, 1003–1037.

Logothetis, N. K. (2003). The underpinnings of the BOLD functional magnetic resonance imaging signal [Review]. *Journal of Neuroscience, 23*(10), 3963–3971.

Logothetis, N. K., Pauls, J., Augath, M., Trinath, T., & Oeltermann, A. (2001). Neurophysiological investigation of the basis of the fMRI signal. *Nature, 412*(6843), 150–157.

Mäkelä, J. P., Ahonen, A., Hämäläinen, M., Hari, R., Ilmoniemi, R., Kajola, M., Knuutila, J., Lounasmaa, O. V., McEvoy, L., Salmelin, R., Salonen, O., Sams, M., Simola, J., Tesche, C., & Vasama, J. P. (1993). Functional differences between auditory cortices of the two hemispheres revealed by whole-head neuromagnetic recordings. *Human Brain Mapping, 1*, 48–56.

McIntosh, A. R., & Gonzalez-Lima, F. (1994). Structural equation modeling and its application to network analysis in functional brain imaging. *Human Brain Mapping, 2*, 2–22.

McIntosh, A. R., Grady, C. L., Ungerleider, L. G., Haxby, J. V., Rapoport, S. I., & Horwitz, B. (1994). Network analysis of cortical visual pathways mapped with PET. *Journal of Neuroscience, 14*, 655–666.

Mechelli, A., Price, C. J., Friston, K. J., & Ishai, A. (2004). Where bottom-up meets top-down: Neuronal interactions during perception and imagery *Cerebral Cortex, 14*, 11, 1256–1265.

Michel, C. M., Murray, M. M., Lantz, G., Gonzalez, S., Spinelli, L., & Grave de Peralta, R. (2004). EEG source imaging. *Clinical Neurophysiology, 115*. 2195–2222.

Miller, R. G., Jr. (1981). *Simultaneous statistical inference*, 2nd ed, New York: Springer.

Mulholland, T. (1969). The concept of attention and the electroencephalographic alpha rhythm. In Evans, C. R., & Mulholland, T. B. (Eds). *Attention in neurophysiology: An International Conference* (pp. 100–127). London: Butterworths.

Murray, M. M., Brunet, D., & Michel, C. M. (2008). Topographic ERP analyses: A step-by-step tutorial review. *Brain Topography, 20*, 249–264.

Näätänen, R. (1992). *Attention and brain function*. Hillsdale, NJ: Erlbaum.

Nunez, P. L. (1981). *Electric fields of the brain*. New York: Oxford University Press.

Ogawa, S., & Lee, T. M. (1990). Magnetic resonance imaging of blood vessels at high fields: In vivo and in vitro measurements and image simulation. *Magnetic Resonance Medicine, 16*, 9–18.

Ogawa, S., Lee, T. M., Kay, A. R., & Tank, D. W. (1990). Brain magnetic resonance imaging with contrast dependent on blood oxygenation. *Proceedings of the National Academy of Sciences USA, 87*, 9868–9872.

Ogawa, S., Menon, R. S., Kim, S. G., & Ugurbil, K. (1998). On the characteristics of functional magnetic resonance imaging of the brain. *Annual Review of Biophysics and Biomolecular Structures, 27*, 447–474.

Ogawa, S., Tank, D. W., Menon, R., Ellermann, J. M., Kim, S. G., Merkle, H., & Ugurbil, K. (1992). Intrinsic signal changes accompanying sensory stimulation: functional brain mapping with magnetic resonance imaging. *Proceedings of the National Academy of Sciences USA, 89*, 5951–5955.

Osterhout, L., & Holcomb, P. J. (1992). Event-related brain potentials elicited by syntactic anomaly, *Journal of Memory and Language, 31*, 785–806.

Pascual-Marqui, R. D. (1999). Review of methods for solving the EEG inverse problem. *International Journal of Bioelectromagnetism, 1*(1), 75–86.

Pascual-Marqui, R. D., Esslen, M., Kochi, K., & Lehmann, D. (2002).Functional imaging with low resolution brain electromagnetic tomography (LORETA): Review, new comparisons, and new validation. *Japanese Journal of Clinical Neurophysiology, 30*, 81–94.

Pascual-Marqui, R. D., Michel, C. M., & Lehmann, D. (1994). Low resolution electromagnetic tomography: A new method for localizing electrical activity in the brain. *International Journal of Psychophysiology, 18*, 49–65.

Paulesu, E., Demonet, J. F., Fazio, F., McCrory, E., Chanoine, V., Brunswick, N., Cappa, S. F., Cossu, G., Habib, M., Frith, C. D., & Frith, U. (2001). Dyslexia: Cultural diversity and biological unity. *Science, 291*, 2165–2167.

Perani, D., Schnur, T., Tettamanti, M., Gorno-Tempini, M., Cappa. S. F., & Fazio, F. (1999). Word and picture matching: A PET study of semantic category effects. *Neuropsychologia, 37*, 293.

Perrin, P., Pernier, J., Bertrand, O., & Echallier, J. F. (1989). Spherical splines for scalp potential and current density mapping. *Electroencephalography in Clinical Neurophysiology, 72*, 184–187.

Pfurtscheller, G. (1992). Event-related synchronization _ERS: An electrophysiological correlate of cortical areas at rest. *Electroencephalography in Clinical Neurophysiology*, *83*, 62–69.

Pfurtscheller, G., & Aranibar, A. (1977). Event-related cortical desynchronization detected by power measurement of scalp EEG. *Electroencephalography in Clinical Neurophysiology*, *42*, 817–826.

Picton, T. W., Lins, D. O., & Scherg, M. (1995). The recording and analysis of event-related potentials. In Boller, F., & Grafman, J. (Eds). *Handbook of neuropsychology* (Vol. 10, pp. 3–73). Amsterdam: Elsevier.

Pylkkanen, L., & Marantz, A. (2003). Tracking the time course of word recognition with MEG. *Trends in Cognitive Science*, *7*, 187–189.

Ray, W. J., & Cole, H. W. (1985). EEG alpha activity reflects attentional demands, and beta activity reflects emotional and cognitive processes. *Science*, *228*, 750–752.

Rif, J., Hari, R., Hämäläinen, M. S., & Sams, M. (1991). Auditory attention affects two different areas in the human auditory cortex. *Electroencephalography in Clinical Neurophysiology*, *79*, 464–472

Roebroeck, A., Formisano, E., & Goebel, R. (2005). Mapping directed influence over the brain using Granger causality and fMRI. *NeuroImage*, *25*, 230–242.

Rugg, M. D., Mark, R. E., Walla, P., Schloerscheidt, A. M., Birch, C. S., & Allen, K. (1998). Dissociation of the neural correlates of implicit and explicit memory. *Nature*, *392*, 595–598.

Sherg, M. (1990). Fundamentals of dipole source potential analysis. In Grandori, F., Hoke, M., & Romani, G. L. (Eds.). *Auditory Evoked Magnetic Fields and Electric Potentials.* (pp. 40–69). Basel: S. Karger.

Silani, G., Frith, U., Demonet, J. F., Fazio, F., Perani, D., Price, C., Frith, C. D., & Paulesu, E. (2005). Brain abnormalities underlying altered activation in dyslexia: A voxel based morphometry study. *Brain, 128* (Pt 10), 2453–2461.

Tettamanti, M., Moro, A., Messa, C., Moresco, R. M., Rizzo, G., Carpinelli, A., Matarrese, M., Fazio, F., & Perani, D. (2005). Basal ganglia and language: Phonology modulates dopaminergic release. *NeuroReport*, *16*(4), 397–401.

Warren, L. R. (1980). Evoked-potential correlates of recognition memory. *Biological Psychology*, *11*, 21–35.

Westfall, P. H., & Young, S. S., (1993). *Resampling-based multiple testing: Examples and methods for p-value adjustment*. New York: Wiley.

Williamson, S. J., & Kaufman, L. (1981). Biomagnetism. *Journal of Magnetic Materials*, *22*, 129–202.

Woldorff, M. G., Gallen, C. C., Hampson, S. A., Hillyard, S. A., Pontev, C., Sobel, D., & Bloom, F. E. (1993) Modulation of early sensory processing in human auditory cortex during auditory selective attention. *Proceedings of the National Academy of Sciences USA*, *90*, 8722–8725.

Woodruff, C. C., Hayama, H. R., & Rugg, M. D. (2006). Electrophysiological dissociation of the neural correlates of recollection and familiarity. *Brain Research*, *1100*, 125–135.

Wright, I. C., McGuire, P. K., Poline, J. B., Travere, J. M., Murray, R. M., Frith, C. D., Frackowiak, R. S .J., & Friston, K. J. (1995). A voxel-based method for the statistical analysis of gray and white matter density applied to schizophrenia. *NeuroImage*, *2*, 244–252.

Yovel, G., & Paller, K. A. (2004). The neural basis of the butcher-on-the-bus phenomenon: When a face seems familiar but is not remembered. *Neuroimage*, *21*, 789–800.

## Appendix: General Notation

**[11C]Raclopride:** Positron-emitting selective dopamine 2 (D2) and dopamine 3 (D3) receptor antagonist
**15O:** Oxygen isotope
**18FDG:** Fluorine-18-fluorodeoxyglucose positron
**AD:** Alzheimer disease
**aMCI:** Amnestic mild cognitive impairment
**BESA:** Brain electrical source analysis procedure
**BOLD:** Blood oxygen level dependent
**CBDS:** Corticobasal degeneration syndrome
**CSD:** Current source density
**CT:** Computed tomography
**DBM:** Deformation-based morphometry
**DCM:** Dynamic causal modeling
**DTI:** Diffusion tensor imaging
**EEG:** Electroencephalogram
**ERD:** Event-related desynchronization
**ERPs:** Event-related potentials
**ERS:** Event-related synchronization
**FDG-PET:** F-18-fluorodeoxyglucose positron emission tomography
**FFA:** Fusiform face area
**fMRI:** Functional magnetic resonance imaging
**gERD:** Generalized ERD
**GCM:** Granger causality mapping
**H215O:** $^{15}$O-labeled water
**ICA:** Independent component analysis
**LORETA:** Low-resolution brain electromagnetic tomography
**MEG:** Magnetoencephalography
**MRI:** Magnetic resonance imaging
**pAD:** Probable Alzheimer disease
**PCA:** Principal component analysis
**PET:** Positron emission tomography
**PFC:** Prefrontal cortex
**PSD:** Power spectral density
**rCBF:** Regional cerebral blood flow
**rCMRglc:** Regional cerebral metabolic rate for glucose
**SEM:** Structural equation modeling
**SPECT:** Single photon emission computed tomography
**SQUIDS:** Superconducting quantum interference devices
**VBM:** Voxel-based morphometry

# 15 Body language

## *Embodied perception of emotion*

*Charlotte B. A. Sinke,*[1,2] *Mariska E. Kret,*[1,3] *and Beatrice de Gelder*[1,4]

[1]Cognitive and Affective Neuroscience Laboratory
Faculty of Social and Behavioural Sciences
Tilburg University
Tilburg, The Netherlands

[2]Department of Cognitive Neuroscience
Maastricht University
Maastricht, The Netherlands

[3]Psychology Department
University of Amsterdam
Amsterdam, The Netherlands

[4]Martinos Center for Biomedical Imaging
Massachusetts General Hospital
Charlestown, Massachusetts

### List of abbreviations

AMG = amygdala; almond-shaped nucleus in anterior temporal lobe
EBA = extrastriate body area; brain area lying in temporal-occipital sulcus which is specifically involved in processing bodies
EEG = electroencephalography; a method to measure electrical activity from the scalp related to cortical activity
ERP = event-related potential; EEG waves time-locked to specific stimuli
FBA = fusiform body area; brain area in the fusiform gyrus that is specifically involved in processing bodies
FFA = fusiform face area; brain area in the fusiform gyrus that is specifically involved in processing faces
FG = fusiform gyrus; part of the temporal lobe that is involved in visual processing
fMRI = functional magnetic resonance imaging; brain imaging method that measures the hemodynamic response (change in blood flow) related to neural activity in the brain
hMT+/V5 = human motion area; brain area specifically processing movement
IOG = inferior occipital gyrus
IFG = inferior frontal gyrus

MEG = magnetoencephalography; a neuroimaging technique that measures magnetic fields produced by electrical activity in the brain
N170 = ERP component originating from lateral occipitotemporal cortex specifically related to a late stage in the early visual encoding of faces
OFA = occipital face area; brain area in inferior occipital gyrus known to be involved in face processing
P1 = very early ERP component related to very early visual processing
PET = positron emission tomography; brain imaging method whereby radioactive tracers are injected into the blood stream
PM = premotor cortex
STS = superior temporal sulcus; posterior part is involved in processing biological motion
TPJ = temporoparietal junction
V1 = primary visual cortex

## 15.1 Introduction

In everyday life, we are continuously confronted with other people. How they behave and move around has a direct influence on us whether we are aware of it or not. In communication, we are generally focused on the face. For this reason, emotion research in the past has focused on faces. Also, facial expressions seem to have universal consistency. However, bodily expressions are just as well recognized as facial expressions, they can be seen from a distance, and are from an evolutionary perspective much older. Body language therefore has a high communicative role albeit we are less aware of it. Models on facial expression processing might also work for understanding bodily expressions. Similar brain regions seem to get activated for both, but although faces show the mental states of people, body postures in addition show an action intention. Therefore, seeing bodies additionally activates motion areas.

In a naturalistic environment, faces never appear alone: they are mostly always accompanied by a body, which influences how the facial expression is perceived. This is also the case for other modalities such as the voice. Which modality is dominant depends on the specific emotion being shown, on the situation, and many other factors. For example, aggression seems to be more pronounced in bodily expressions, whereas shame or disgust can clearly be seen from the face. Also the context, including other people or not, can facilitate recognition of emotions. Moreover, we do not live in a static world; dynamic stimuli give us, just as in the real world, more information. We also would like to put forward that brain responses to emotional expressions are not driven by external features alone but are determined by the personal significance of expressions in the current social context. For example, individual differences such as personality type and gender play an important role. Moreover, body language of people interacting can tell us much about their relationship.

We argue that the nature of emotion perception cannot be fully understood by focusing separately on social, cultural, contextual, individual, or interpersonal factors. The perception of an emotion is embodied, and its bodily grounded nature provides a foundation for social communication. "What you see is what you get," does not apply here. People do not "see" the same, nor do they attend to the same.

Furthermore, perception and recognition of bodily expressions do not require full attention nor do they require that the visual stimulus is consciously seen. This is most evident from patients with hemianopia.

All these topics are discussed in this chapter. They show us that being able to recognize emotional meaning from others is vital and that body language is of crucial importance in normal communication. This is clearly impaired in disorders such as autism. Therefore, investigations of bodily expressions will enrich basic clinical research and can lead to the development of new observational and diagnostic tools.

## 15.2 Similarities and differences in neurofunctional basis of faces and bodies

For several years the neural correlates of body shape (Downing, Jiang, Shuman, & Kanwisher, 2001) and perception of bodily expressions (de Gelder, Snyder, Greve, Gerard, & Hadjikhani, 2004) have been the focus of experimental investigations. Although more or less neglected in the past in favor of faces, it is now increasingly believed that the perception of bodies has a special influence on our behavior. To be able to do this, they must be processed from other objects distinctly.

The major concept used to argue for the specificity of processing is that of configuration. There is clear evidence that both faces and bodies are processed configurally, as a whole, rather than as a collection of features. This has been shown with the "inversion effect": recognition of faces and bodies presented upside-down is relatively more impaired than inverted objects (Reed, Stone, Bozova, & Tanaka, 2003). Besides behaviorally, this effect can also be investigated psychophysically by looking at electrophysiological recordings. With electroencephalography (EEG), electrical activity coming from firing neurons is picked up at the scalp through electrodes. By averaging brain activity to certain events, event-related potentials (ERPs) are formed. One such ERP component is the N1, which is thought to reflect a late stage in the structural encoding of the visual stimulus (Bentin, Allison, Puce, Perez, & McCarthy, 1996; Eimer, 2000) and originates from the lateral occipitotemporal cortex which houses the fusiform gyrus (FG). In the case of face processing, the N1 peaks at a different latency (around 170 ms after stimulus onset and hence called the N170) from that for objects. The latency of the N170 is delayed when presented faces are inverted, which shows the involvement of FG in processing faces configurally. The N1 peak for body processing also differs from objects; it ranges from 154 to 228 ms after stimulus onset (Gliga & Dehaene-Lambertz, 2005; Meeren, van Heijnsbergen, & de Gelder, 2005; Righart & de Gelder, 2007; Stekelenburg & de Gelder, 2004; Thierry et al., 2006; van Heijnsbergen, Meeren, Grezes, & de Gelder, 2007) and it also shows an inversion effect. Does this mean there is no difference between face and body processing?

No, it does not. Although EEG has a very high temporal resolution and can therefore tell us a lot about the timing of processing, it is hard to link a specific brain area to the found activation. A method better suited to do this is magnetoencephalography (MEG). This was recently done for investigation of the earliest onset of the electrophysiological inversion effect for different stimulus categories (Meeren, Hadjikhani, Ahlfors, Hamalainen, & de Gelder, 2008). They indeed found that the cortical distribution of this early effect was highly category specific. Different time courses of activation were observed in the common neural substrate in FG. Furthermore, faces activated the inferior occipital gyrus (IOG; also named occipital face area (OFA)), whereas for bodies the effect was observed in the posteriodorsal medial parietal areas (precuneus/posterior cingulate). Hence, whereas face inversion modulates early activity in face-selective areas in the ventral stream, body inversion evokes activity in dorsal areas, suggesting different early cortical pathways for configural face and body perception.

In addition to this early processing in perceiving faces and bodies, more general processing on longer time scales can be investigated with functional magnetic resonance imaging (fMRI). With this method, a distinction has actually been found in the FG between faces and bodies, thereafter called fusiform face area (FFA) and fusiform body area (FBA) (Schwarzlose, Baker, & Kanwisher, 2005). Furthermore, bodies seemed also to be processed in another area: the extrastriate body area (EBA) (Downing et al., 2001). This area lies very close to the human motion area (hMT+/V5), and given that bodies imply action, this finding is not peculiar. Besides, the superior temporal sulcus (STS) and premotor cortex (PM) also get activated for bodies (Grèzes, Pichon, & de Gelder, 2007); the former is known to be involved in biological motion (Bonda, Petrides, Ostry, & Evans, 1996), the latter also being a motor area.

When directly comparing the neural correlates of faces and bodies, the sparse evidence points to a broader network for the perception of bodies, probably due to the action component involved in those. It is remarkable that the literature on isolated face and body perception is more extensive compared to the knowledge of the more ecologically valid combined perception of a face on a body. The few studies available addressing this issue consistently point to a strong mutual influence (Aviezer, Hassin, Ryan, Grady, Susskind, & Anderson, 2008; Meeren, van Heijnsbergen, & de Gelder, 2005; Van den Stock, 2007).

## 15.3 Emotional modulation of body selective areas

That faces and bodies are processed in a distinct way, being special classes of objects, has probably to do with their ecological value. We are experienced in recognizing many different facial identities, and being able to react appropriately to intentions stated in bodies has survival value. Important sources of information about someone's intentions are facial and bodily expressions. To be able to react quickly to these, they must be effectively processed in the brain.

Evidence was found for fast automatic processing of emotional body language. Fear expressed by the body affected the response of the P1 component at 100–120 ms after stimulus onset and the N170 component also showed a difference (van Heijnsbergen et al., 2007). This means that processing of the emotion is faster than identifying a body.

This emotional processing partly takes place in the face and body areas, suggesting a better representation of the faces and bodies. Several studies have reported emotional modulation of face-selective areas, fusiform face area (FFA), and occipital face area (OFA; Breiter, Etcoff, Whalen, Kennedy, Rauch, & Buckner, 1996; van de Riet, Grèzes, & de Gelder, 2009; Vuilleumier, Armony, Driver, & Dolan, 2001). However, this effect may be dependent on age (Guyer, Monk, McClure-Tone, Nelson, Roberson-Nay & Adler, 2008), attachment style (Vrticka, Andersson, Grandjean, Sander, & Vuilleumier, 2008), personality type, and gender of the observer and the observed (Kret, Pichon, Grèzes, & de Gelder, 2011). So far, only a few studies have investigated the effects of emotional information provided by body expressions on activation of body areas in the brain. The first functional magnetic resonance imaging (fMRI) study addressing this issue observed an increased activation of FG and amygdala (AMG) for fearful body expressions (Hadjikhani & de Gelder, 2003). A follow-up experiment additionally showed the involvement of motor areas (de Gelder et al., 2004). Also when directly comparing neutral and emotional faces and bodies (van de Riet et al., 2009), we observed that emotional bodies activate (sub)cortical motor-related structures, such as the inferior frontal gyrus (IFG), caudate nucleus, and putamen which probably has to do with being able to respond quickly to emotional bodies.

Although our findings of emotional modulation of FBA have been replicated (Peelen, Atkinson, Andersson, & Vuilleumier, 2007), emotional modulation of EBA is uncertain. We did not observe a difference between neutral and emotional body images (van de Riet et al., 2009) but our data with dynamic body expressions do show emotional modulation (Grèzes, Pichon & de Gelder, 2007; Kret, Pichon, Grèzes, & de Gelder, 2011b; Pichon, de Gelder, & Grèzes, 2008; Sinke, Sorger, Goebel, & de Gelder, 2010).

## 15.4 Affective gist of the scene influences the perception of emotions

Normally, we do not see isolated people, but we see them in a context. How does this influence our perception of the bodily expression of a single individual?

### *15.4.1 Emotional context*

Because of repetitive co-occurrence of objects or co-occurrence of a given object in a specific context, our brain generates expectations (Bar & Ullman, 1996; Palmer, 1975). A context can facilitate object detection and recognition (Boyce, Pollatsek, & Rayner, 1989; Palmer, 1975), even when glimpsed briefly and even when the background can be ignored (Davenport and Potter, 2004). Joubert, Fize, Rousselet, and Fabre-Thorpe (2008) also observed that context incongruence induced a drop in correct hits and an increase in reaction times, thus affecting even early behavioral responses. They concluded that object and context must be processed in parallel with continuous interactions possibly through feedforward coactivation of populations of visual neurons selective to diagnostic features. Facilitation would be induced by the customary coactivation of "congruent" populations of neurons, whereas interference would take place when conflicting populations of neurons fire simultaneously. Bar (2004) proposes a model in which interactions between context and objects take place in the inferior temporal cortex.

Just as recognizing objects is not independent from other cues such as context, emotion perception does not proceed on information from one cue (such as facial expressions) alone (Hunt, 1941). Knowledge of the social situation (Aviezer et al., 2008; Carroll & Russell, 1996), body posture (Meeren et al., 2005; Van den Stock et al., 2007), other emotional faces (Russell & Fehr, 1987), voice (de Gelder & Vroomen, 2000), or linguistic labels (Barrett, Lindquist, & Gendron, 2007) influences emotion perception and even which emotion is seen in the structural configuration of the participants' facial muscles. In line with the evolutionary significance of the information, the effects of the emotional gist of a scene may occur at an early level. We previously showed scene context congruency effects on facial expressions in behavioral responses but also in EEG measurements. It could be observed when participants had to explicitly decode the emotional expression of the face (Righart & de Gelder, 2008) but also when they focused on its orientation (Righart & de Gelder, 2006). This indicates that it reflects an early and mandatory process and suggests a perceptual basis. Looking at an EEG, we see that the presence of a fearful expression in a fearful context enhanced the face-sensitive N170 amplitude as compared to a face in a neutral context. This effect was absent for contexts-only, indicating that it resulted from the combination of a fearful face in a fearful context (Righart & de Gelder, 2006). That scenes are indeed important is also shown in two recent fMRI studies where participants interpreted facial expressions differently and different brain areas were activated depending on the context (Kim, Somerville, Johnstone, Polis, Alexander, & Shin, 2004; Mobbs, Weiskopf, Lau, Featherstone, Dolan, & Frith, 2006).

### *15.4.2 Social emotional context*

Does it influence our emotional reaction when we watch a single individual fleeing from danger while bystanders are passively standing there? Do we ignore the social scene to focus only on the emotion of the target figure or are we unwittingly influenced by the social scene viewing individual action through the filter it provides us? Studies on crowd behavior (McDougall, 1920) indicate that social scenes provide a context in which individual actions are better understood prompting an adaptive reaction in the observer. Using point-light displays, Thornton and Vuong (2004) have shown that the perceived action of a walker depends upon actions of nearby "to-be-ignored" walkers. Another point-light study by Clarke and colleagues demonstrates that the recognition of a person's emotional state depends upon another person's presence (Clarke, Bradshaw, Field, Hampson, & Rose, 2005).

A recent study by Kret and de Gelder (2010) report that the social group in which we encounter a person, and especially her bodily expressions, influence how we perceive the body language of this single individual. In this study, images of emotional body postures were briefly presented as part of social scenes showing neutral or emotional group actions. These were more accurately and quickly recognized when the actions in the scenes expressed an emotion congruent with the bodily expression of the target figure. These studies show the importance of a social (emotional) scene. However, other processes than the ones measured may contribute to the observed effects, for example, the tendency to automatically mimic and synchronize facial expressions, vocalizations, postures, and movements with those of another person and to converge them emotionally (de Gelder et al., 2004; Hatfield, Cacioppo, & Rapson, 1994). Similar brain areas are involved when subjects experience disgust (Wicker, Keysers, Plailly, Royet, Gallese, & Rizzolatti, 2003) or pain (Jackson, Meltzoff, & Decety, 2005), as when they observe someone else experiencing these emotions. Such a process may contribute to observers' ability to perceive rapidly ambiguity between a person's body language and its social (emotional) context. Such incongruity may create a conflict in emotional contagion processes triggered by the target figure and help to explain the slower and less accurate reaction in the observer.

### *15.4.3 Static versus dynamic*

Research performed with facial and bodily pictures have contributed a lot to our understanding of how our brain processes these stimuli. However, in real life, we are confronted with moving people. Although static body postures already imply motion, dynamic stimuli obviously contain more information, which helps in better understanding someone's intentions and being able to react appropriately to these. Point-light display studies showed that biological motion is quickly detected (Johansson, 1973). A few neuroimaging studies report the importance of movement in processing emotional expressions (see, for example, Decety & Chaminade, 2003; Grosbras & Paus, 2006; LaBar, Crupain, Voyvodic, & McCarthy, 2003). Adolphs, Tranel, and Damasio (2003) report that a patient with a ventral pathway lesion is able to read emotion from dynamic, but not from static facial expressions.

In healthy subjects, Sato, Kochiyama, Yoshikawa, Naito, and Matsumura (2004) found that the AMG, IOG, and FG were more activated by dynamic than static fearful facial expressions. Studies of bodily expressions also report better recognition rates for dynamic versus static stimuli (Atkinson, Dittrich, Gemmell, & Young, 2004; de Meijer, 1989). A recent brain imaging study looked at the perception of angry and neutral hand and face movements (Grosbras & Paus, 2006). The authors reported that regions known to be involved in action and emotion generation in oneself are also activated when perceiving action and emotion in the faces and hands of others. Furthermore, they reported an interaction between emotion and body part: when hand actions were performed with emotion, a region in the supramarginal gyrus responded mostly to this. Because this region had been implicated before as being involved in getting attention toward a limb (Rushworth, Krams, & Passingham, 2001), it seems here that the emotion in the hand movement increased this attention.

This study, however, was not designed to detect specifically what additional information is contributed by dynamics. Two studies that tried to do this used 3-s videoclips of someone opening a door in either a neutral or in a fearful (Grèzes et al., 2007) or angry way (Pichon et al., 2008). From each movie, one frame at which the emotion was at its peak was taken and also presented for 3 s. Not surprisingly, dynamic versus static body expressions (irrespective of the emotional content) caused motor resonance: bilateral activations of PM and parietal cortex, STS, and FG. Most interestingly, an interaction was observed between emotion and motion in STS and right PM. In humans, STS, parietal, and PM are involved in action observation and probably also in action understanding (Grèzes & Decety, 2001), so inasmuch as these areas represented the emotional action in this study, they could also be involved in emotion understanding.

## 15.5 Individual differences

### *15.5.1 Gender*

One aspect that has so far not received much attention in the studies of facial and bodily expressions concerns the role of gender in emotional processing. Some isolated findings indicate that there may be gender differences in emotional processes. Females tend to score higher than males on tests of empathy, social sensitivity, and emotion recognition (see Hall, 1978 and McClure, 2000 for reviews). But whereas females show more facial mimicry in response to emotional movie fragments, they did not report experiencing more emotion than males, which suggests an expressive, rather than an experiential difference (Kring & Gordon, 1998). Testosterone level is a good predictor of the presence of an anger trait, aggressive behavior, and dominance (van Honk & Schutter, 2007), and at the neuronal level, AMG response to fear and anger signals (Derntl, Windischberger, Robinson, Kryspin-Exner, Gur, & Moser, 2009). Aleman and Swart (2008) report stronger activation in the IFG and STS in men than women in response to faces denoting interpersonal superiority.

A different issue is whether the gender of the person we observe influences us differently depending on our own gender. When we think of the interpersonal superiority effect in male observers as reported by Aleman and Swart (2008), it probably does. Except for very interesting work on gender stereotypes for different emotions, this question is hardly explored in the field of social neuroscience. Armony and Sergerie (2007) studied memory for fearful, happy, and neutral expressions in relation to the gender of the observer. They report that the hemispheric laterality of AMG for memory of facial expressions was a function of the sex of the subjects and the sex of the faces being remembered. The left AMG was more active for successfully remembered female fearful faces in women, whereas in men the right AMG was more involved in memory for male fearful faces. These results demonstrate a subtle relationship between the observer and the stimulus.

A recent study by Kret et al. (2011a) reveals how face- and body-specific areas are modulated by gender. Two event-related FMRI experiments, using an oddball task, were used to record female and male participants' brain activity while they observed videos showing fear, anger, or neutral signals expressed by female and male actors. In the first experiment, short video fragments of the angry and neutral expressions were used, in the second fearful and neutral expressions. The AMG was modulated more by facial than bodily expressions. FG was involved in processing body stimuli, more than in processing faces. Threatening body expressions, whether fearful or angry, modulated activity in hMT+/V5-EBA and the parietal and somatosensory cortex (which may play a role in action understanding). We also found significant influences of the gender of the actors and of the observers. A higher activation of EBA and STS was observed for threatening male versus female actors. Male observers showed more activation for threatening versus neutral bodies in many visual processing areas, more so than female observers and especially to male body expressions. These results are in line with previous studies that show male observers are more reactive to threatening signals than female observers (Aleman & Swart, 2008).

Human emotion perception depends to an important extent on whether the stimulus is a face or a body and also on the gender of the observer and observed. Therefore, these gender effects can also be seen in the neurofunctional mechanisms of emotion.

### *15.5.2 Personality differences*

"Embodied cognition," a concept that has recently been getting a lot of attention in cognitive science, suggests that our mind and thus our perception is shaped as much by our body and how we physically interact with the environment as by passive sensory experience. Increased vigilance and enhanced autonomic activity are part of an adaptive response to threat. In otherwise healthy individuals this can become maladaptive when stress is too great. In various pathological conditions the anxiety response is disproportionate to the stress, either because of a misinterpretation of threat, or because of hyper- or hyporesponsiveness at any of a variety of points in the complex network of neural pathways that serve the stress response. Imaging techniques offer unique opportunities to explore the neurofunctional basis of personality differences and indeed show that perceiving emotions is greatly regulated by top-down processes being different from person to person.

People suffering from social phobia or anxiety generally show increased AMG activity when confronted with threatening faces (for a meta-analysis see Etkin & Wager, 2007). However, the role of the AMG in depression is less clear. Whereas some studies report increased AMG response for threatening versus neutral expressions related to depressive symptoms (Canli, Cooney, Goldin, Shah, Sivers, & Thomason, 2005; Peluso, Glahn, Matsuo, Monkul, Najt, & Zamarripa, 2009), others report a decrease in activity (Thomas, Drevets, Whalen, Eccard, Dahl, & Ryan, 2001), or no difference at all (Davidson & Dalton, 2003; Lee, Seok, Lee, Cho, Yoon, & Lee, 2008). Several studies report decreased cortico-limbic connectivity in depression in response to emotional stimuli (Anand, Li, Wang, Lowe, & Dzemidzic, 2009; Drevets, 1998; Fossati, Hevenor, Graham, Grady, Keightley & Craik, 2003) but antidepressant treatment shows reciprocal effects (Anand, Li, Wang, Gardner, & Lowe, 2007). Decreased activation in the anterior cingulate cortex has been reported in depression as well (Davidson & Dalton, 2003; Fossati et al., 2003).

Recognition of another's emotion does not suffice for proper communication. The orbitofrontal cortex (OFC) regulates appropriate social responses (Kringelbach, O'Doherty, Rolls, & Andrews, 2003; Rolls, 2000). Socially anxious people are afraid of possible scrutiny and negative evaluation by others. Not surprisingly, many studies find an overactive frontolimbic system (including OFC, insula, and AMG) in this group during threat perception (Shah, Klumpp, Angstadt, Nathan, & Phan, 2009; Straube, Mentzel, & Miltner, 2005). Moreover, the OFC has been consistently involved in the pathophysiology of major depressive disorder and bipolar disorder (Davidson & Dalton, 2003; Drevets, 2007).

People with type D ("distressed") personality (21% of the general population) have higher scores on depression and anxiety scales (Denollet, Schiffer, Kwaijtaal, Hooijkaas, Hendriks & Widdershoven, 2009). They suffer from emotional distress ("negative affectivity"), which they consciously suppress ("social inhibition"). This personality type is associated with a negative prognosis in disease and a range of somatic effects. A recent study by van de Riet and colleagues (2009) showed a correlation between the negative affectivity subscale and AMG hypoactivation for fearful facial and bodily versus neutral expressions. These findings were later replicated and extended by Kret, Denollet, Grèzes, and de Gelder (2011). So, even small personality differences in the normal population account for a different perception of threat. However, this study focused only on the AMG as the region of interest and neglected other possibly interesting effects that could have been detected in a whole brain analysis. Moreover, this study used static stimuli.

In a follow-up study, we aimed to reveal neural correlates of type D personality and perceiving dynamic threatening facial and bodily expressions. We observed a negative correlation in the temporal pole and cingulate cortex on both subscales. Furthermore, a negative correlation was observed between negative affectivity and activation in brain areas commonly involved in emotion: AMG, FG, insula, STS, and IFG. The right OFC correlated negatively with social inhibition. Also interesting is the relation between social inhibition and increased activation following threat in the anterior intraparietal sulcus, left TPJ, STS, right IFG, secondary somatosensory cortex, and left OFC. These regions are all involved in the action goal of the observed (see, for a recent meta-analysis, Van Overwalle & Baetens, 2009). When observing action, we need to take the other's perspective which we do by activating our mirror and mentalizing system. The mirror system (anterior intraparietal sulcus and PM) is engaged in perceiving and executing motions of body parts and is important for understanding action and emotion (Rizzolatti & Craighero, 2004). TPJ plays an important role in our mentalizing system and computes the orientation or direction of the observed behavior to predict its goal (Van Overwalle & Baetens, 2009). Observing as well as imitating facial expressions activates the IFG (Carr, Iacoboni, Dubeau, Mazziotta, & Lenzi, 2003). People who tend to inhibit socially are likely to overactivate the mirror and mentalizing system.

Taking the other's perspective is not enough; we need to empathize and reason how to act. The OFC is connected with areas that underlie emotional function and empathy (Hynes, Baird, & Grafton, 2006) and interprets somatic sensations (Bechara, Damasio, Tranel, & Anderson, 1998) mediated by internally generated somatosensory representations that simulate how the other person would feel when displaying an emotion (Adolphs, 2002). Without these representations, appropriate reactive behavior would be difficult. Rauch, Savage, Alpert, Miguel, Baer, and Breiter (1995) used positron emission tomography (PET) to measure the changes in right cerebral blood flow in phobic patients provoked by exposure to the feared object. They observed significant increases during the symptomatic compared with the control state in OFC and somatosensory cortex. The complex connections between the OFC and areas involved in emotion suggest implications for its role in anxiety disorders (Fischer, Andersson, Furmark, & Fredrikson, 1998). We hypothesize that people with high scores on social inhibition prefer to avoid social situations because it gives them too much cognitive stress.

## 15.6 Perceiving interactions

Trying to get additional information going from static to dynamic facial and bodily expressions, including a context and taking into account gender stereotypes, there is another step to take to get to even more naturalistic situations. This is the perception of a person interacting with another person. The interplay between them can inform us about their relationship.

In previous stimuli creation, actors always looked into the camera. Therefore, an emotional expression had an immediate impact on the observing participant. In a direct confrontation, it makes sense that you want to react immediately. But what happens when the threat is not directed toward you? This question has been studied recently by Sinke et al. (2010). In this study, we wanted to investigate how the brain reacts to a situation that is threatening for one of the two persons involved. For this study, we created 3-s videoclips in which a male actor grabbed the handbag of a female actor. He did this either in a very aggressive way whereby the woman expressed fear, or in a teasing way, as if the two knew each other. The actors faced each other and did not look toward the observer. When you walk on the street you may have your thoughts on an upcoming deadline instead of on the people on the other side of the street. Will you then still be able to recognize a threat?

To investigate this second question, three small dots, presented only for 40 ms, were added to each movie. Participants in the first task had to look explicitly to the bodies and categorize the situation as threatening or teasing. In the other task condition, they had to monitor the randomly appearing dots and categorize their color. Results showed first of all that the AMG showed heightened activation for the threatening interactions as compared to the teasing ones. The AMG seems to act as some kind of warning signal and possibly passes information through to other regions. Also, during unattended threat, more processing took place in body-sensitive visual regions in FG, middle occipitotemporal gyrus, and STS than teasing interactions. Furthermore, this heightened activation for unattended threat was paired with better behavioral performance on the dot task during threatening interactions. It seemed as if the threat heightened their attention and because the dots were always placed somewhere on the bodies, they were able to perceive them better. Another finding was that although the threat was clearly not directed toward the observer, regions known to be involved in action observation (IFG, TPJ, and inferior parietal lobe) and preparation (PM, putamen) showed increased activation for threat. In conclusion, bodily expressions are easily recognized even though your attention is not explicitly on the situation and the threat is not directed toward you, which has high survival value.

## 15.7 Bodies processed without attention and visual awareness

Studies with hemianopia patients have shown that perception or recognition of bodily expressions does not require full attention. Patients with striate cortex lesions or an attentional disorder can react to a visual stimulus even though they have not consciously seen it. Patients with left hemispatial neglect due to a lesion in the right parietal cortex fail to direct attention to stimuli in their left visual field. However, when the stimulus is an expressive in contrast to a neutral face or body or a neutral object, they are better able to perceive it.

The clearest example of being able to process emotional signals has been given by patients with lesions to their primary visual cortex (V1). Under stringent testing conditions, they were able to discriminate between visual properties of stimuli they could not consciously see. This phenomenon is called "blindsight." Later, it was shown that they were also able to guess correctly the emotional valence of facial stimuli presented in their blind visual field, so-called "affective blindsight" (de Gelder, Vroomen, Pourtois, & Weiskrantz, 1999). In the first behavioral study only moving stimuli but not still images of facial expressions appeared to support affective blindsight. If movement were the critical aspect to support nonconscious discrimination of different emotional expressions, one would expect blindsight also for other attributes that rely on movement. However, blindsight was only observed for emotional facial expressions and not facial speech (de Gelder, Vroomen, Pourtois, & Weiskrantz, 2000). Other facial attributes such as personal identity or gender were also tested with negative results, suggesting that neither movement nor nonemotional facial attributes are per se determinants of the phenomenon.

More directly, in later research affective blindsight also emerged very clearly when still images of facial expressions were used, especially when tested with indirect methodologies (Anders, Birbaumer, Sadowski, Erb, Mader & Grodd, 2004; Pegna, Khateb, Lazeyras, & Seghier, 2005). Still unknown is whether affective blindsight is induced by nonconscious processing of overall face configuration or by individual key features. There is evidence that the eye region is most salient in conveying emotion information, and that the most ancient parts of our visual and emotion systems in the brain seem tuned to detect this simple signal rather than the whole face configuration (Kim et al., 2004; Morris, deBonis, & Dolan, 2002).

Aside from facial expressions, other stimulus categories have been used to test whether affective blindsight could be extended to other stimuli. Thus far, the most studied categories are affective scenes and bodily expressions. Generally, negative results have been reported for scenes, suggesting that the appraisal of the emotional content of complex pictures requires cognitive and semantic processing that depends on conscious visual perception (de Gelder, Pourtois & Weiskrantz, 2002). On the other hand, behavioral and neuroimaging results have shown that affective blindsight for bodily expressions may be at least as clearly established as that previously reported for facial expressions, and sustained by a partly overlapping neural pathway (de Gelder & Hadjikhani, 2006). This implies that implicit processing of emotions in blindsight is nonspecific for faces but specific for biologically primitive emotional expressions in general.

## 15.8 Conclusion

There are important similarities and differences in the neurofunctional basis of faces and bodies. Both are very strong cues. They grab our attention and can even be processed without attention and visual awareness. Whereas it is widely accepted that the FG plays a role in the perception of emotions, whether from the face or body, emotional modulation of the EBA is still under discussion. The scene in which we perceive emotions can facilitate our recognition, and the presence of other people expressing the same emotion naturally helps us perceive another's emotion correctly. Moreover, in a natural social scene, we see people interacting with each other. The perception of emotions is not a pure bottom-up process. Several top-down processes such as knowledge of the social situation, gender, and personality type play a role as well. In real life, people express their emotions in a dynamic way. This movement component adds information, thereby facilitating recognition. To conclude, the perception of emotion is not so straightforward and involves many different kinds of processes.

## References

Adolphs, R. (2002). Recognizing emotion from facial expressions: Psychological and neurological mechanisms. *Behavioral Cognition Neuroscience Review, 1*, 21–61.

Adolphs, R., Tranel, D., & Damasio, A. R. (2003). Dissociable neural systems for recognizing emotions. *Brain Cognition, 52*(1), 61–69.

Aleman, A., & Swart, M. (2008). Sex differences in neural activation to facial expressions denoting contempt and disgust. PLoS ONE *3*(11)): e3622.

Anand, A., Li, Y., Wang, Y., Gardner, K., & Lowe, M. J. (2007). Reciprocal effects of antidepressant treatment on activity and connectivity of the mood regulating circuit: An fMRI study. *Journal of Neuropsychiatry and Clinical Neuroscience, 19*(3), 274–282.

Anand, A., Li, Y., Wang, Y., Lowe, M. J., & Dzemidzic, M. (2009). Resting state corticolimbic connectivity abnormalities in unmedicated bipolar disorder and unipolar depression. *Psychiatry Research, 171*(3), 189–198.

Anders, S., Birbaumer, N., Sadowski, B., Erb, M., Mader, I., & Grodd, W. (2004). Parietal somatosensory association cortex mediates affective blindsight. *Nature Neuroscience, 7*(4), 339–340.

Armony, J. L., & Sergerie, K. (2007). Own-sex effects in emotional memory for faces. *Neuroscience Letters, 426*, 1–5.

Atkinson, A. P., Dittrich, W. H., Gemmell, A. J., & Young, A. W. (2004). Emotion perception from dynamic and static body expressions in point-light and full-light displays. *Perception, 33*(6), 717–746.

Aviezer, H., Hassin, R., Ryan, J., Grady, G., Susskind, J., & Anderson, A. (2008). Angry, disgusted or afraid? Studies on the malleability of emotion perception. *Psychological Science, 19*, 724–732.

Bar, M. (2004). Visual objects in context. *National Review of Neuroscience, 5*(8), 617–629.

Bar, M., & Ullman, S. (1996). Spatial context in recognition. *Perception, 25*(3), 343–352.

Barrett, L. F., Lindquist, K. A., & Gendron, M. (2007). Language as context in the perception of emotion. *Trends in Cognitive Sciences, 11*, 327–332.

Bechara, A., Damasio, H., Tranel, D., & Anderson, S. W. (1998). Dissociation of working memory from decision making within the human prefrontal cortex. *Journal of Neuroscience, 18*(1), 428–437.

Bentin, S., Allison, T., Puce, A., Perez, E., & McCarthy, G. (1996). Electrophysiological studies of face perception in humans. *Journal of Cognitive Neuroscience, 8*, 551–565.

Bonda, E., Petrides, M., Ostry, D., & Evans, A. (1996). Specific involvement of human parietal systems and the amygdala in the perception of biological motion. *Journal of Neuroscience 16,* 3737–3744.

Boyce, S. J., Pollatsek, A., & Rayner, K. (1989). Effect of background information on object identification. *Journal of Experimental Psychology: Human Perception and Performance, 15*(3), 556–566.

Breiter, H. C., Etcoff, N. L., Whalen, P. J., Kennedy, W. A., Rauch, S. L., & Buckner, R. L. (1996). Response and habituation of the human amygdala during visual processing of facial expression. *Neuron, 17*(5), 875–887.

Canli, T., Cooney, R. E., Goldin, P., Shah, M., Sivers, H., & Thomason, M. E. (2005). Amygdala reactivity to emotional faces predicts improvement in major depression. *Neuroreport, 16*(12), 1267–1270.

Carr, L., Iacoboni, M., Dubeau, M. C., Mazziotta, J. C., & Lenzi, G. L. (2003). Neural mechanisms of empathy in humans: a relay from neural systems for imitation to limbic areas. *Proceedings of the National Academy of Sciences of the United States of America, 100*(9), 5497–5502.

Carroll, J. M., & Russell, J. A. (1996). Do facial expressions signal specific emotions? Judging emotion from the face in context. *Journal of Personality and Social Psychology, 70*(2), 205–218.

Clarke, T. J., Bradshaw, M. F., Field, D. T., Hampson, S. E., & Rose, D. (2005). The perception of emotion from body movement in point-light displays of interpersonal dialogue. *Perception, 34*(10), 1171–1180.

Davenport, J. L., & Potter, M. C. (2004). Scene consistency in object and background perception. *Psychological Science, 15,* 559–564.

Davidson, R. J., & Dalton, K. (2003). Dysfuction in the neural circuitry of emotional face processing in individuals with autism. *Psychophysiology, 40*, s3.

Decety, J., & Chaminade, T. (2003). Neural correlates of feeling sympathy. *Neuropsychologia, 41*(2), 127–138.

de Gelder, B., & Hadjikhani, N. (2006). Non-conscious recognition of emotional body language. *Neuroreport, 17*(6), 583–586.

de Gelder, B., Pourtois, G., & Weiskrantz, L. (2002). Fear recognition in the voice is modulated by unconsciously recognized facial expressions but not by unconsciously recognized affective pictures. *Proceedings of the National Academy of Sciences USA, 99*(6), 4121–4126.

de Gelder, B., Snyder, J., Greve, D., Gerard,.G., & Hadjikhani, N. (2004). Fear fosters flight: A mechanism for fear contagion when perceiving emotion expressed by a whole body. *Proceedings of the National Academy of Sciences USA, 101*(47), 16701–16706.

de Gelder, B., & Vroomen, J. (2000). The perception of emotions by ear and by eye. *Cognition and Emotion, 14*(3), 289–311.

de Gelder, B., Vroomen, J., Pourtois, G., & Weiskrantz, L. (1999). Non-conscious recognition of affect in the absence of striate cortex. *Neuroreport, 10*(18), 3759–3763.

de Gelder, B., Vroomen, J., Pourtois, G., & Weiskrantz, L. (2000). Affective blindsight: Are we blindly led by emotions? Response to Heywood and Kentridge (2000). *Trends in Cognitive Science, 4*(4), 126–127.

de Meijer, M. (1989). The contribution of general features of body movement to the attribution of emotions. *Journal of Nonverbal Behavior, 13*, 247–268.

Denollet, J., Schiffer, A. A., Kwaijtaal, M., Hooijkaas, H., Hendriks, E. H., & Widdershoven, J. W. (2009). Usefulness of type D personality and kidney dysfunction as predictors of interpatient variability in inflammatory activation in chronic heart failure. *American Journal of Cardiology, 103*(3), 399–404.

Derntl, B., Windischberger, C., Robinson, S., Kryspin-Exner, I., Gur, R. C., & Moser, E. (2009). Amygdala activity to fear and anger in healthy young males is associated with testosterone. *Psychoneuroendocrinology, 34*(5), 687–693.

Downing, P. E., Jiang, Y., Shuman, M., & Kanwisher, N. (2001). A cortical area selective for visual processing of the human body. *Science, 293*(5539), 2470–2473.

Drevets, W. C. (1998). Functional neuroimaging studies of depression: The anatomy of melancholia. *Annual Review of Medicine, 49*, 341–361.

Drevets, W. C. (2007). Orbitofrontal cortex function and structure in depression. *Annals of the New York Academy of Science, 1121*, 499–527.

Eimer, M. (2000). The face-specific N170 component reflects late stages in the structural encoding of faces. *Neuroreport, 11*(10), 2319–2324.

Etkin, A., & Wager, T. D. (2007). Functional neuroimaging of anxiety: A meta-analysis of emotional processing in PTSD, social anxiety disorder, and specific phobia. *American Journal of Psychiatry, 164*(10), 1476–1488.

Fischer, H., Andersson, J. L., Furmark, T., & Fredrikson, M. (1998). Brain correlates of an unexpected panic attack: A human positron emission tomographic study. *Neuroscience Letters, 251*(2), 137–140.

Fossati, P., Hevenor, S. J., Graham, S. J., Grady, C., Keightley, M. L., & Craik, F. (2003). In search of the emotional self: An fMRI study using positive and negative emotional words. *American Journal of Psychiatry, 160*(11), 1938–1945.

Gliga, T., & Dehaene-Lambertz, G. (2005). Structural encoding of body and face in human infants and adults. *Journal of Cognitive Neuroscience, 17*, 1328–1340.

Grèzes, J., & Decety, J. (2001). Functional anatomy of execution, mental simulation, observation, and verb generation of actions: A meta-analysis. *Human Brain Mapping, 12*(1), 1–19.

Grèzes, J., Pichon, S., & de Gelder, B. (2007). Perceiving fear in dynamic body expressions. *Neuroimage, 35*(2), 959–967.

Grosbras, M. H., & Paus, T. (2006). Brain networks involved in viewing angry hands or faces. *Cerebral Cortex, 16*(8), 1087–1096.

Guyer, A. E., Monk, C. S., McClure-Tone, E. B., Nelson, E. E., Roberson-Nay, R., & Adler, A. D. (2008). A developmental examination of amygdala response to facial expressions. *Journal of Cognitive Neuroscience*.

Hadjikhani, N., & de Gelder, B. (2003). Seeing fearful body expressions activates the fusiform cortex and amygdala. *Current Biology, 13*(24), 2201–2205.

Hall, J. A. (1978). Gender effects in decoding nonverbal cues. *Psychological Bulletin, 85*, 845–857.

Hatfield, E., Cacioppo, J. T., & Rapson, R. L. (1994). *Emotional contagion*. Cambridge: Cambridge University Press.

Hunt, W. A. (1941). Recent developments in the field of emotion. *Psychological Bulletin, 38*, 249–276.

Hynes, C. A., Baird, A. A., & Grafton, S. T. (2006). Differential role of the orbital frontal lobe in emotional versus cognitive perspective-taking. *Neuropsychologia, 44*(3), 374–383.

Jackson, P. L., Meltzoff, A. N., & Decety, J. (2005). How do we perceive the pain of others? A window into the neural processes involved in empathy. *Neuroimage, 24*(3), 771–779.

Johansson, G. (1973). Visual perception of biological motion and a model for its analysis. *Perception & Psychophysics, 14*, 201–211.

Joubert, O. R., Fize, D., Rousselet, G. A., & Fabre-Thorpe, M. (2008). Early interference of context congruence on object processing in rapid visual categorization of natural scenes. *Journal of Vision, 8*(13), 1–18.

Kim, H., Somerville, L. H., Johnstone, T., Polis, S., Alexander, A. L., & Shin, L. M. (2004). Contextual modulation of amygdala responsivity to surprised faces. *Journal of Cognitive Neuroscience, 16*(10), 1730–1745.

Kret, M. E., & de Gelder, B. (2010). Social context influences recognition of bodily expressions. *Experimental Brain Research, 203*(1), 169–180.

Kret, M. E., Denollet, J., Grèzes, J., & de Gelder, B. (2011). The role of negative affectivity and social inhibition in perceiving social threat: An fMRI study. *Neuropsychologia, 49*, 1187–1193.

Kret, M. E., Pichon, S., Grèzes, J., & de Gelder, B. (2011a). Men fear other men most: Gender specific brain activations in perceiving threat from dynamic faces and bodies. An fMRI study. *Frontiers in Emotion Science, 2, 1–11.*

Kret, M. E., Pichon, S., Grèzes, J., & de Gelder B. (2011b). Similarities and differences in perceiving threat from dynamic faces and bodies. An fMRI study. *NeuroImage, 54*, 1755–1762.

Kring, A. M., & Gordon, A. H. (1998). Sex differences in emotion: Expression, experience, and physiology. *Journal of Personality and Social Psychology, 74*, 686–703.

Kringelbach, M. L., O'Doherty, J., Rolls, E. T., & Andrews, C. (2003). Activation of the human orbitofrontal cortex to a liquid food stimulus is correlated with its subjective pleasantness. *Cerebral Cortex, 13*(10), 1064–1071.

LaBar, K. S., Crupain, M. J., Voyvodic, J. T., & McCarthy, G. (2003). Dynamic perception of facial affect and identity in the human brain. *Cerebral Cortex, 13*(10), 1023–1033.

Lee, B. T., Seok, J. H., Lee, B. C., Cho, S. W., Yoon, B. J., & Lee, K. U. (2008). Neural correlates of affective processing in response to sad and angry facial stimuli in patients with major depressive disorder. *Progress in Neuropsychopharmacology and Biological Psychiatry, 32*(3), 778–785.

McClure, E. B. (2000). A meta-analytic review of sex differences in facial expression processing and their development in infants, children, and adolescents. *Psychological Bulletin, 126*, 424–453.

McDougall, W. (1920). *The group mind.* New York: G.P. Putnam's Sons.

Meeren, H. K., Hadjikhani, N., Ahlfors, S. P., Hamalainen, M. S., & de Gelder, B. (2008). Early category-specific cortical activation revealed by visual stimulus inversion. *PLoS ONE, 3*(10), e3503.

Meeren, H. K., van Heijnsbergen, C. C., & de Gelder, B. (2005). Rapid perceptual integration of facial expression and emotional body language. *Proceedings of the National Academy of Sciences USA, 102*(45), 16518–16523.

Mobbs, D., Weiskopf, N., Lau, H. C., Featherstone, E., Dolan, R. J., & Frith, C. D. (2006). The Kuleshov effect: The influence of contextual framing on emotional attributions. *Social Cognitive Affect in Neuroscience, 1*(2), 95–106.

Morris, J. S., deBonis, M., & Dolan, R. J. (2002). Human amygdala responses to fearful eyes. *Neuroimage, 17*(1), 214–222.

Palmer, L. A., & Rosenquist, A. C. (1975). Single-unit studies in the cat. *Neuroscience Research Program Bulletin, 13*(2), 214–220.

Peelen, M. V., Atkinson, A. P., Andersson, F., & Vuilleumier, P. (2007). Emotional modulation of body-selective visual areas. *Social, Cognitive and Affective Neurosciences, 2*, 274–283.

Pegna, A. J., Khateb, A., Lazeyras, F., & Seghier, M. L. (2005). Discriminating emotional faces without primary visual cortices involves the right amygdala. *Nature Neuroscience, 8*(1), 24–25.

Peluso, M. A., Glahn, D. C., Matsuo, K., Monkul, E. S., Najt, P., & Zamarripa, F. (2009). Amygdala hyperactivation in untreated depressed individuals. *Psychiatry Research, 173*(2), 158–161.

Pichon, S., De Gelder, B., & Grèzes, J. (2008). Emotional modulation of visual and motor areas by still and dynamic body expressions of anger. *Social Neuroscience 3*(3), 199–212.

Rauch, S. L., Savage, C. R., Alpert, N. M., Miguel, E. C., Baer, L., & Breiter, H. C. (1995). A positron emission tomographic study of simple phobic symptom provocation. *Archives of General Psychiatry, 52*(1), 20–28.

Reed, C. L., Stone, V. E., Bozova, S., & Tanaka, J. (2003). The body-inversion effect. *Psychology Science, 14*(4), 302–308.

Righart, R., & de Gelder, B. (2006). Context influences early perceptual analysis of faces: An electrophysiological study. *Cerebral Cortex, 16*(9), 1249–1257.

Righart, R., & de Gelder, B. (2007). Impaired face and body perception in developmental prosopagnosia. *Proceedings of the National Academy of Sciences of the United States of America, 104*(43), 17234–17238.

Righart, R., & de Gelder, B. (2008). Recognition of facial expressions is influenced by emotional scene gist. *Cognitive Affect in Behavioral Neuroscience, 8*(3), 264–272.

Rizzolatti, G., & Craighero, L. (2004). The mirror-neuron system. *Annual Review of Neuroscience, 27*, 169–192.

Rolls, E. T. (2000). The orbitofrontal cortex and reward. *Cerebral Cortex, 10*(3), 284–294.

Rushworth, M. F., Krams, M., & Passingham, R. E. (2001). The attentional role of the left parietal cortex: The distinct lateralization and localization of motor attention in the human brain. *Journal of Cognitive Neuroscience, 13*(5), 698–710.

Russell, J. A., & Fehr, B. (1987). Relativity in the perception of emotion in facial expressions. *Journal of Experimental Psychology: General, 116*(3), 223–237.

Sato, W., Kochiyama, T., Yoshikawa, S., Naito, E., & Matsumura, M. (2004). Enhanced neural activity in response to dynamic facial expressions of emotion: An fMRI study. *Brain Research and Cognitive Brain Research, 20*(1), 81–91.

Schwarzlose, R. F., Baker, C. I., & Kanwisher, N. (2005). Separate face and body selectivity on the fusiform gyrus. *Journal of Neuroscience, 25*(47), 11055–11059.

Shah, S. G., Klumpp, H., Angstadt, M., Nathan, P. J., & Phan, K. L. (2009). Amygdala and insula response to emotional images in patients with generalized social anxiety disorder. *Journal of Psychiatry and Neuroscience, 34*(4), 296–302.

Sinke, C. B. A., Sorger, B., Goebel, R., & de Gelder, B. (2010). Tease or threat? Judging social interactions from bodily expressions. *NeuroImage, 49*(2), 1717–1727.

Stekelenburg, J. J., & de Gelder, B. (2004). The neural correlates of perceiving human bodies: An ERP study on the body-inversion effect. *Neuroreport, 15*(5), 777–780.
Straube, T., Mentzel, H. J., & Miltner, W. H. (2005). Common and distinct brain activation to threat and safety signals in social phobia. *Neuropsychobiology, 52*(3), 163–168.
Thierry, G., Pegna, A. J., Dodds, C., Roberts, M., Basan, S., & Downing, P. (2006). An event-related potential component sensitive to images of the human body. *Neuroimage, 32*(2), 871–879.
Thomas, K. M., Drevets, W. C., Whalen, P. J., Eccard, C. H., Dahl, R. E., & Ryan, N. D. (2001). Amygdala response to facial expressions in children and adults. *Biological Psychiatry, 49*, 309–316.
Thornton, I. M., & Vuong, Q. C. (2004). Incidental processing of biological motion. *Currents in Biology, 14*(12), 1084–1089.
van de Riet, W. A. C., Grèzes, J., & de Gelder, B. (2009). Specific and common brain regions involved in the perception of faces and bodies and the representation of their emotional expressions. *Social Neuroscience, 4*(2), 101–120.
Van den Stock, J., Righart, R., & de Gelder, B. (2007). Body expressions influence recognition of emotions in the face and voice. *Emotion, 7*(3), 487–494.
van Heijnsbergen, C. C., Meeren, H. K., Grèzes, J., & de Gelder, B. (2007). Rapid detection of fear in body expressions, an ERP study. *Brain Research, 1186*, 233–241.
van Honk, J., & Schutter, D. J. (2007). Testosterone reduces conscious detection of signals serving social correction: Implications for antisocial behavior. *Psychology and Science, 18*(8), 663–667.
Van Overwalle, F., & Baetens, K. (2009). Understanding others' actions and goals by mirror and mentalizing systems: A meta-analysis. *Neuroimage, 48*(3), 564–584.
Vrticka, P., Andersson, F., Grandjean, D., Sander, D., & Vuilleumier, P. (2008). Individual attachment style modulates human amygdala and striatum activation during social appraisal. *PLoS One, 3*(8), e2868.
Vuilleumier, P., Armony, J. L., Driver, J., & Dolan, R. J. (2001). Effects of attention and emotion on face processing in the human brain: An event-related fMRI study. *Neuron, 30*(3), 829–841.
Wicker, B., Keysers, C., Plailly, J., Royet, J. P., Gallese, V., & Rizzolatti, G. (2003). Both of us disgusted in my insula: The common neural basis of seeing and feeling disgust. *Neuron, 40*(3), 655–664.

# 16 Risk assessment and decision making

*Leslie R. Pendrill*
SP Technical Research Institute of Sweden
Borås, Sweden

## 16.1 Introduction

One of the principal motives for making any measurement is to provide objective evidence on which decisions of conformity of entities of any kind (product, service, etc.) to specifications can be based. This chapter deals with decisions of conformity based on measurements specifically with persons, either where measurements are made of a person or where a person can be considered as a measurement instrument. A brief introduction to conformity assessment is followed by two main sections, dealing, respectively, with uncertainty and with the treatment of risk assessment associated with uncertainties when making decisions.

Special aspects of measurements with persons include the complexity of the subject of measurement, ranging from objective to more subjective measures and including perception, interpretation, and cognition. Uncertainties, which are often appreciable, need to be accounted for in multivariate measurement, exposure/stimulus, and hazard/response. Variability is relatively large, both for each individual as well as between different individuals. Basic concepts of quality-assured measurement familiar in "traditional" metrology in engineering and physics, such as traceability to reference standards and measurement uncertainty, can nevertheless be applied when measuring humans, as has been explored in one of the main thrusts of the EU project MINET (2009). Indeed such concepts of quality-assured measurement are essential in any situation—such as health care and in the control room—where a human being can often be the most critical or the weakest link in the overall measurement system.

The MINET network has the ambition to advance the measurement of multi-dimensional phenomena that are mediated by human interpretation or perception, to be able to advance the frontiers of the science of measurement, and to respond to future requirements for measuring properties such as comfort, naturalness, perceived quality, feelings, body language, and consciousness. At the same time, one is aware of and is trying to bridge the gap between an engineering tradition which is criticized for a far too instrumental view of operators and the humanistic and behavioral science tradition all too preoccupied with issues centered on human operators. The

MINET network consists of a unique mix of physicists, engineers, medical scientists, neurologists, psychologists, and sociologists (EU NEST, 2007).

MINET is investigating how "generic" metrological issues of (1) measurement concepts and terminology, (2) measurement techniques, (3) measurement uncertainty, and (4) decision making and impact assessment can be applied specifically to measurement of persons in terms of man as a measurement instrument and measuring man. This has been studied among others in a series of MINET Think Tanks (2009) and presented in an Internet-based online MINET Repository (2009).

Conformity assessment provides confidence that requirements have been met and is often essential for reasons of public interest, public health, safety, and order, protection of the environment, the consumer and in ensuring fair trade. Assessment is often based on measurement data (EU Commission, 2004, 2005, 2006; Codex 2004). Measurements with persons, either where measurements are made of a person or where a person can be considered as a measurement instrument, are the focus of this chapter.

Measurement and testing of entities provide valuable, often quantitative, evidence on which decisions of conformity can be based. Many tests are, however, made in practical situations where time and resources are limited. A balance has to be struck between expenditure on inspection and the potential costs associated with various risks, to both the supplier and customer, associated with incorrect decisions arising from limited measurement accuracy and test uncertainties (ILAC, 1996; Williams & Hawkins, 1993; Thompson & Fearn, 1996; AFNOR, 2004; Pendrill, 2007).

Two main sections of this chapter deal, respectively, with uncertainty (Section 16.2) and with the treatment of risk assessment associated with uncertainties when making decisions (Section 16.3). A discussion in terms of utility of common rules in conformity assessment based on measurement is given. The methodology is of general applicability but is illustrated in the present work with examples when measurements and decisions are made with persons. Optimum strategies for the supplier are illustrated in terms of minimizing production and testing costs, while at the same time maintaining satisfactory levels of customer satisfaction.

The application of a unified approach is a step toward establishing clearer procedures for setting and specifying tolerances and associated uncertainties, and in facilitating acceptance of conformity by both customer and supplier, even in measurements of perception and cognition.

## 16.2 Measurement of human performance and reliability

The presence of a human operator can be a major factor in determining the overall performance and reliability of a measurement system. It is therefore important to describe, measure, assess conformity, and improve the performance and reliability of a human as an essential component in any system, alongside other key components.

The performance capability and reliability of a human as a component of a measurement system can be described in ways somewhat similar to the description of other key components of the system. The classic model of a measurement system (MSA, 1995) is shown in Figure 16.1, where the object is the entity to be measured;

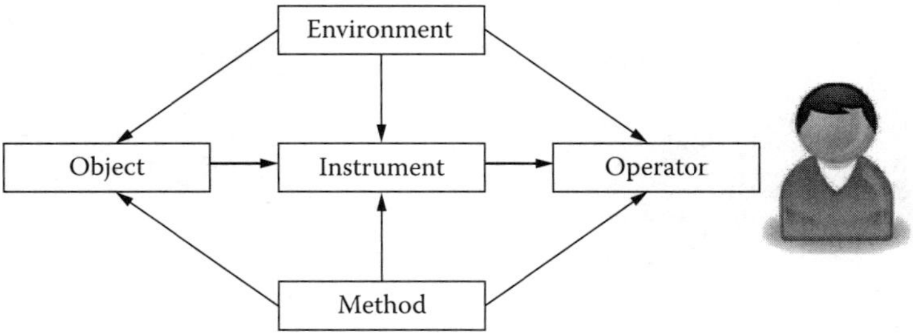


*Figure 16.1* Man as the operator in a measurement system.

and a human operator monitors and controls the object by interpreting information signals from the object communicated via a measurement instrument. These three basic elements—object, instrument, and operator—can all be influenced in different ways by the actual environment of measurement as well as the chosen measurement method.

The same basic measurement system model can also be applied in assessing the capability and reliability of a human, by introducing man as one or other of the basic elements of the system. A useful distinction in measurements concerning humans is to either view a human as the object one makes measurements on or as a measurement instrument:

- *Measuring Man:* Measures of human body language and consciousness can be important factors in assessing human performance and reliability, in other words, human alertness, stress, and health (Section 16.2.1).
- *Man as Measurement Instrument:* Human performance and reliability can be understood in terms of human perception of one's surroundings in terms of perceived comfort, naturalness, quality, feelings, and so on—human awareness (Section 16.2.2)—in creating and maintaining a correct mental model of the system.

In this chapter, we use this distinction repeatedly and describe these two cases in the following sections.

### *16.2.1 Measuring man*

In the case of *measuring man*, the measurement object in the measurement system (Figure 16.2) is a person and one often aims to assess human performance, health, and reliability. This covers disciplines that include physiology, psychology, psychophysics, psychometrics, and sociology. In making measurements on man himself, for instance when attempting to assess the performance of an individual in a control room, a wide range of measurement techniques can be employed, from functional magnetic resonance imaging (fMRI) of brain activity to self-reporting from the human measurement object himself. With all the complexity this implies and

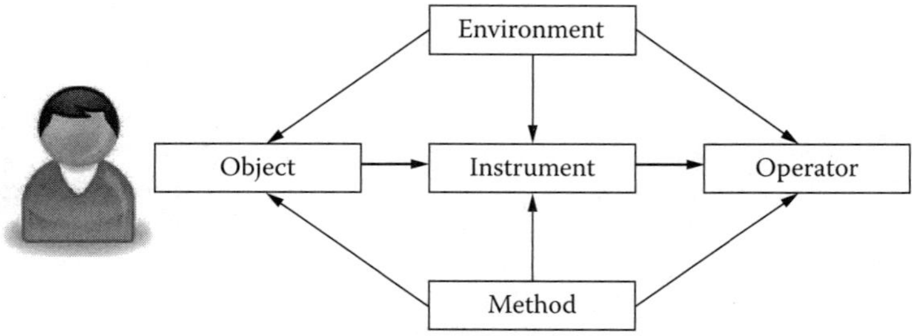


*Figure 16.2* Measuring man.

*Table 16.1* Information and measurement

| *Element* | *Person* | *Uncertainty* | *Information* | *Communication* |
|---|---|---|---|---|
| Object | Measuring man | Hazard and exposure | "Ambiguity": nonspecific, one-to-many relation, variety, generality, diversity, and divergence | Act of measurement (or more generally of transmitting a message) will reduce our ignorance or uncertainty |
| Instrument | Man as instrument | Measurement | "Vagueness": fuzziness, unclearness, indistinctness, etc. | Uncertainty reflects certain loss of information when communicating message from transmitter to receiver |
| Operator | Man as operator | Measurement | Lack of knowledge or skill | Act of measurement will reduce our ignorance or uncertainty—Bayes' theorem |

where the measurement object may react differently each time the measurement is made, uncertainties can in many cases be expected to be appreciable.

Table 16.1 summarizes different categories of uncertainty in perceptive measurement. Measurement uncertainty will often be a dominant factor, as an essential factor for quantifying the quality of the measurements and in making decisions of conformity, and reflecting limitations in measurement knowledge. On the other hand, hazard (or response) uncertainty can be a main concern when measuring man.

### 16.2.1.1 *Example: Different measurements of human fatigue*

Fatigue is highly relevant for operators as a parameter when measuring man. In a recent study of driver alertness in a vehicle (Schleicher, Galley, Briest, & Galley,

2008), two different measurement methods were employed to gauge the level of fatigue. In addition to a self-assessment by the driver of his own level of alertness at various times during a particular drive, a novel measurement technique was used, involving video monitoring of the eye movements, including blinks and saccades. When comparing the measurement results from two methods such as in this case (Schleicher et al., 2008), it is important in assessing apparent differences in alertness estimates obtained by the two methods to ensure that each method can be traced to common reference standards. In addition, it is difficult to judge the significance of any differences in results of the two methods unless measurement uncertainties for both sets of measurement results are not only calculated and displayed in any comparative presentation but also interpreted in terms of consequence and impact.

### *16.2.1.2 Example: Risks of exposure and toxicity in measurements with persons*

An example of conformity assessment when measuring man concerns the case where uncertainties in levels of exposure and in levels of toxicity have to be weighed together in assessing overall risks when making measurements with persons. In such cases, as illustrated in Figure 16.3, estimates of the probability risk of exposure are plotted together with the predicted increase in risk of toxicity with increasing exposure/dose. The dotted lines beside each main curve in Figure 16.3 represent the estimated uncertainties in each cumulative probability curve for exposure and toxicity. The overall impact on human health is determined by a combination of the risk of exposure and the risk of toxicity for each level of exposure. We return below (Section 16.3.2) to a general approach to introducing measures of impact and risk in conformity assessment in measurements with man.

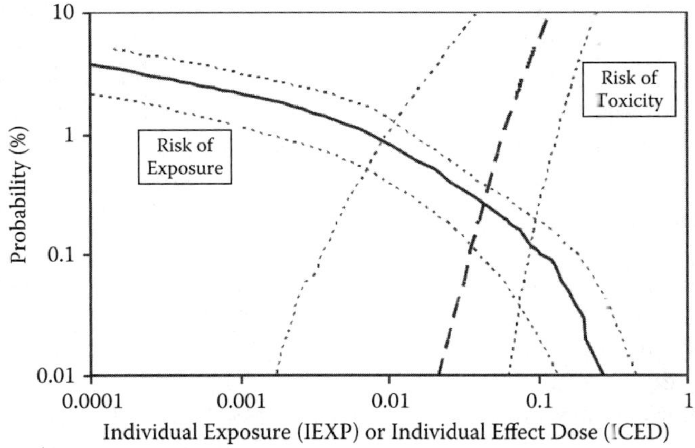


*Figure 16.3* Plotting the risk of exposure against the risk of toxicity over a range of exposure levels. Reproduced from van der Voet and Slob (2007), with permission.

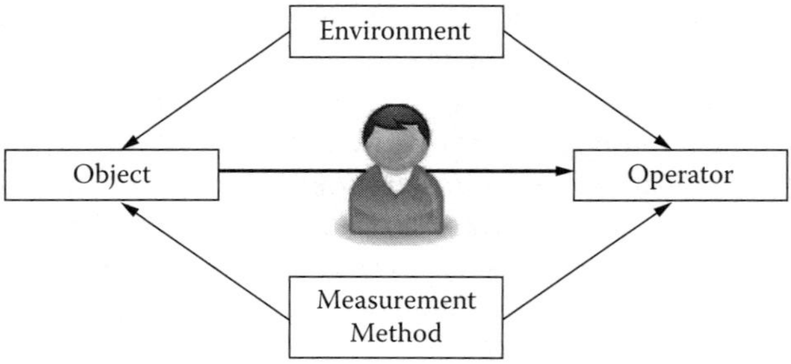


*Figure 16.4* Man as a measurement instrument.

### 16.2.2 Man as a measurement instrument

The instrument in the measurement system (Figure 16.4) can in some cases be replaced by a person as is of interest, for instance, when aiming to understand human performance and reliability as a critical element in any system. An example of the latter is a series of paintings of the Houses of Parliament in London made by the famous artist Monet (Baker and Thornes 2006): a comparison with actual instrumental measurements of the appearance and profile of the buildings reveals some considerable variation in Monet's perception, both from painting to painting but also with reality! Measurement uncertainty is a prime issue when the person is himself acting as a measurement instrument.

When man is the measurement instrument, we have exchanged the traditional measurement instrument, which often is considered as objective, with a subjective human and perception with the five senses. Measured quantities include perceived comfort, naturalness, quality, feelings, and human awareness. An extra dimension is that the human instrument (as with the human object above) might be highly variable with time and it will sometimes be difficult to repeat measurements under similar conditions. In this type of work, the calibration of the perceived intensity of various stimuli might be challenging (Berglund and Harju, 2003), although there is a long tradition in some areas, such as in vision and hearing, of quality-assured measurement in photometry and acoustics, respectively, where explicit allowance for the human physiological response is already included.

#### *16.2.2.1 Example: Operator reaction time*

In a control room, a human may well intervene by taking the role of a measurement instrument in measuring a particular characteristic of an object to be studied (such as the system to be controlled or the display of an instrument in a control panel console).

One example is measurement and assessment of human performance response time in the case of a signaler's intervention in a rail incident in the United Kingdom. Despite being identified in the incident investigation as a major factor, more recent research (Stanton and Baber, 2008) has shown that the 18-second response time of the signaler is in no way exceptionally long and that there is a wide variability of human response times when interpreting and acting on, for example, alarm signals on instrument displays among different individuals and under different circumstances. In such cases, key factors indicating the level of quality of measurement, such as measurement method accuracy and measurement uncertainty when determining human reaction times, can be crucial in making objective and correct decisions of conformity.

### *16.2.2.2 Example: Risks in nuclear waste storage*

A panel of experts was asked to estimate the overall probability for a certain event with increasing values of an influence parameter $x$ in estimating the risks with long-term nuclear waste storage (Helton, Johnson, Sallaberry, & Storlie, 2006). As noted by these authors, the experts did not necessarily have to formulate estimated probability distribution functions (PDF) but only how the cumulative probabilities (CDF) vary in their judgment. An acceptable procedure is then to take an average of the different operating characteristic curves for the various experts in order to get a consensus value.

The tool can also be employed when uncertainties are based not on probability theory, but also on evidence theory (plausibility and belief) and possibility theory (possibility and necessity) (Helton et al., 2006). Curves such as shown in Figure 16.5

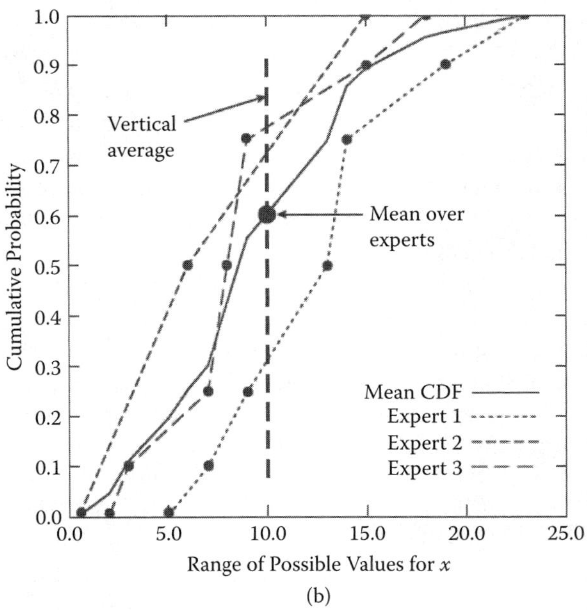


*Figure 16.5* Operating characteristics judged on a number of experts. Reproduced from Helton et al. (2006), with permission.

(called operating characteristics or power curves in traditional statistical significance testing; Montgomery, 1996) arise where there is a distribution—either intrinsic or apparent—in quantity values; without such a distribution, associated, for example, with uncertainty due to a less than complete knowledge of exact response or exact level of exposure, probabilities would show sharp limits where, for instance, the risk of exposure would fall abruptly to zero at a particular exposure level.

An account of statistical significance testing (Montgomery, 1996), including the derivation of operating characteristics (power curves) from probability distribution functions, is deferred to later in this chapter (Section 16.3).

### *16.2.3 Measurement scales and measurement uncertainty in perception*

With measurement techniques so diverse, ranging from fMRI to self-reporting, and from objective to more subjective judgments, perceptive measurements cover a large variety of classes. In order to treat these measurements correctly there is a variety of scales: ordinal, interval, and ratio (nominal scales are not usual referred to as measurement). For the different scales there are different permissible operations and different appropriate statistics.

Much effort has been expended in the metrology community over the past decade or so in giving guidance about, and harmonizing how to evaluate, measurement uncertainty (JCGM 100, 2008). Any measurement system (consisting of an instrument, operator, method, environment, and the object itself, as shown in Figure 16.1) is not perfect and errors caused by limitations in the quality of the particular measurement system at hand can affect the result of any measurement. Measurement uncertainty here refers to situations where time and resources are limited so that not all measurement errors are fully evaluated and corrected for; that is, limited measurement quality can lead to an apparent variability in measurement data. Measurement uncertainty can be evaluated in different ways, with probability theory being one of the dominant schools. Special aspects of the evaluation of measurement uncertainty with persons include subjectivity and that uncertainties, which are often appreciable, need to be accounted for in multivariate measurement (Emardson, Jarlemark, & Floberg, 2005; van der Heijden & Emardson, this volume).

Apart from measurement uncertainty, other forms of uncertainty will be of concern in general conformity assessment. For instance, in making decisions of conformity about, say, environmental exposure of persons to some stimulus (noise, poison, etc.), there will be uncertainties both in the actual levels of exposure and of potential hazards that certain levels of exposure can mean for persons, which may of course vary from case to case and from person to person, as exemplified above (Section 16.2.1.2). In measurements with persons it is important to distinguish between uncertainties in the actual levels of exposure and hazard and between these and measurement uncertainties in each of these quality characteristics.

Various kinds of uncertainty can be regarded as examples of a more general treatment of information theory, as summarized in Table 16.1. In a probabilistic approach to measurement uncertainty, it is interesting to note in the context of measurements with persons that use of Bayes' theorem allows the inclusion of prior measurement knowledge by the operator, in which the actual measurement enables an updating of knowledge about the measurement value. Prior knowledge complements a regular statistical frequentist kind, by adding a more experience-based evidence (where corresponding methods of evaluation of measurement uncertainty are termed type A and type B, respectively, in the GUM approach).

Accepting that uncertainty of all kinds is often associated with limited communication of information, Klir and Folger (1988) emphasize that to deal adequately with uncertainty in human communication, it is necessary to account for three aspects of information:

*Syntactic:* Relationship among signs employed for communication
*Semantic*: Relationship between signs and the entities for which they stand, that is, meaning of signs
*Pragmatic*: Relationship between signs and their utility

As discussed in the context of conformity assessment and decision making (Section 16.3.2), it has been found useful not only to employ syntactic and semantic types of information, but also to include pragmatic measures of utility in assessing risks associated with uncertainty.

## 16.3 Conformity assessment and measuring man

The aim of conformity assessment of a type of entity is to assess conformance of actual values of a characteristic with respect to specification limits (Montgomery, 1996; Joglekar 2003). Dispersion in characteristic entity values will be due to actual variability in the manufacturing process when the product is made. Subsequent entity variability will be due to wear and tear during the product lifetime.

The various tools of statistics can be used in different ways in conformity assessment; they can be used to describe actual variability as well as enable modeling of probable variability. Such statistical modeling is useful in cases where actual variability is not known, where prior knowledge needs to be included, and when predictions are made in advance in order to plan for measurements in the best way.

In evaluating production variations of quantity $\eta = X$ in the entity (or product) space, measurements made multilaterally might be on repeated items in a production process or by taking a sample of the population of items subject to conformity assessment. The corresponding probability distribution function PDF, $g_{entity}(x)$, will have a form determined ideally (in the absence of measurement or sampling uncertainty) by the intrinsic quantity variations of prime interest in conformity assessment.

Measurement quality variations, expressed with a measurement uncertainty PDF $g_{test}$, may partially mask observations of actual entity dispersion. As such, measurement variability is just one, and it is hoped, a relatively minor, source of uncertainty that needs to be accounted for when making decisions of conformity. A general challenge is to find methods that can be used reliably to separate these different variability components. Uncertainties associated with entity variability and stimulus variability will often be of dominant concern. Overall decisions of conformity will need to account for each of these different kinds of uncertainty in order to assess commensurate risks correctly (van der Voet and Slob, 2007).

Independently of whether conformity assessment is made of objects or persons, it is important to specify the assessment target as clearly as possible: *global* conformity denotes the assessment of populations of typical entities, whereas *specific* conformity assessment refers to inspection of single items or individuals (Rossi and Crenna, 2006). Specification limits are often set in conformity assessment on actual values of a characteristic of a type of entity.

### *16.3.1 Uncertainties and risks of incorrect decision making*

An important factor in making decisions of conformity assessment is to allow for the risks of incorrect decision making arising from uncertainty. Test results clearly inside or outside the regions of permissible values can lead readily to unambiguous decisions about conformity or nonconformity.

Uncertainty can lead to:

- Correctly conforming human operators being incorrectly failed on inspection
- Nonconforming human operators being incorrectly passed on inspection

particularly when a test result is close to a specification limit. As shown in Figure 16.6(a), a test result, apparently within limits, might actually be nonconforming in as much as the tail of the probability distribution function extends slightly beyond the limit. An example is an assessment of compliance with specified minimum reaction times for a human in a control room, as exemplified in the case of the railway signaler (Section 16.2.2.1).

Uncertainty can also lead to ambiguity when assessing the significance in general of an apparent difference in pairs of measurement results, for instance, as obtained from two different measurement methods (see example of driver fatigue, Section 16.2.1.1). As shown in Figure 16.6(b), two measurement results can be examined as to whether they are significantly different by assessing the distance in entity value separating the two distributions' PDF.

There is, as is well known, a complete set of statistical significance tests for distributions of individual and average values, as well as tests of variances. These include for variables the *t*-test and Normal tests to determine whether an unknown population mean differs from a standard population mean, and the $\chi^2$-test and *F*-test to determine whether an unknown population standard deviation is greater or less than a standard value (Ferris, Grubbs, & Weaver, 1946: Montgomery, 1996). Corresponding tests when sampling by attribute (i.e., binary decisions such as go/no-go yielding percent nonconforming, for example) can be based on the binomial and Poisson distributions (Joglekar, 2003). The comparison and significance testing of multiple populations can be tackled by conducting analysis of variance (ANOVA; Joglekar, 2003).

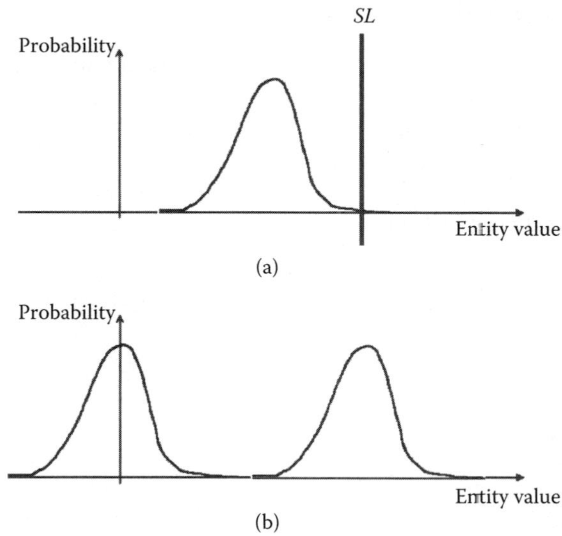


*Figure 16.6* Comparing a distribution (PDF) of entity values: (a) with a specification limit, SL; (b) between two sets of observations.

Risks and the consequences of incorrect decision making in conformity assessment of human performance and reliability in control rooms should be evaluated. They can be minimized by setting limits on maximum permissible measurement uncertainties and on maximum permissible consequence costs.

### *16.3.2 Introducing impact and cost into conformity assessment risks*

"Utility … is only a description of the subjective judgement of the decision-maker… . It thus does not appear to be measurement" (Finkelstein, 2005). But we would argue that utility *does* become a key factor in conformity assessment based on pragmatic measurement with persons. In general, the impact of a wrong decision in conformity assessment is expressed as a risk *Risk*, defined as the probability $p$ of the wrong decision occurring multiplied by the cost (utility) $C$ of the consequences of the incorrect decision:

$$Risk = p \cdot C \tag{16.1}$$

In this section, new expressions for decision-making risks including costs are presented, together with a novel tool—the operating cost characteristic curve—as an extension of traditional statistical tools, with the addition of an economic decision-theory approach. Complementarity with the optimized uncertainty methodology (Thompson and Fearn, 1996) is emphasized in the concluding remarks.

### *16.3.3 Conformity assessment by variable*

Inspection by variable involves measurement of the magnitude $y_m$ of a characteristic of an item (ISO 3951-1 2005). Taking account of varying costs/impact for different quantity values in the case where product cost value varies with unit quantity value with the cost function C(η), leads to the following:

*Customer's cost risk*:

$$C_{specific}(y_m) = \int_{\eta < L_{SL}} C(\eta) \cdot g_{test}(\eta | y_m) \cdot d\eta \tag{16.2}$$

with $y_m \geq L_{SL}$.

*Supplier's cost risk:*

$$C^*_{specific}(y_m) = \int_{\eta \geq L_{SL}} C^*(\eta) \cdot g_{test}(\eta | y_m) \cdot d\eta \tag{16.3}$$

with $y_m < L_{SL}$ for specific conformity assessment involving the inspection of an entity with respect to a (lower) specification limit $L_{SL}$. The integral in Equation (16.2), for instance, corresponds to the tail of the probability distribution function extending slightly beyond the specification limit illustrated in Figure 16.6(a) for a test result apparently within limits.

An incorrect accept on inspection of a nonconforming object will lead to customer costs associated with an out-of-tolerance product. Overall costs, consisting of a sum of testing costs and the costs associated with customer risk (Equation 16.2), can be calculated with the expression:

$$E(y_m, \sigma) = D(y_m, \sigma) + C(y_m) = \frac{D}{\sigma^2} + \int_{\eta \notin R_{PV}} C(\eta) \cdot g(\eta | y_m) \cdot d\eta \tag{16.4}$$

with $y_m \in R_{PV}$, where $R_{PV}$ denotes the region of permissible entity values, where test costs $D$ are modeled as varying inversely to the squared dispersion σ. Expression (16.4) can be applied to both specific and global conformity assessment (Pendrill, 2007).

Overall costs E($y_m$,σ), according to (16.4) can be plotted over either of the following:

1. A range of quantity values of $L_{SL} - h \cdot \sigma \leq y_m \leq L_{SL} + h \cdot \sigma$ for a given test dispersion σ, and guard-band factor $h$, yielding an "operating cost characteristic" analogous to the traditional, probability-based operating characteristic.
2. A range of test uncertainties σ for a given quantity value $y_m \geq L_{SL}$, the so-called "optimized uncertainty curve."

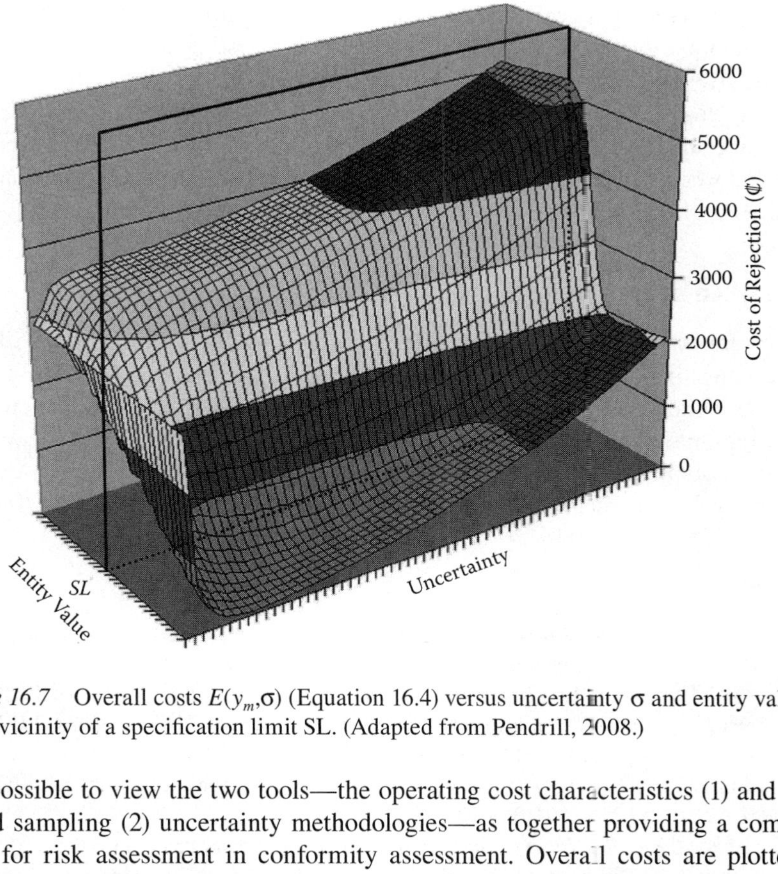


*Figure 16.7* Overall costs $E(y_m,\sigma)$ (Equation 16.4) versus uncertainty $\sigma$ and entity value $y_m$ in the vicinity of a specification limit SL. (Adapted from Pendrill, 2008.)

It is possible to view the two tools—the operating cost characteristics (1) and optimized sampling (2) uncertainty methodologies—as together providing a complete basis for risk assessment in conformity assessment. Overall costs are plotted in three dimensions, shown in Figure 16.7, where at each entity value on the operating characteristic curve, the corresponding optimized uncertainty curve would cross in the orthogonal direction. The U-shaped optimized uncertainty curve (case 2 above, where the costs of testing are balanced against the costs of incorrect decision making) is clearly visible along the uncertainty axis of the 3-D plot in Figure 16.7. In this way, the optimum uncertainty required at specific conformity assessment points, such as those for customer and supplier risk, can be identified across the full range of entity values.

## 16.4 Conclusions

Having agreed on appropriate descriptors of human performance and reliability and how to measure and assess them, a next step would be to consider ways of improving these. An example of how the effects of training can be measured and improve human performance and reliability in control room situations is Sauer, Burkolter, Kluge, Ritzmann, and Schüler (2008).

The work presented here extends traditional significance testing to include utility and economic assessments of the costs of measuring, testing, and sampling together with the costs of incorrect decision making. This provides the decisionmaker with a more complete and arguably more relevant assessment of expectations and risks additionally including measures of impact, importance, and consequence. This is especially important when assessing perceptive or cognitive measurements where a human being can often be the most critical or the weakest link in the overall measurement system.

## Acknowledgments

Thanks are owing for discussions about the performance of the testing of different measurement instruments to Håkan Källgren, Jan-Erik Elander, Jonatan Westerberg, and other colleagues at SP. The author has also benefited from participation in the Joint Committee for Guides in Metrology (JCGM), Working Group 1. This work has been partially financed by grant 38:10 National Metrology of the Swedish Ministry of Industry, Employment and Communication.

## References

AFNOR (2004). Metrology and statistical applications: Use of uncertainty in measurement: Presentation of some examples and common practice, FD x07-022, 2004.

Baker, J. & Thornes, J. E. (2006). Solar position within Monet's Houses of Parliament. *Proceedings of the Royal Society A, 462*, 3775–3788, doi: 10.1098/rspa.2006.1754.

Berglund, B., & Harju, E.-L. (2003). Master scaling of perceived intensity of touch, cold and warmth. *European Journal of Pain, 7,* 323–334 Special Issue dedicated to Ulf Lindblom, doi:10.1016/S1090-3801(03)00043-0.

Codex (2004). *General guidelines on sampling* (codex alimentarius commission FAO/WHO of the United Nations, CAC/GL 50-2004), www.codexalimentarius.net/download/standards/10141/CXG_050e.pdf.

Emardson, T. R., Jarlemark, P. O. J., & Floberg, P. (2005). Uncertainty evaluation in multivariate analysis: A test case study. *Journal of Mathematical Modelling and Algorithms, 4,* 289–305, doi: 10.1007/s10852-005-9005-2.

EU Commission (2004). MID *Measurement instrument directive PE-CONS 3626/04* MID 2004/22/EC (2004),
http://europa.eu/eur-lex/pri/en/oj/dat/2004/l_135/l_13520040430en00010080.pdf.

EU Commission (2005). Metrology, pre-packaging, http://ec.europa.eu/enterprise/prepack/metrol_requir/inmetrolog_requir_en.htm; OIML 2004 R 87 Quantity of product in prepackages; OIML 2004 E 4 The statistical principles of the metrological surveillance of the net content of prepackages as laid down by the CEE 76/211 Directive, International Recommendation, International Organisation of Legal Metrology (www.oiml.org).

EU Commission (2006). N560-2 EN 2006-0906 Annex to A Horizontal Legislative Approach to the Harmonisation of Legislation on Industrial Products, European Commission, http://ec.europa.eu/enterprise/newapproach/review_en.htm.

EU NEST (2007). Measuring the impossible projects. ftp://ftp.cordis.europa.eu/pub/nest/docs/1-nest-measuring-290507.pdf.

Ferris, C. D., Grubbs, F. E., & Weaver, C. L. (1946). Operating characteristics for the common statistical tests of significance. *Annals of Mathematical Statistics, 17,* 178–197.

Finkelstein L (2005). *Measurement,* 38, 267–274.

GUM (2008). *Evaluation of measurement data: Guide to the expression of uncertainty in measurement*, JCGM 100:2008 (GUM 1995 with minor corrections), http://www.bipm.org/en/publications/guides/gum.html.

Helton, J. C., Johnson, J. D., Sallaberry, C. J., & Storlie, C. B. (2006). Survey of sampling-based methods for uncertainty and sensitivity analysis. *Reliability Engineering and Safety Systems, 91,* 1175–1209.

ILAC (1996). *Guidelines on assessment and reporting of compliance with specification*, Guide no. 8.

ISO 3951-1 (2005). *Sampling procedures for inspection by variables—Part 1*, ISO Geneva (CH).

JCGM 100 (2008). *Evaluation of measurement data—Guide to the expression of uncertainty in measurement, GUM 1995 with minor corrections.*

JCGM WG1 (2009). *Evaluation of measurement data—The role of measurement uncertainty in deciding conformance to specified requirements, draft GUM Supplement JCGM 106* April.

Joglekar, A. M. (2003). *Statistical methods for Six Sigma in R&D and manufacturing.* Hoboken, NJ: Wiley.

Klir, G. J., & Folger, T. A. (1988). *Fuzzy sets, uncertainty and information.* Englewood Cliffs, NJ: Prentice-Hall.

MINET (2009). http://minet.wordpress.com.

MINET Repository (2009). http://minet3repository.wordpress.com/.

MINET Think Tanks (2009). http://lesliependrill.wordpress.com/minet-wp3-think-tanks/.

Montgomery, D. C. (1996). *Introduction to statistical quality control.* Hoboken, NJ: Wiley.

MSA (1995). Measurement system analysis MSA. Chrysler Corp, Ford Motor Company and General Motor Corporation, Reference manual, 2nd edition.

Pendrill, L. R. (2006). Optimised measurement uncertainty and decision-making when sampling by variables or by attribute. *Measurement, 39,* 829–840, Advanced Mathematical Tools for Measurement in Metrology and Testing, http://dx.doi.org/10.1016/j.measurement.2006.04.014.

Pendrill, L. R. (2007). Optimised measurement uncertainty and decision-making in conformity assessment, *NCSLi MEASURE*, 2(2), 76–86.

Pendrill, L. R. (2008). Operating 'cost' characteristics in sampling by variable and attribute. *Accredited Quality Assurance, 13,* 619– 631, doi: 10.1007/s00769-008-0438-y.

Pendrill, L. R., & Källgren, H. (2006a). Decision-making with uncertainty in attribute sampling. *Advanced Mathematical and Computational Tools in Metrology VII* in Series on Advances in Mathematics for Applied Sciences 72, pp. 212– 220, Singapore: World Scientific.

Pendrill, L. R., & Källgren, H. (2006b). *Exhaust gas analysers and optimised sampling, uncertainties and costs, Accredited Quality Assurance 11,* 496–505, doi: 10.1007/s00769-006-0163-3. http://dx.doi.org/10.1007/s00769-006-0163-3.

Pendrill, L. R., & Källgren, H. (2008). Optimised measurement uncertainty and decision-making in the metering of energy, fuel and exhaust gases. *Izmeritelnaya Technika (Measurement Techniques), 4,* 18–22, April. doi: 10.1007/s11018-008-9047-8.

Rossi, G. B., & Crenna, F. (2006). A probabilistic approach to measurement-based decisions. *Measurement, 39,* 101–119.

Sauer, J., Burkolter, D., Kluge, A., Ritzmann, S., & Schüler, K. (2008). The effects of heuristic rule training on operator performance in a simulated process control environment. *Ergonomics, 51,* 953–967, doi: 10.1080/00140130801915238.

Schleicher, R., Galley, N., Briest, S., & Galley, L. (2008). Blinks and saccades as indicators of fatigue in sleepiness warnings: Looking tired? *Ergonomics, 51* (7 July), 982–1010, doi: 10.1080/00140130701817062.

Stanton, N. A., & Baber, C. (2008). Modelling of human alarm response times: A case study of the Ladbroke Grove rail accident. *Ergonomics, 51*(4), 423–440, doi: 10.1080/00140130701695419.

Thompson, M., & Fearn, T. (1996). What exactly is fitness for purpose in analytical measurement? *Analyst, 121,* 275–278.

van der Heijden, G. & Emardson, R. (this volume). Multivariate measurements. In B. Berglund, G. B. Rossi, J. T. Townsend, & L. R. Pendril (Eds.). *Measurement With Persons: Theory, Methods, and Implementation Areas* (pp. 125–142). New York: Psychology Press.

van der Voet, H., & Slob, W. (2007). Integration of probabilistic hazard characterization. *Risk Analysis, 27,* 351–371.

Williams, R. H., & Hawkins, C. F. (1993). The economics of guardband placement. *Proceedings, 24th IEEE International Test Conference*, Baltimore, MD, Oct. 17–21.

# Author Index

## C

## F



## G

## H

## I



## J

## K



## L

## M

## N



## O

## P



## Q



## R

## S

## T

## U



## V



## W

## Y



## Z

# Subject Index

## B

## E

## F



## G

## H



## I

## M

## N

# P

## Q



## R

## T

## U

## V

## W



## Y